The
Hormone
Balance
Bible

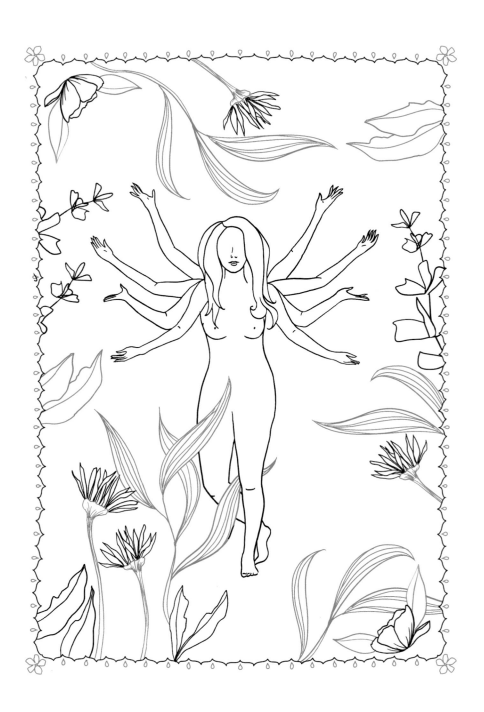

The Hormone Balance Bible

A HOLISTIC PLAN TO CREATE
LIFELONG HEALTH

SHAWN TASSONE, MD, PhD

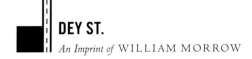

DEY ST.
An Imprint of WILLIAM MORROW

THE HORMONE BALANCE BIBLE. Copyright © 2021 by Shawn Tassone. All rights reserved. Printed in Canada. No part of this book may be used or reproduced in any manner whatsoever without written permission except in the case of brief quotations embodied in critical articles and reviews. For information, address HarperCollins Publishers, 195 Broadway, New York, NY 10007.

HarperCollins books may be purchased for educational, business, or sales promotional use. For information, please email the Special Markets Department at SPsales@harpercollins.com.

FIRST EDITION

Designed by Paula Russell Szafranski
Illustrations by Peggy Dean

Library of Congress Cataloging-in-Publication Data has been applied for.

ISBN 978-0-06-295854-9

21 22 23 24 25 TC 10 9 8 7 6 5 4 3 2 1

This book is dedicated to my mother

and all the women who have shared their stories

over the past 20 years.

CONTENTS

Foreword by Dr. Izabella Wentz

As a woman who has had her own health challenges, and as a pharmacist who is an advocate for women's health, I've found that in many cases, women with health struggles are dismissed by modern medicine. They are told that feeling tired and irritable, gaining weight, having thinning hair, and experiencing sleep troubles are "normal" things that they should just get used to. While these symptoms may be common, I assure you that they are not normal, that you do not have to live with them, and that you can feel calm, fit, beautiful, well rested, and balanced once more.

The guiding principle of *The Hormone Balance Bible* is that "normal is not always normal." Even if your lab test results indicate "normal," that may not be *your* normal. I love how Dr. Tassone empowers you to listen to your own gut—you know your body better than anyone.

If you've read either of my *New York Times* bestselling books, *Hashimoto's: The Root Cause* and *Hashimoto's Protocol*, you may be aware that I also struggled with my own health journey for many years. I know what it's like to search for answers on how to regain or improve your health. You may be experiencing fatigue, weight gain, mood swings, hair thinning, insomnia, irregular periods, water retention, stretch marks, or recurrent miscarriages—and are tired of being told by multiple physicians that your test results are fine, or that you're "just getting older." I, too, was told these same things when I was only twenty-six years old.

I've been there, done that, and then wrote a book on how to feel human again with Hashimoto's, the leading cause of hypothyroidism. I lost almost a decade on my quest for answers because those answers were outside the conventional medical paradigm. While my journey was thyroid-related, it's important to note that any hormone-related issues can affect other hormones. *The Hormone Balance Bible* discusses not only thyroid imbalances but also imbalances with estrogen, testosterone, cortisol, and progesterone.

If you, too, are struggling with issues related to the various hormone imbalances that commonly affect women, I want you to know you've come to the right place. The book you have in your hands can be your guide to feeling better. I wish I had crossed paths with Dr. Shawn Tassone earlier in my journey. Dr. Tassone is a physician who truly looks beyond conventional medicine and uncovers the many layers of healing, to help you feel your best. With his training, knowledge, and comprehensive approach that shines from his twenty years of experience with over fifty thousand patients, Dr. Tassone has done in this book what other hormone books have not been able to do. He has bridged the gap between conventional and alternative medicine in a manner that is well researched and self-guided, and that *works*. He reminds us that with the guidance of an integrative physician, patients have a proactive means of correcting and self-regulating their hormonal imbalances. He truly follows his own tenet that medicine is better with an engaged patient and a passive physician.

Sadly, women's voices are not always heard by the medical community these days; studies have shown that we wait longer in the emergency room before we receive pain medications, and it takes seven years on average before we obtain a diagnosis of endometriosis. As a scientist, I love the fact that Dr. Tassone has the depth and understanding of the research on all these topics—his background in integrative medicine and his graduate degree in philosophy confirm he knows how to vet relevant research.

One of the things I appreciate most about Dr. Tassone, however, is that he truly listens. He is someone with decades of experience listening to women's stories and helping women get their health back. Thanks to this critical (but often rare) skill, as well as the women who have trusted him with their health, Dr. Tassone has been able to develop the first integrative hormonal-mapping system.

Dr. Tassone's new book, *The Hormone Balance Bible*, will provide you with an easy way to identify and understand your hormone type through an in-depth discovery of twelve different hormonal imbalance profiles, characterized as easy-to-relate-to archetypes—with each delivering a complete protocol broken down into six simple steps for care and treatment. I absolutely love the heroine's journey in each of the twelve archetypal stories. I'm certain you'll find yourself in more than one of these, but with the gentle guidance provided in both the book and an eye-opening quiz, you will land on the archetype that best fits. I suggest that you read each one, because the circle of women in your life may come to mind as the experiences, stories, symptoms, and answers begin to make sense and help you recognize not only yourself, but also someone you know.

Over the years, I have seen that when women don't feel well, they give up their power to others, their doctors, and other professionals who all mean well, but might not have the knowledge or experience needed to truly help. This book puts the power in your hands.

It's time for you to shed your symptoms and uncover your true self once more.

I encourage you to turn the page and start your healing journey today.

—Dr. Izabella Wentz, PharmD, FASCP
New York Times bestselling author of
Hashimoto's: The Root Cause and *Hashimoto's Protocol*

INTRODUCTION

Hormones, the Invisible Driving Forces of
Women's Lives

W hat's *your* problem?" I yelled at my mother.

My mother and I often battled when I was a teenager, and on this occasion, she had made what I considered a particularly snarky comment. Okay, I will admit that it may have been my teenage ego getting the better of me.

"Forget to take your pill?" I quipped.

I grew up as the only child of a single mother, and to say that we were close would be an understatement. I was as privy to my mother's personal struggles as she was to mine, and among my mother's struggles that I recall most clearly were a series of significant gynecological issues that she endured in the 1980s, beginning when she was in her thirties and I was a teenager. My mother suffered chronic pelvic pain—pain that eventually became so severe that her doctors could no longer tell her to just endure it, though they were at a loss for a diagnosis. She had wild mood swings and could easily go from laughing to being tense and tearful in what seemed like seconds. My teenage self thought she was overreacting to things, and I would tell her, which would launch us into yet another verbal battle. But I also knew how often she was in pain, so I mostly tried to tolerate the days when she was short-tempered with me. I knew she often felt lousy. Hormone testing was limited at that time, and her doctors eventually decided it was best to perform a hysterectomy, removing her uterus and one of her ovaries. This caused an immediate drop in her estrogen levels, for which they prescribed the popular hormone replacement therapy (HRT) drug of the time, Premarin. As a teenager, I understood little of what was happening to my mother, and I knew next to nothing about women's hormones. I also had no idea what was in the little pill her doctor had prescribed for her, or what side effects would come along with it. I assumed that her suffering began and ended with her hormones, and that hormones were the problem. At that time, a woman's hormones seemed to be blamed for just about anything that couldn't be explained otherwise.

FOR CENTURIES, WESTERN MEDICINE AND SOCIETY AT LARGE have tended to connect a woman's mood and emotional state, as well as her physical state, with her hormones. In the Victorian era, for example, "hysteria" (which shares its root, *hyster*, with "hysterectomy") was a medical diagnosis that emerged to describe a neurotic condition in women caused by a disfunction of the uterus. "She must be on her period" has become the modern equivalent of diagnosing a woman with hysteria, a dismissive way of equating negative mood or emotion with hormonal function. Hormones are also occasionally connected with positive emotion, for example, that blissful state or "glow" that we associate with certain happy pregnant women. But whether we are talking about negative or positive emotion, attributing emotional state to hormones significantly oversimplifies their effects on the female body and discounts a vast array of alternate explanations for why someone may be feeling one way or another.

As a teenager affected by my mother's experiences, I didn't have any reason to question the assertion that hormones were the cause of both physical pain and emotional suffering. Now, of course, I clearly see how oversimplifying the story told by what are actually symptom groupings can lead to overlooking the true cause of a disorder. And I believe that this kind of oversimplification is a bit sexist. We don't make the same assertions about men's emotions. No one has ever said to me, "Hey, Shawn, you seem down. How's your testosterone?" Although science supports the distinction between men's and women's hormones to a degree—men produce lower levels of most hormones than women do, and the psychological impact of those hormones tends to be less significant—the fact remains that a woman's internal experience and behavior may be no more reduced to hormonal activity than a man's.

YOUR JOURNEY THROUGH *THE HORMONE BALANCE BIBLE* begins with this realization: There is nothing wrong with you. You are not broken. You may have come to this book because you are experiencing hormonal issues of one kind or another, and your hormones may not be in their ideal balance, instead operating at levels and in ways that are disrupting your routine and causing you suffering and discomfort. But again, this does not mean there is anything wrong with you. In fact, it means you are completely normal. Patients seek out my help at every stage of life, from premenstrual challenges that bring pain and sometimes severe cramping that can make anyone feel miserable, to infertility challenges and birth control preferences to endometriosis, adrenal fatigue, and burnout to the many forms of malaise that women feel when hormones aren't performing as they should.

For women who are entering perimenopause or menopause, discomfort and imbalance may be related to the fact that as humans, our biological evolution has failed to keep pace with the medical advancements that prolong our lives. Life expectancy in the United States has roughly doubled over the past two hundred years. Whereas American women living in the nineteenth century could expect to die before they had to deal with menopause, their twenty-first-century counterparts are living to an average age of eighty-one. Think about that. Women's ovaries cease producing estrogen around the age of fifty. But with women living three decades beyond this, that's practically an additional lifetime of trying to live and function optimally without estrogen production. This calls for a strategy if you want to continue living with vitality, which I know we all want! Add to that the array of lifestyle choices that women have today. Some choose to start families at a young age and savor their freedom later. Others delay having children or choose not to have them at all. Women today choose how they want to pace their lives based on their goals and desires, and they deserve this same level of choice when it comes to physical and hormonal health—at every age and stage of life.

Statistically speaking, American women, including many of my patients, are now having children later in life than their mothers and grandmothers did. It's not uncommon today for a woman to be in perimenopause or menopause and have a five-year-old child. Women are amazingly strong and resilient, but the body simply has not evolved to support many of the physical and emotional demands of motherhood later in life, and patients often come to see me after pushing themselves for long periods of time beyond what their bodies can reasonably support. But we do have strategies that can optimize what our hormones offer us as a resource, rather than viewing them as a drain on our energy, mental clarity, and sexual health.

Trying to live a busy life with your hormones out of balance or depleted is a bit like driving your car down the road with the gas tank close to empty. Eventually, you're going to run out of gas. You can try to keep going by revving the engine a bit, and this may carry you along for another half mile or so. But inevitably, your car (body) is going to stop. Then you're sitting there by the side of the road with your tank empty, but you're somehow still expected to keep going at sixty miles per hour. How are you going to do this?

The answer is: You can't. It's impossible. But here's the great news: Your car is just out of gas. You need to fill it up to carry on, and then you'll be on your way. In other words, it is a temporary state. There are many things you can do to address hormonal imbalances. But very few women realize that this is possible when it comes to their hormones—that they can utilize their hormones to their full advantage while correcting the imbalances that are making them feel drained and depleted. Women often consider their hormones a bother rather than an asset.

If you take only one thing away from this book, I want it to be this: You are completely normal, even when your hormones are out of balance. There is nothing wrong with you. The trouble is that you are living a busier and longer life than the one to which your hormones have evolutionarily adapted. This is not a problem, per se. But it does call out that you may want to take advantage of the medical *and* nonmedical interventions that can help you navigate any change in your hormonal state. Remember that your hormones are in an almost constant state of change throughout your adolescent and adult life.

These interventions, which I will present in this book, are unlikely to extend your life or make you a different person. But they can help to alleviate symptoms that are negatively affecting your quality of life. These interventions will help you sleep better. They will improve your sex life and increase your desire. And they will give you back some of the enjoyment of life that may have gone missing.

When I discuss hormonal health with my patients, I often tell them the story of my ninety-five-year-old Italian grandmother who jokes that she took a "just rub some dirt on it and walk it off" approach to the hormonal shifts and discomfort that came along with menopause. Now, it may be that she doesn't remember menopause all that well, or it may be that she genuinely took a "no pain, no gain" approach to push through it—she was of a different generation, after all. Whatever the case, and regardless of a woman's age or stage of life, there is simply no reason hormonal issues should spell discomfort or the need to live with pain.

We know so much more about hormonal health today than we did in my grandmother's day, or even in my mother's day. We have many more choices, and we have access to so much more information, which should empower us. Just as you would put effort into understanding the importance of a healthy diet and exercise, you can *choose* to play an active role in understanding the way hormones function in the body, assessing and working to alleviate the negative impact of hormonal imbalances. Today's health choices are affordable and accessible to any woman who chooses to take on this vital aspect of her health and well-being. The eye-opener here is that *everything about your hormonal health touches every other aspect of your life through quality of living.*

Finding Your Hormonal Balance

It may surprise you to learn that all women, regardless of background, genetics, or body type, have the same hormones. These hormones include estrogen, progesterone, testosterone, cortisol, cortisone, thyroid, DHEA, melatonin, and vitamin D. However, the exact levels of each of these hormones vary from one person to the next, and every woman has a unique balance point, which I will refer to as the hormonal balance point throughout this book. This balance point keeps the body working at its best both physiologically (in terms of body function) and psychologically (in terms of mental and emotional state). Determining the exact levels of each hormone that will keep a woman's body within a range of balance may involve a process of trial and error, both in addressing symptoms and in evaluating hormone levels through testing, which may reveal more subtle hormonal influences on a particular mind or body function. Your hormonal balance point will be different from your mother's and your sister's and your girlfriend's. In the coming chapters, I will go into specific detail about each hormone and how they perform together to create that balance, as well as give you a better understanding of what is happening when there is an imbalance.

Often, when a patient comes to me for a consult, she will say that she has had her hormones tested and that her levels are "normal." "Well," I ask, "do you feel normal?" The answer is typically no. Physicians often tell patients that their hormone levels are normal because they fall within clinically established "normal" ranges. But within this broader range, one woman's normal may be completely different from another's; a certain level of a particular hormone may make one woman feel sick but another woman feel great.

Take testosterone, for example. In women, the "normal" range for free testosterone (the active form of testosterone in your body) is 0.2 to 6.4 nanograms per milliliter (ml).[1] This means anyone whose testosterone levels fall within this range may be regarded as "just fine." But often a patient who comes to me with "normal" levels of testosterone will complain of low libido, or falling asleep at work at four in the afternoon, or feeling too weak to work out. This same patient might also show signs of osteopenia, the precursor to osteoporosis. If this patient's testosterone level were 0.2 pg/ml, for example, which I see in roughly 90 percent of my patients, I could increase her levels *thirtyfold*, and she would still be within the clinically normal range. However, that change could be a game changer for *her* because she is likely to feel much better, have lots more energy, and be excited about her sexual satisfaction again. If her symptoms were caused by a testosterone deficiency, even a fivefold increase would likely go some distance toward relieving them.[2]

The *Hormone Balance Bible* Method

When a new patient comes into my office with a gynecologic problem, before I do an exam, I will ask her to list the top five issues affecting her, both physically and emotionally, that she wants to address through our work together. My goal is to help each of my patients find her new hormonal balance by determining what it is about her physiological and emotional experiences that she wants to change. When my patients make this list, some common desires are "Have more energy" and "Feel more joy day to day." Less frequently, though still common, might be "Increase low libido" or "Lose fat around my waist." As we embark on our journey together in this book, I want you to make your own list of the top five ways, both physically and emotionally, that you would like to feel better. Be as specific as you can with your answers. These five answers will point us in the direction of your own hormonal balance point, the point toward which we are working together. We will return to this list and reassess later in the book.

Your Hormonal Balance Point —Goals

1 ....

....

2 ....

....

3 ....

....

4 ....

....

5 ....

....

Introducing the Hormonal Archetypes

While the hormonal balance point in every woman's body is unique, in over twenty years practicing medicine and listening to women tell their stories, I have discovered that patients tend to fall into a number of consistently identifiable groups, which I call Hormonal Archetypes:

The
Queen

The
Nun

The Unbalanced
Heroine

The
Warrior

The
Mother

The
Underdog

The
Wisewoman

The
Overachiever

The
Workaholic

The
Chairwoman

The
Saboteur

The
Philosopher

You'll be introduced to each of these in chapter four, with detailed information and an online diagnostic quiz that you can use to determine which of the archetypes you might be. With that said, there is overlap between the archetypes because the state of our hormones is fluid, and it is possible to migrate from one archetype to another as your hormones fluctuate. The Hormonal Archetypes go beyond physical symptoms to also address the emotional and spiritual experiences shared by women who identify with each archetype, and I use these as a holistic framework for treating my patients and understanding a woman's health needs and experiences.

Some of the archetypes center on single hormones. The Queen, for example, is characterized by her high estrogen level. Low progesterone levels cause trouble for the Unbalanced Heroine, and excess testosterone drives the Warrior. Other archetypes are characterized by combinations of imbalances. The Mother tends to be both estrogen dominant and progesterone deficient, because she is naturally a Queen and Unbalanced Heroine. None of the archetypes are meant to serve as any woman's permanent conception of her permanent hormonal makeup. You may find yourself in more than one overlapping archetype. Many women have dominant archetypes in regard to their full experience, and secondary ones that also fit in smaller ways. Women's archetypes also change over time. In the short and long term, hormonal imbalances tend to be fluid. Patients I've treated for two decades have sought my help for everything from progesterone deficiency to menopause, and their archetypes have shifted along the way.

The archetype framework is not intended to be a means to an end so much as a means to a beginning—the beginning of a journey along which you will learn not only about your body and its functioning but also about your larger life. These archetypes are designed to help you understand how your hormones affect your feelings and drive your behavior, and also how they amplify or detract from your innate and learned personality traits. Careful assessments of hormone levels and their attendant symptoms reveal how the archetypes work in combination and which aspects of each archetype drive a woman's symptomology and her current approach to life.

The SHINES Protocol

How do we put these insights from the Hormonal Archetype framework to work for you?

The answer is the SHINES protocol, a multifaceted approach that combines medical and nonmedical interventions in a comprehensive program you may tailor to suit your specific needs. I developed these interventions during my twenty years as a practitioner of integrative medicine, working with women to improve their physical health while helping them achieve spiritual, emotional, and energetic balance.

The SHINES protocol, divided by archetype, will be fully presented in specific detail in chapter five. Each individual protocol is composed of six modalities, which work separately and together to support the optimal functioning of body and mind. It's useful to conceive of the following six elements as interconnected and working in concert to promote overall wellness.

SPIRITUAL PRACTICE

A spiritual practice is one that inspires introspection, stillness, and inner peace. It need not be religious, though it can be. Contemplative prayer can have centering, healing effects. Meditation—guided or unguided—can also be a helpful restorative practice, as can acupuncture.

HORMONE MODULATION

Hormone modulation—or "biohacking," as many healthcare practitioners now refer to it—is the practice of increasing or decreasing certain hormone levels by taking prescription oral, transdermal, or suppository medications. Whether hormone modulation is right for your archetype depends on the severity of the underlying imbalance and the potential related effects of intervention. Ongoing monitoring by a physician will also help determine appropriate dosing and duration of treatment.

A note on nonprescription hormonal supplements: While there are some over-the-counter (OTC) hormone modulation therapies available, including DHEA, progesterone, and pregnenolone-based options, I recommend that any biohacking be supervised by a physician.

INFOCEUTICALS

Infoceuticals are energetic remedies that include energetic healing modalities and essential oils. They represent any approach that deals with your energetic field.

NUTRITION

For each of the twelve archetypes, there are foods to seek out and others to avoid, as well as preparation techniques to embrace and others to steer clear of. In some cases, traditionally "healthy" foods turn out to be undesirable, and "less healthy" foods turn out to be not so bad for you. In each case, the focus is on the impact certain foods can have on hormonal imbalances and/or on their problematic downstream effects.

EXERCISE

Exercise figures prominently into the SHINES protocols for each archetype. Activities of various types and levels of intensity can positively influence different archetypes, improving strength, balance, and circulation, as well as mental clarity.

SUPPLEMENTS

Dietary supplements are an important aspect of the SHINES method, and I encourage my patients to incorporate these into their broader strategy for hormonal balance.

The message implicit in the SHINES protocol is this: True hormonal health requires action. It requires you to be an active participant in your health journey. This is why I consistently remind my patients that the journey toward hormone health is about rewriting your story. The strategies outlined in this book, including hormone assessment, lifestyle changes, and medical intervention, are not a means to an end. They are a beginning, part of a lifelong practice.

Find Your Hormone Type

Please use this code to locate the Hormone-Typing Quiz. By taking this quick assessment, you can determine your Hormonal Archetype, and use this book most effectively. It is important to note, however, that your Hormonal Archetype will change throughout your life, so valuable information can be found by reading the descriptions and treatment plans for every archetype in this book.

Shawn
TASSONE MD PhD
ONEmind • **ONE**body • **ONE**medicine

Western Medicine Is Not Enough

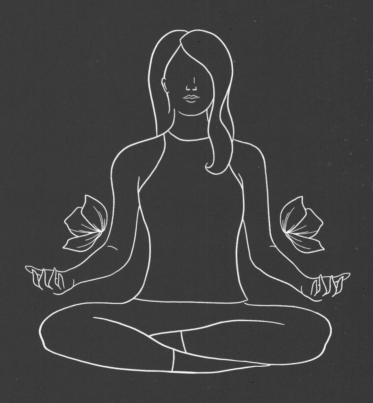

In the introduction, I told you a bit about my mother and the health issues she was going through during my snarky teen years. But that certainly isn't the whole story. In many ways, my mother was an inspiration to me. We were a family of three (counting my stepfather), so we were exceptionally close. I knew from a young age that I wanted to practice medicine. I understood early on that getting to the root cause of a problem could help you more easily solve it. Watching my mother suffer made me determined to find answers. Once I was in medical school, I chose to specialize in obstetrics and gynecology in large part because of the ongoing health challenges my mother faced. When I was a second-year resident, my mother was having pain in her right side, which turned out to be ovarian cancer. As she battled cancer, I watched as the disease and the treatments took a collective toll on her body, and I recall feeling distinctly that I couldn't help her and wanted more: As a son, I wanted more time with my mother. As a physician, I wanted more treatment options, more information about what was happening to her, and more *possibilities*. Over the course of her treatments, my mother's hair fell out, she couldn't sleep, her joints ached, she was weak, and she was in constant pain. Her battle continued until she eventually entered hospice care, slipped into a coma, and passed away. I was emotionally devastated, and I also found myself discouraged by the limitations of what Western medicine had been able to offer her.

My medical training and career took shape during my mother's health struggles, and what I went through with my mother indelibly affected the way I practice medicine and care for my patients today. Early on in my career, I made two enduring commitments that continue to guide my work as a physician. First, I made a firm commitment that I would never allow myself to be as limited in my treatment of patients as a doctor as I felt throughout my mother's health struggles. I knew there had to be more options and more that could be done to ease suffering, find solutions, and heal.

The second commitment I made came after my mother's death, as I became profoundly aware that she was—as we all are—so much more than the body that encased her being. This led me to the realization that there is so much more to health than traditional medical interventions allow for. And so I committed to pushing the boundaries of traditional Western medicine and to learning everything I possibly could about the way the mind, body, and spirit work together to determine our health, and whether we are just surviving or thriving.

Not long after my mother's death, and coming to these two big realizations, I was sitting in a spa in Sedona, Arizona, and I casually picked up a copy of Andrew Weil's book *8 Weeks to Optimum Health*, which offers practical strategies for improving health using a holistic approach. This was 2005, and up to that point in my career, when treating patients, I had relied solely on what I was taught in medical school and residency. Weil's book, however, opened my eyes to the potential of healing powers that exist beyond the traditional Western scope. Fascinated, I immediately decided to apply to Weil's program on integrative medicine at the University of Arizona; I was accepted, and I trained there for two years. And integrative medicine is what I practice with my patients to this day.

It is important to note that integrative medicine is not practiced in opposition to traditional Western medicine. Rather, integrative medicine is viewed as an additional layer of knowledge, practice, and expertise that allows doctors so trained to combine Western training, knowledge, and various board certifications (such as mine in obstetrics and gynecology) with the best of other healing modalities.

As I've stated, I'm not a fan of limitations or rules. When a patient comes to me concerned about a particular symptom, which may signal imbalance or disease in the body, I of course want to alleviate that symptom. But a symptom is only part of the story, one piece of the bigger picture of that patient's overall health. This is why I am drawn to the philosophy of integrative medicine, which aims to understand the bigger picture of a patient's overall health while also treating individual ailments and symptoms. Integrative medicine also holds that when internal and external issues affecting the body—such as lifestyle choices, physical and emotional trauma, and periods of intense stress—aren't addressed, they often manifest as health problems. Integrative medicine seeks to make a patient more attuned to the needs of her body and to how lifestyle choices and external factors may be affecting her health. The ultimate goal is to show a patient how to create the best internal and external ecosystem to support her individual needs. Nowhere is this more relevant than with hormonal health, because a woman's hormones are in constant flux due to her monthly cycle, her life stage, even the way her blood sugar rises and falls throughout the day.

Integrative and functional medicine have grown in popularity in recent years because these approaches give us so many more options than traditional Western medicine alone does. Women today are juggling so much that a treatment method addressing the many facets of life affecting her naturally appeals. But perhaps the biggest reason so many women are turning to integrative medicine for answers is that they want to be heard. In my approach, every symptom and every individual experience is key to unlocking a patient's individual health story.

Before We Begin: Debunking Some Popular Myths About Hormone Modulation

Many of us think of hormones as only affecting us as we age. But hormonal health begins at puberty and continues throughout life. Additionally, many tend to think of hormones as *causing* problems in the mind and body, while overlooking the many opportunities to *optimize* health and well-being offered by hormonal modulation. At every age, the body is constantly changing, as are our hormones. This book provides a grand tour of your hormonal makeup. I encourage you to approach these pages with a beginner's mind, which means you will let go of judgment and approach this topic with openness and curiosity. In order to do that, let's dismantle some biases and misinformation you may have adopted or considered along the way.

Hormones have been misunderstood, misrepresented, and vilified for decades. As a result, there are a number of misconceptions about how to approach optimal hormone health. Some of these concern testing. Others concern interventions. Still others are about potential health risks when weighed against benefits. Let's consider . . .

MYTHS AROUND HORMONE TESTING

IT COSTS A SMALL FORTUNE

A common misbelief is that hormone testing is prohibitively expensive. This is not necessarily the case. If you are working with a physician, they may bill your insurance for most blood serum– or urine-based tests (in addition to the cost of your visits). Although some innovative tests on the market—tests that are more comprehensive and precise than their traditional counterparts—are not covered by insurance, when clients are looking to minimize out-of-pocket costs, I always recommend blood (serum) testing if it is covered by health insurance. Although not the most nuanced test, it does reveal certain imbalances and can therefore serve as a starting point for you and your physician.

I do recommend hormonal testing if you suspect that you have an imbalance, and before you embark on any kind of hormonal treatment program. As a physician who is concerned about the danger of overprescribing hormones and raising a client's levels to a supraphysiologic (greater-than-normal) point, the more precise the test, the more useful the results, and the closer you are to a solution. This said, a thorough examination of your symptoms can also be a valid means of determining your Hormonal Archetype and is to be carefully considered along with test results. So, if the financial aspect of testing is your concern, your doctor should be able to identify any significant issues by conducting a proper medical history, a blood serum test, and a physical, and by asking the right questions.

ONCE YOU HAVE YOUR HORMONES TESTED, YOU NEED TO HAVE THEM RETESTED EVERY SIX TO EIGHT WEEKS

Often, once a client and I have completed her initial hormone health assessment, she'll ask, "So, should I plan on coming back for more testing in a few weeks? And a few weeks after that?" This is a reasonable question, of course. But the reality is, 90 percent of the time, we do a test in the very beginning, develop a holistic management protocol, and the client's symptoms improve. So long as this improvement continues, I recommend retesting only once per year. The reason for this is that you are not simply the results of your tests. You are also a conglomerate of symptoms and experiences that needs to be looked at when talking about hormones.

Of course, a woman's hormone levels may shift. Old symptoms may also reemerge, or new ones may take hold. If a patient begins to notice a shift in symptoms, I retest, and we reassess the management protocol we've developed. But again, unless a client tells me that her condition has deteriorated, I recommend annual assessments.

TESTING IS ONLY FOR WOMEN IN MENOPAUSE

Women of all ages are affected by hormonal imbalance and may benefit from hormone-level assessments. I test women in their twenties who seek help for irregular or missed periods, for example, given that this may be symptomatic of polycystic ovarian syndrome (PCOS). I also recommend hormone testing for young women struggling with decreased libido and fatigue. While hormones may not be the root cause, a screening will reveal whether hormones are a factor and how hormone modulation may help. The bottom line is that if you are not feeling your best, whether mentally or physically, it's never a bad idea to screen for hormone imbalances. Even if a woman is taking birth control pills, tests can still reveal variations that are worth taking a closer look at.

ESTROGEN MODULATION IS DANGEROUS

In Western culture, we have come to fear estrogen. Specifically, we have been told that it can lead to various female cancers, notably breast and endometrial cancers. While estrogen in excessive levels can cause issues, normal levels are essential for many women to live a productive life. More than this, some types of estrogen may be of minimal risk even in those women with a history of breast cancer. Testing can reveal all of a woman's estrogen levels (estradiol, estrone, and estriol), including metabolites, and determine whether her production of the hormone is excessive or deficient. There is definitely reason to respect estrogen as a prescription because there are indeed estrogen-sensitive cancers of the breast and uterus, but to say solely estrogen causes cancer is a bit untrue. If estrogen caused cancer, then every woman would get cancer because you all have estrogen in your body. Cancer is caused by so many factors, like genetics, diet, lack of exercise, where you live, how you live, and habits like excessive smoking and alcohol consumption. If you have a cancer cell that has an estrogen receptor, then it can definitely stimulate that cancer. Also, we know that excessive amounts of unopposed estrogen without the benefit of having protective progesterone can have increased risks of uterine cancer, which is why we don't utilize unopposed estrogen unless you have had a hysterectomy.

SEEKING HELP FOR HORMONE IMBALANCES IS A SIGN OF WEAKNESS

I have come up against this belief time and time again. Some women have the attitude that if their hormones are creating uncomfortable symptoms, they should tough it out and find a way to "self-correct" rather than complain. Even women who come to me for help can be resistant to medically treating their hormonal imbalances, thinking of treatment as the "easy way out." As if suffering through hormonal issues is an inevitable rite of passage for women and they should bear it as a natural part of being female. Some of these women point to their mothers' difficult experiences, or their sisters', insisting that they, too, should prepare themselves to power through the changes ahead.

But going back to the fact that each woman has her own "normal" and unique hormonal balance point, why should you have to suffer just because others have? This is your story. Understand that your internal ecosystem is constantly changing, often driven by (or at least due in some part to) your hormones. You can access health strategies and treatments that not only will alleviate uncomfortable symptoms, but can optimize your overall health through hormonal balance. There is no personal weakness here. Own it, take on your health issues, and don't feel bad about it. Seeking help is not an admission of weakness. There are resources that can reduce your suffering and help you feel more energized and more engaged in your life. Take advantage of them and be the woman you want to be.

EVERY WOMAN SHOULD HAVE THE HORMONES OF A TWENTY-YEAR-OLD

It seems that everywhere we look, from magazines to books to TV and movies, we're bombarded by messages telling us that we should want to look and feel younger, sending us in search of mythical fountains of youth. But when it comes to hormonal issues, some women have more difficulty in their twenties than they do later. For others, these issues develop as they get older. But for all people, the reality is the same: We age. Our bodies change, and we must adapt and change with them.

The important question is this: *What is normal for you right now?* Understanding that your body is in a constant state of change can help you realize that your hormonal state is always fluctuating. You are not living with the exact same body you had when you were twenty. Your body changes as you age, and your hormones need to function differently within your body as these changes occur. This book is engineered to help you support and sustain the hormonal balance that works best for you at any given time—meeting the needs of the changes in your body *now*. And it will also be a valued resource that you can return to again during changes in the future.

HORMONES ARE *ALWAYS* THE PROBLEM

Keep in mind that not *every* physical malfunction is about hormonal imbalance. Feeling overheated does not always mean you are having a hot flash. Perhaps a new medication is making you flush, or perhaps it was that glass of wine. Night sweats? Maybe your blankets are too thick. Weight gain? Perhaps you're being less vigilant about your diet. Decreased libido? Maybe you're not getting along with your partner.

Let's look at weight gain for a moment. In some cases, as difficult as this can be for patients to hear, when a woman enters perimenopause or menopause, her body simply wants to hold on to some extra weight. This means that even if you eat healthy and work out like a fiend, you still may not be able to shed those additional pounds. The body may hold on to a little extra fat for a number of reasons: to strengthen your bones, for example, which begin to weaken when your estrogen levels drop. Despite what a magazine cover may tell you, having drastically low body weight at fifty may not be achievable—or desirable.

This is why building the full picture of a woman's health story is important before assuming that any health occurrence or complication is hormonal.

FIXING HORMONAL IMBALANCE IS DIFFICULT

This should not be the case if you are working with a physician who is an expert on hormonal issues. It is important to find someone with sufficient knowledge and experience to guide you through hormonal testing and to develop a comprehensive approach for dealing with symptoms. So do your research on the physician you're consulting, and make sure that they have not only the credentials but the *experience* necessary to help you. Finding the right doctor is key to building an approach that works.

In 80 to 90 percent of my patients' cases, we get it right the first time. Occasionally, a woman will present with a particularly complex case that requires extra time and investigation. But even in such a case, we are able to nail down an assessment and a tailored protocol within a few visits. The majority of cases require just one visit. And if all goes according to plan, we proceed with occasional follow-ups by phone or email and annual in-person reassessments.

BALANCING YOUR HORMONES IS AS EASY AS TAKING A PILL

As straightforward a process as hormone modulation may be, it is not as easy as taking a prescription. Adjusting the levels of any given hormone can ameliorate some symptoms, but if an excess or deficiency is a symptom of a larger problem, addressing a specific imbalance won't be the end game. In fact, it might be just the beginning.

Remember: Taking a holistic approach to hormone health is a process. It requires dedicated work on multiple fronts—physiological, psychological, and spiritual. It isn't just about changing your hormones; it's about changing your life. You have to be willing not only to look at what's imbalanced in your body and your life more generally, but also to do something about it. And then keep doing it.

Hormones are a tricky business, and they can be influenced by external stimuli and internal stimuli alike. You might feel good for a while, but then feel worse. And when this happens, you need to be willing to come back to the table and reassess. You also need to be willing to look at the various other components that influence your overall health—including diet, exercise, any energetic or spiritual practices, and other lifestyle factors.

None of this is easy. But all of it is worth it.

2 Our Hormones, Ourselves

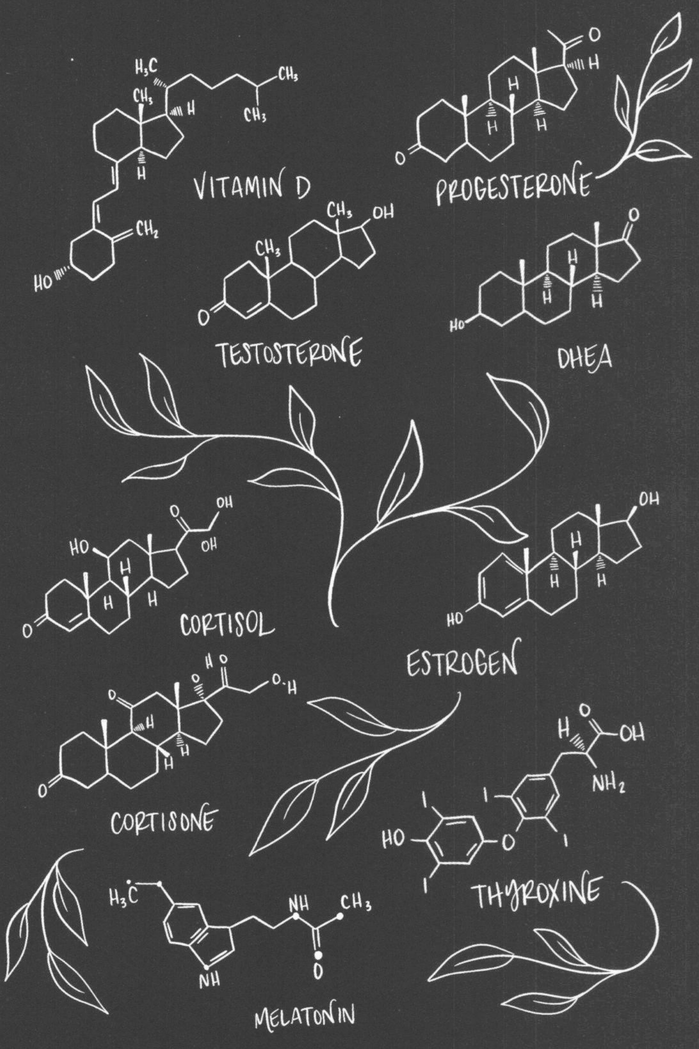

VITAMIN D

PROGESTERONE

TESTOSTERONE

DHEA

CORTISOL

ESTROGEN

CORTISONE

THYROXINE

MELATONIN

A few years ago, a patient named Barbara[1] came to see me in the office. She was in her late forties at the time, and I had an idea of what her symptoms might be and what kind of help she might be seeking, and I began by asking her a few questions to get us started. She told me she was having trouble sleeping, had too little energy, and was finding it increasingly difficult to get out of bed. Before long, she began to cry, and our conversation quickly veered to the circumstances of her personal life. Although she genuinely believed that her hormones were imbalanced and she wanted my help, she was also grieving the loss of her husband, who had died just six months before.

Now, I think many of us would look at this situation and say that this woman's symptoms were likely caused by her grief, not by a hormone imbalance. But the reality is that the grief itself could have *caused* an imbalance. Or perhaps she had been living her life very differently since the death of her spouse, and she either gained or lost weight, which then threw her hormones out of whack. I tested her levels and discovered she was low in progesterone, which helps you sleep, and testosterone, which helps maintain your energy levels. I prescribed progesterone for her to take at night and testosterone for the morning. I also recommended a supplement of hops (see page 463) to see if that would help her sleep. She was seeing a therapist and actively addressing the emotional and spiritual aspects of her recovery. I was pleased that she was referred to me for help with hormonal management. I asked her to come back and see me a few months later.

When I saw Barbara next at her follow-up appointment, she reported feeling better. Her sleep had improved, as had her energy levels. She said she still struggled to get out of bed each morning, and she was tearful as she told me this. But she also said she felt she was heading in the right direction and wanted to continue taking the hormones I had prescribed. I suggested that her grief was likely still causing some of her symptoms and would take time to shift. I also tested her hormone levels again. These had changed slightly, and I adjusted her dosages accordingly.

I didn't hear from Barbara until roughly a year after that follow-up. She called and told me she hadn't come back to see me again because she'd been feeling much better, as well as could be expected. But recently she had been feeling poorly again. She wasn't sleeping. She was suffering panic attacks. "What's changed in your life?" I asked. "What's going on?"

As it turned out, Barbara had entered into a new romantic relationship. She told me she was feeling strange about it—guilty, really, because she felt as if she were betraying her late husband. This, I thought, could account for her trouble sleeping. But I did not rule out a change in her hormone levels. Our hormones are influenced by our behavior even as they influence it themselves. The two factors are inevitably intertwined.

In Barbara's case, it turned out her levels had changed again, and I made the appropriate adjustments to her medications. But balancing her hormones alone did not improve Barbara's symptoms, make her happier in her daily life, or help her enjoy her relationship with her new partner. These improvements in her life did not take place until she had time to move through her grief and find the energy to feel restored. She made other changes. She began to pursue her long-standing interest in music and became involved in her local arts community. She began a regular yoga practice. She also became well versed in essential oils, discovering her passion for this natural approach to wellness. Hormones are only part of your internal and external ecosystem. That is why a holistic approach to your symptom story is so crucial.

It has been seven years since I first met Barbara. Today, at age sixty, she is a dynamo. She looks and feels great, and she is fully enjoying her life day to day, including her relationships with her partner and grandchildren. And while I am entirely confident that hormones have helped her, I also know that her discovery of spiritual, intellectual, and physical practices has helped bring her peace and find inner equilibrium. During one of our last conversations, Barbara told me that when her husband was dying, he told her, "Whenever you find a penny on the ground, that's me thinking of you." These days, I watch for her Facebook posts of all the pennies she's found. "I was feeling sad," she writes, "and there one was." This has become a vehicle for dealing with her grief, one rooted in spirituality and faith in an enduring connection with her late husband, and what a blessing it has been.

In finding her own zest for life, Barbara has become a beacon for other women enduring their own struggles. Many have come to see me on her recommendation. "Go see Dr. Tassone," Barbara tells them. "He's good at figuring things out." But the reality is, *she* is good at figuring things out. And with some guidance and understanding, and a comprehensive, actionable protocol, you will be, too.

What Do Hormones *Do*, Anyway?

As simplistic as it sounds, here's the truth: In women, hormones do almost everything. Every organ in a woman's body is equipped with estrogen receptors, for example, and estrogen and other hormones drive the organs' functionality. Although the human body can survive with depressed levels of some hormones (and in the absence of certain others), it can't function very well. Hormones influence the quality of your life experiences. They are what make those experiences enjoyable and uniquely your own. As I've mentioned, you have a hormonal "signature," which comprises the concentrations of the various hormones your body creates and the way they influence your physiological, psychological, and emotional experiences. Your hormone signature is a vital part of what makes you . . . you. That's why on some level—large or small—you know when your hormones are "off": You don't quite feel like yourself; sometimes you feel like a complete stranger.

HOW DO HORMONES WORK?

Think of each of your hormones as a key, and your organs' receptor cells as locks. As hormones travel throughout your body via your bloodstream, they encounter locks into which only they fit. When they successfully "unlock" these receptors, they begin to exert their effects. Estrogen will unlock receptor cells in your breast tissue, for example, and stimulate growth. When estrogen reaches your uterus, the hormone will unlock that organ's receptor cells and stimulate the growth of the uterine lining. When progesterone comes along, it will unlock different uterine receptors and block the estrogen's effects, halting the growth of the uterine lining and stabilizing the existing lining.

Each of the following nine hormones plays a critical role in a woman's body and is featured in one or more of the twelve archetypes. Later, you will find tables that detail where each is made, what function it serves, and what happens when it's out of balance:

Estrogen

Progesterone

Testosterone

Cortisol

Cortisone

Thyroid

DHEA

Melatonin

Vitamin D

HOW HORMONES WORK TOGETHER

Imagine your body as a watch. Behind its face, a series of interconnected gears keeps its hands moving at the right pace. Your hormones are these gears, and their running at the right pace determines whether this watch keeps the right time. When one or more of these gears—your estrogen or progesterone, for example—begins to slow down or speed up, all the pieces of the larger machine to which they're connected are affected, as are all the pieces connected to those. This downstream effect may not stop the watch altogether. But when it causes the watch's hands to move a little too slowly or a little too fast, the watch begins to tell the wrong time.

Suppose, for example, that your estrogen gear starts moving too rapidly, driven by birth control pills, or excess body fat, or polycystic ovarian syndrome (PCOS). This causes the sex-hormone-binding globulin (SHBG) gear to move too quickly, which in turn makes the testosterone gear slow down. This could have a negative impact on your libido, energy level, and mood.

If, on the other hand, your triiodothyronine (T3) gear begins moving too slowly, your brain will send a message to your pituitary gland to produce more thyroid-stimulating hormone (TSH) in an attempt to make more T3. If the thyroid cannot respond adequately to the stimulation, this can cause weight gain and potentially increase estrogen levels, causing you to possibly become insulin resistant. Suffice it to say, the hormonal axis is not simply an orchestra that might sound fine if one section isn't working. When one system is off, it can affect others and throw off the entire harmony of the person.

As patients work with me to address their hormone imbalances, they quickly learn that this is not about fixing one problem with one prescription. Your hormone health is intricately linked to your complete health. How well you feel overall is greatly influenced by your hormones. For example, if your follicle-stimulating hormone (FSH) and luteinizing hormone (LH) levels suggested that your estrogen gear was moving slowly, treatment with estrogen to turn the FSH and LH gears down or off might well be our first step. But then we would turn to nutrition to help bring down your blood sugar levels and to exercise to help you lose some weight while we work on your insulin production. We would look at supplementation, including a product called DIM (diindolylmethane), a food-based compound that helps process and eliminate estrogen metabolites. We would also consider whether spiritual practices or alternative healing methods would help improve the flow of energy through your body.

Hormone Essentials: A Quick Guide

When imbalances begin to take hold, the impact may vary depending on the degree of imbalance and the situation. Your watch may be an hour off, or it may lag just a few imperceptible seconds behind. But the point is, it's off, and at some point, you will notice the discrepancy. When you do, it's time to consider the various forces at work within this intricate machine, figure out how its different gears are affecting one another, and determine what physical and psychological effects this is having on you.

I've created the following tables to give you easy access to each of the hormones that affect your life, day in and day out. As you learn about hormones, they become less intimidating and more just another aspect of your health. These tables tell you where in the body each hormone is produced, what function it serves, and what happens when it's out of balance.

Estrogen (estrone, estradiol, estriol)	
Where and how is it made?	In the ovaries, fat cells, and through aromatization of testosterone
What is its function?	*Women have estrogen receptors in every cell, so its effects are far-reaching:* Increases good cholesterol (HDL) Decreases bad cholesterol (LDL) Preserves bone density Affects the skin Maintains body temperature Maintains vaginal lubrication and the vaginal mucosal lining Thickens the uterine lining
What happens when it's out of balance?	*Menopausal-type symptoms:* Night sweats Irritability Mood swings Vaginal dryness Absence of menstruation Mental fogginess Breast sensitivity Weight gain

(continues)

Progesterone

Where is it made?	In the ovaries, adrenal glands, and placenta
What is its function?	Sex hormone Metabolites are critical to the production of other steroids Deflects physiological aspects of estrogen Diuretic Stabilizes and thickens the lining of the uterus Pregnancy hormone Slows down or relaxes smooth muscle Inhibits lactation May reduce inflammation in patients with brain trauma Enhances function of serotonin receptors in brain Upregulates GABA receptors and can help with sleep Natural anti-inflammatory
What happens when it's out of balance?	Insomnia Headaches Neurochemical imbalances Water retention Slowing of bowels, constipation Anxious feelings PMS symptoms

Testosterone (dihydrotestosterone)	
Where is it made?	In the ovaries and adrenal glands
What is its function?	Binds to androgen receptors Drives bone and muscle growth Accelerates metabolism Can break down into estradiol Maintains libido
What happens when it's out of balance?	Female-pattern baldness Diminished libido Lethargy Progressive wastage of muscle Change of metabolic rate Mood-related symptoms: anxiety, depression In high levels: acne, hair growth, and deepening of the voice Low levels can contribute to hair thinning

(continues)

Cortisol	
Where is it made?	In the adrenal glands
What is its function?	Stress hormone Counters insulin Prevents sodium loss and helps regulate potassium Regulates body's pH Increases sugar in the blood Reduces inflammation Aids memory function Helps control blood pressure
What happens when it's out of balance?	Adrenal problems, burnout In high levels: high blood sugar levels (which is why stress causes weight gain) In high levels: atrophy of the hippocampus Increased gastric acid Fatigue Weight loss or weight gain Stretch marks Inability to respond to external stressors

Cortisone	
Where is it made?	In the adrenal glands. Comes from cholesterol
What is its function?	Glucocorticoid Affects blood sugar levels Decreases inflammation
What happens when it's out of balance?	Cortisol breaks down into cortisone Long-term problems with sugar levels Diabetes Osteoporosis Decreased menstruation Depression and/or anxiety Increased blood pressure Suppressed immune system

(continues)

Thyroid Hormone (thyroxine [T4] and triiodothyronine [T3])	
Where is it made?	In the thyroid gland
What is its function?	Metabolic furnace Controls lipid and carbohydrate metabolism Responsible for growth in children Regulates heart rate Regulates body temperature
What happens when it's out of balance?	Sluggishness (from effect on nervous system) Infertility if not controlled, or if there's too little Irregular periods Inability to tolerate cold or heat Weight gain or weight loss

A note on thyroid disease versus thyroid hormone imbalance: It is important to distinguish hypothyroidism and hyperthyroidism from a thyroid hormone imbalance. The first two signal a malfunctioning of the thyroid gland itself, caused by an autoimmune disease, radiation treatment, or other conditions. This malfunction requires treatment that falls outside the scope of the SHINES protocol. Hashimoto's thyroiditis, a condition in which the immune system attacks the thyroid gland, is an example of an illness that a hormone test may help diagnose but that also requires specialized intervention.

DHEA (dehydroepiandrosterone)

Where is it made?	In the adrenal glands
What is its function?	Precursor to estrogen and testosterone Breaks down into estrogen and testosterone Lipid profile
What happens when it's out of balance?	In low levels: sluggishness, fatigue Can be bought over the counter Conversion into estrogen and testosterone (but you don't know how much of it converts)

(continues)

Melatonin

Where is it made?	In the pineal gland (at night), which self-regulates its production unless we change our physiology by staying awake at night. Melatonin production is also linked to cortisol levels, both of which change as we age and impact sleep patterns and other body functions.
What are its characteristics and functions?	Helps us get to sleep Strongest antioxidant in the body Light changes it—red light won't stimulate it Water-soluble Crosses the placenta and helps signal the baby's biological clock as well as the mother's While no archetype is ascribed to melatonin, per se, it is featured in the SHINES protocol for pacifying the Queen
What happens when it's out of balance?	Insomnia Headaches In women who work night shifts: higher levels of breast cancer In low levels: heart disease

Vitamin D
(D2 and D3, discovered during the last decade as most important types)

Where is it made and what is it?	In the kidneys
	Body makes its own vitamin D in the skin
	Converted in liver and then kidneys into vitamin D
	Equally important as the other hormones
	Fat-soluble
What is its function?	Bone health
	May be beneficial in prevention of heart disease, depression, hypertension, and influenza

Finding the Right Health Specialist

Often, patients are exasperated and exhausted when they come in to see me for the first time because they feel unheard. Modern medicine has conditioned both doctor and patient to hurry through a visit rather than spending time and paying attention to the details of how symptoms are making a patient feel. But I believe that taking the time to listen and communicate is essential, because understanding a patient's story is key to unlocking the mysteries of her hormone health. I want to encourage you to use this book as a guide to understanding your own hormone story. One of the primary characters in your story is the hormone health specialist who will work with you as you embark on this journey. It is incredibly important to partner with a practitioner who will really listen and pay attention to all the facets of your hormonal experiences.

The first step is to find a specialist you like and trust. Do some research into "hormone specialists," and you will find there is a wide variety of practitioners using this term to describe their expertise and services. Some are physicians, some are nurse practitioners, and still others are health coaches. Be a savvy consumer. Make sure you consult a medical professional who has experience managing hormonal imbalances over the long term. Also, make sure you feel comfortable asking them questions, whether these are about testing, symptoms you are experiencing, medications you're taking, your diet and exercise regime, any supplements you think may prove helpful, your mood, your energy levels, or your sex drive. Confirm for yourself that you're able to bring your questions into their office and that you leave with helpful advice, even if their help is a referral to another qualified health provider who may be better equipped to help with your specific needs.

You may find physicians like myself, generally OB/GYNs, who

specialize in hormones. But there are also internal medicine specialists who focus on treating women's hormone imbalances. We are constantly learning from our patients and also from other doctors and researchers innovating in this space. In my office, I see thousands of women a year, multiple times each year, and work with them to track their hormone levels over time and adjust and readjust their management plans.

"Hormones" has become a bit of a buzzword these days that helps with searchability online. There are doctors and nurse practitioners who consult and prescribe to patients seeking hormone help (and who may even work in hormone "clinics"), but who are also new to the field and relatively inexperienced when it comes to holistically managing women's hormone health. You will also find OB/GYNs who have treated hundreds or even thousands of women and call themselves hormone specialists. But some of these doctors may specialize in obstetrics rather than gynecology, a focus that may limit their perspective on women's long-term hormone health. OB/GYNs who specialize in gynecology may have broader knowledge of hormones' functionality over the course of a woman's life, but lack experience treating hormonal imbalances, per se. Especially where this requires a multidimensional (medical and nonmedical) integrative approach.

Whether you are considering a doctor, a nurse practitioner, or a health coach, it is important to ask what kind of training and experience this person has in hormone health. Some are well versed in scientific innovations around women's hormone health and the various nonmedical treatments available. But just because a healthcare specialist focuses on women's health does not mean they have expertise in hormone regulation. This can be especially true with health coaches; it's important to determine whether a coach's knowledge base and/or perspective is limited by the scope of their education or experience.

You have everything to gain by finding the right healthcare specialist to work with as you begin to balance your hormones and put effort into your hormonal health. Expect your provider to engage with you—to validate you in some instances and challenge you in others. Expect meaningful dialogue that provides you with concrete takeaways and action steps. Expect to make progress, and to feel guided and supported as you do.

Tips for Finding the Right Hormone Specialist

1. Ask your primary care physician for a recommendation.

Often your primary care physician (PCP) will know the level of expertise of other physicians in the area. It is a reflection on your PCP if they refer you to someone who isn't up to snuff, so they will you refer to those people whom they think are good at what they do. And their patients will likely have reported back to them with ongoing results.

2. Ask your friends for recommendations.

If you have friends who are seeing hormone specialists and experiencing positive results, ask them to refer you. Keep in mind that the more referrals you get for the same person, the better that referral could potentially be.

3. Ask your compounding pharmacist for recommendations.

Pharmacies are not allowed to give doctors monetary kickbacks, so if they recommend a physician, it is most likely because that physician has a good reputation. They also see patients monthly when they pick up their prescriptions and preparations, and often know if those customers are satisfied with good results. I also suggest that you avoid overreliance on your pharmacist because many of them charge a fee to evaluate labs, which is fine to gather information, but they cannot treat you or prescribe medications.

4. Read reviews.

Typically, I don't like online reviews, but if your provider has many happy patients who are saying they've never felt better, then that's a good indication of a provider who knows hormones. Of course, there are almost always a few outliers who post bad reviews, because everyone experiences individual results. But chances are, if there are lots of good and great reviews, this is a knowledgeable and caring physician or other qualified healthcare specialist.

5. Find a provider who uses bioidentical hormones/ compounded hormones.

Prescriptive bioidentical hormones are man-made, chemically identical hormones acting exactly like those your body produces and may have better side effect profiles than synthetic hormones. Compounding hormones are a customized combination of hormones made by a compounding pharmacist based on a physician's prescription. If your physician doesn't want to use compounded hormones, there are prescriptive bioidenticals made by larger pharmaceutical companies.

6. Avoid a provider who uses hormone pellets.

The use of these pellets doesn't mean they are a poor physician, but in my opinion, it means they don't have a depth of knowledge about hormones. Pellets are protocol-driven, not individualized, and I believe they are the worst method of hormone replacement for women. I have been vocal about this for years, for many reasons, and I highlight ten of these reasons

(continues)

later in the book on page 348. The summation of my opinion is that hormone pellets are for animals, not women, so suffice it to say that my advice is to stay away from them.

7. Don't trust a specialist who says "everything looks normal" or who does not listen to you.

You wouldn't be seeing a specialist if you felt normal. If you feel poorly and your test results show numbers on the lower end of the "normal" range, this might not be *your* normal, and your healthcare practitioner should understand this. The partnership you create with your specialist is crucial. You want someone who can listen to the story of what you are experiencing, because it is within the story that the answer is often found. Your story is not told by the results of any one lab test. It is the full complement of what you are experiencing that points in the right direction. Choose a knowledgeable practitioner who is interested in your story and invested in how you feel, not just interested in addressing your symptoms.

8. Don't trust someone who charges inordinately high fees for office visits or testing.

Some physicians ask that patients pay out of pocket up front; there is nothing wrong with this. But if a physician's fees are unusually high, you may want to question that. Just because something costs more doesn't mean that it is better. Some clinics charge large amounts to give the illusion of quality.

9. Don't trust a specialist who tries to "upsell" you on supplements or programs.

There is nothing wrong with investing in high-quality supplements or programs, but if the larger effort of the clinic is to sell you these supplements and programs with little regard for treating your health issues, you likely have not found the right place.

10. Trust your instincts.

You know when something is out of balance and when it merits your attention and the advice of an experienced health provider. You can equally rely on your instincts to tell you if you've found the right guide who will help you get where you want to go. And don't be shy. Come ready with your questions and concerns.

There's a Test for That

Now that you have a plan for finding the right hormone specialist to work with, the next step, with the help of your physician, is having your hormonal levels tested. There are three types of hormone testing out there: blood serum–based testing, saliva-based testing, and urine-based testing. In this section, we're going to look at the strengths and weaknesses of each of these and discuss how sensitive, specific, and useful their results can be. I am asked many times a month, "When is the best time to test?" The best answer is cycle day 21, with day 1 being the beginning of your bleeding.

BLOOD SERUM TESTING

Blood serum testing measures total hormone levels in the serum, or plasma, part of the blood. Importantly, blood serum testing makes no distinction between a hormone's bioavailability (how much of any particular hormone is active in the body) and nonbioavailability (how much is present but not active). This means that an abundance of bound hormones (which are inactive) can make levels appear normal or even high, masking functional deficiencies. For example, a test for total testosterone doesn't tell you how much of that testosterone is biologically active in your body. You need to know the level of free testosterone in your blood to know the actual amount of active testosterone.

STRENGTHS

The primary strength of blood serum testing is that it's a **direct measure of what is in your blood at any given time**. You don't have to account for your hormones having been secreted across membranes before they appear in your saliva or filtered through your kidneys before they appear in your urine. In your blood, your hormone levels simply are what they are. Blood serum testing is an extremely accurate means of determining hormone levels because it measures what is literally in your body at the time of the test. It is also widely regarded as the **best tool for determining bioidentical dosages** of oral estriol and sublingual hormone treatments.

An added advantage of blood serum testing is that when ordered by a physician, it's typically **covered by insurance**. Saliva and urine testing, while still affordable, are generally not covered.

WEAKNESSES

A notable weakness of blood serum testing is that it **provides only a snapshot in time**. You will know what your hormone levels were at the moment the needle entered your arm, but that is all. Given that the levels of various hormones can significantly rise and fall during the course of a day, you'll want to retest your blood on a regular basis. (This is why saliva-based testing is better for measuring cortisol: It is far easier to take several saliva samples during a 24-hour period, which is important for cortisol in particular.)

If you're going to rely on blood serum testing, I recommend **retesting every six to eight weeks**. This is especially important if you are taking hormone medications or supplements. Blood testing works well if you're taking oral estrogens, DHEA, patches, pellets, or injections. But the results are a little less predictable if you're taking medications that either cause your hormone levels to peak quickly and then recede or take time to enter your system. For example, oral progesterone poses a challenge for blood serum testing because it causes significant fluctuations in your progesterone levels. Sublingual troches, vaginal and anal suppositories, and transdermal creams can also lead to misleading results, given how long it takes the medication to be absorbed into your system. In order to mitigate the impact of inconsistent levels on test results, I encourage my patients to standardize the time of day they take their medications and the time they have their blood tested and to keep these times consistent.

Despite the fact that blood serum–based hormone testing is FDA approved and widely used among physicians (I recommend it to many of my own patients), **this method also falls short when it comes to metabolites** (see below). Blood tests can't tell you whether your body is generating more protective or potentially carcinogenic metabolites.

The thing to remember about blood serum testing is that getting a good read on your hormone levels may require multiple data points (meaning multiple tests). This can be done—it just requires an experienced doctor and a dedicated patient.

What Are Metabolites?

For the purpose of elimination, each of the sex hormones—estradiol, estrone, estriol, progesterone, and testosterone—is broken down by enzymes. The resulting metabolites, the products of this breakdown, can have both positive and negative effects on the body, so an experienced practitioner will be able to both assess their activity using a urine-based test known as a DUTCH test (see page 54) and make recommendations based on this process in your body. This test is the *only* method of measuring metabolites currently available for wide-

(continues)

scale use. Your physician will be able to interpret your results for you. A good question to ask might be: "Are metabolites playing any role in my hormone profile?"

This process involves two steps: hydroxylation and methylation. In some cases, women's bodies fail to methylate properly, a condition commonly associated with the lack of a gene called MTHFR. When this malfunction occurs, the body may produce metabolites associated with certain health risks.

For example, each of the three types of estrogen—estradiol, estrone, and estriol—can be broken down into metabolites associated with an increased risk of breast cancer and heart disease (especially estrone), and elevated levels of homocysteine, a condition that can result in early heart attack and stroke. To screen for cancer risk, some hormone specialists use the ratio between two estrone metabolites: 2-hydroxyestrone and 4-hydroxyestrone. A decrease in the ratio of these metabolites is associated with an increased risk of breast and cervical cancers, which is something you and your physician can address.

The production of metabolites rarely results in any obvious symptoms, but measuring them can give you valuable insight into processes beyond hormone production and into your overall well-being.

SALIVA TESTING

Saliva testing is an easy and noninvasive way of assessing your hormone levels. Samples are easy to collect at your doctor's office, at work, or at home, and when stored properly, are stable for several weeks. Results are highly accurate (92 to 96 percent), and relative to other methods, saliva testing is also very affordable.

Unlike other forms of testing, saliva tests measure the levels of your "unbound" (bioavailable) hormones. These are the hormones present in your bloodstream that are not bound to proteins, which means they are therefore free to bind with receptor cells and exert their effects. (Unlike "bound"—nonbioavailable—hormones, unbound hormones are small enough to pass through the cell membranes of the salivary glands when your blood is filtered through them.) In general, roughly 5 percent of a given hormone will be bioavailable, while the remaining 95 percent will be bound.

STRENGTHS

Saliva testing can **reveal trends in estrogen and progesterone levels during the menstrual cycle.** (Taking samples ten times during a twenty-eight-day cycle is a reasonable standard.) While this type of testing is not sufficiently sensitive to generate precise measurements of the levels of either of these hormones, it can reveal patterns that may indicate certain underlying issues.

An important strength of saliva-based testing is that it's **widely regarded as the gold standard for measuring cortisol levels.** When samples are taken throughout the course of a day, saliva shows the rise and fall of cortisol levels in your system, data that can help your physician determine what is driving over- or underproduction of this hormone.

WEAKNESSES

The primary weakness of saliva-based testing is that it **does not measure estrogen sufficiently accurately to differentiate between pre- and postmenopausal symptoms.** For example, saliva testing is not useful for measuring estradiol, the primary estrogen physicians and other hormone specialists tend to want to assess. Because levels of estradiol are 1,000 times less concentrated in saliva than they are in urine, you may have far higher levels of estradiol in your bloodstream than your saliva indicates.[2]

Saliva-based testing is also **very hard to standardize**. Everyone secretes hormones into their saliva differently, so it is impossible to establish "normal" ranges. Just as important, the test cannot accurately measure hormones in patients using hormone treatments administered via vaginal or anal suppository, or in patients using hormone-replacement patches, pellets, injections, or transdermal creams. All of this has to do with the rate at which women absorb these medications into their bloodstream and the rate at which they release hormones into their saliva.

Hormone metabolites pose yet another challenge to saliva-based testing. Because saliva-based testing does not distinguish between hormones and their metabolites, it may seem that there are higher levels of an active hormone than there actually are.

Measuring estrogen metabolites is an important aspect of assessing and improving hormonal health. Before excretion, each of the three types of estrogen are broken down into metabolites, some of which are associated with an increased risk of heart disease and certain cancers. There are ways to help tip the ratio of "good" to "bad" metabolites in a healthier direction, and measuring the levels of these metabolites is the first step (which can be done via urine testing, which will be discussed on page 53).

A final shortcoming of saliva-based testing (and perhaps the most obvious one) is that **results can be skewed by food, drink, or hormone-based medications**. If you've recently rinsed your mouth with mouthwash or had a cup of coffee, for example, your results may be off. This weakness is even more important to consider if you're taking an oral hormone medication or supplement.

If saliva-based testing seems like the best option for you, be sure that you deal with a reputable lab or service provider that will help ensure you get the most useful results possible. Also, make sure you provide a sufficient number of samples for each 24-hour period the test covers.

Last, it's a good idea to repeat saliva testing at least every eight weeks. This way, you have the best chance of uncovering trends in your levels. Certainly, if you begin taking hormone medications and/or supplements, you will want to repeat whatever test you take on a regular basis.

URINE TESTING

This form of testing requires collecting multiple samples over a 24-hour period. This accounts for a full day of hormone secretion, avoiding the possibility that the measurement will capture only a peak or depressed point in the secretory cycle.

Urine testing measures your level of unbound (bioavailable) hormones, and the results tend to correlate well with symptoms patients report on questionnaires. This form of testing also tends to accurately measure changes in hormone levels brought about by hormone supplementation.

STRENGTHS

One of the key advantages of urine-based testing is that it **measures estrogen metabolites** (though not those of progesterone), which neither saliva- nor blood serum–based options can. It also **reliably measures hormone levels in women using patch-, pellet-, or injection-based hormone therapies.**

WEAKNESSES

There are some drawbacks to urine-based testing. Perhaps the most obvious is that it's cumbersome to collect urine samples over a 24-hour period. But just as important, **both oral medications and vaginal or anal suppositories can skew results.** When hormones are taken by mouth, levels of those hormones in the urine may be falsely elevated due to first-pass metabolism by the liver. Experts recommend not taking DHEA or oral estrogen on the day of testing.

Transdermal medications also pose a challenge. Test results will vary depending on the rate at which your body absorbs the medication and the timing of its application.

Urine-based testing is better at measuring overall progesterone levels in women taking oral progesterone than both saliva- and blood serum–based options, but it **does not reveal progesterone metabolites.** This is a significant drawback. **Testosterone readings can also be falsely low** in patients who have certain genetic metabolic defects. This is another reason your test results must be considered along with your symptoms while working with a hormone-knowledgeable physician.

Due to the impact of first-pass metabolism on test results, 24-hour urine testing is **not recommended for determining dosages of oral estrogen or most sublingual hormone medications.**

A final consideration is that urine-based testing is **not generally covered by insurance** and can be costly.

DRIED URINE TEST FOR COMPREHENSIVE HORMONES (DUTCH TEST)

The DUTCH test, which uses dried urine, is an innovative, easy-to-administer, and highly comprehensive method of measuring hormones and metabolites.

STRENGTHS

Of all the tests available, the DUTCH test is the most extensive and accurate. It offers **readings of adrenal hormones, including cortisol and melatonin, as well as sex hormones.** It also **reveals your hormones' metabolites,** which means it will tell you if you're properly methylating your estrogen, progesterone, and other hormones.

Like blood serum testing and traditional urine testing, the DUTCH test **works well in women taking patch-, pellet-, or**

injection-based hormone treatments. It is also best in class for measuring progesterone (and its metabolites) in women taking oral progesterone medications or supplements. When it comes to **vaginal and anal suppositories,** only this test **avoids contamination** in addition to giving reliable readings of hormone and metabolite levels.

Specimen collection is easier than for traditional 24-hour urine testing. Patients supply four samples taken during a 24-hour period, sending the air-dried strips to the vendor for assessment.

WEAKNESSES

The DUTCH test is **not appropriate for patients with abnormal creatinine excretion or other kidney issues.** The test also suffers from similar limitations to traditional urine testing when it comes to measuring estrogen levels in women who take oral estrogen. **Due to first-pass metabolism by the liver, estrogen levels may appear falsely high.** Readings of **testosterone levels may be similarly affected.**

As with traditional urine testing, the DUTCH test is **not recommended for determining dosages of oral estrogen or most sublingual hormone medications.** Test results are too timing-dependent to be useful.

Transdermal creams pose a challenge for the DUTCH test (as they do to all testing methods). Some application techniques have been shown to yield more accurate results, however. This is worth discussing with your physician.

A final consideration is that the DUTCH test is **not covered by insurance.** The cost of the test is approximately $350.

Additional information about the DUTCH test is available at https://dutchtest.com. If you decide to go with this test, I recommend discussing testing with your physician or healthcare specialist. You will certainly want to review your results with someone who can tell you what they reveal and work with you to develop an appropriate management plan. Also, the best way to override the relatively few limitations of the DUTCH test is to repeat it at certain intervals. Again, your physician will help you determine how often.

Determining Your Hormonal Archetype with the Hormone-Typing Quiz

3

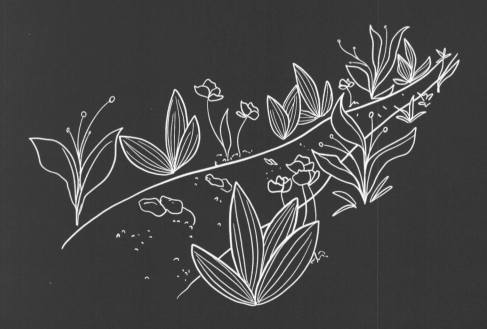

n my approach to treating patients and measuring hormonal health, I look beyond test results and symptoms. These are my data points, but it is also essential to consider each woman's unique health "story" before determining a course of treatment. In my practice, over years of listening to the stories of how hormonal fluctuations and symptoms were affecting my patients' lives, I began to realize that my patients could benefit immensely from thinking of their health challenges in an archetypal way.

What do I mean by "archetypal way"? Archetypal psychology was first introduced by Swiss psychiatrist Carl Jung in the 1920s, and further developed throughout the second half of the twentieth century. In the psychological tradition, archetypes refer to shared, deep-seated patterns of thinking and behavior exhibited by human beings across cultures. Psychological archetypes can provide a framework for understanding broader human experience as applied to one's own unique experience. By talking about archetypes in the context of hormonal health, you can begin to build a narrative that allows you to see your hormonal health as more than just a group of symptoms or the way you feel at any given time. Archetypes allow you to see yourself as a heroine in your own story, a woman who takes charge of her own health and destiny. So many times, when I start working with women, their words are focused on frustration, pain, and discomfort. Of course, that is typically why they have sought my help, and I listen carefully to what they describe so that I can then help them begin their story of action, recovery, and ultimately victory as they navigate through their hormonal needs.

Over her lifetime, every woman will undergo a series of transformational journeys, and her hormones will in many ways be at the center of these journeys. For many women, pregnancy and menopause will be the most life-changing of these hormonal journeys, but other hormonal shifts and imbalances, large and small, can kick off smaller side journeys. I like to borrow from author and teacher Joseph Campbell's classic conception of the "monomyth" as a way to view the hormonal journeys my patients experience. Each journey begins with a woman living in the *ordinary world*, in her natural state, when she is called to *adventure*. Now, you may be thinking, "A hormonal journey? That does *not* sound like an adventure I want to be on!" But stay with me. A woman's hormones touch every aspect of her life, and her life choices in turn influence and affect her hormones in a kind of continuous dance. This is why hormone regulation is so well served by "story": Once a woman chooses to own her hormonal "story" and adds the narrative that begins to make connections, it is easier to view the journey as an adventure. She becomes an active participant in the story, one with the power to change it, rewrite it, and chart its course. In fact, our work in this book is to help you, the reader, become the "heroine" of your own story.

Over many years and through countless experiences with patients, I have developed the twelve Hormonal Archetypes presented in this chapter. These archetypes provide a framework for understanding the origins and effects of the hormonal imbalances that you may experience in your lifetime, and for navigating the ebb and flow of these imbalances as a "heroine's journey" that you can own and lead. The archetypes also provide us with a holistic opportunity for treating hormonal imbalance and looking at these issues in terms of physical, emotional, and spiritual well-being.

These archetypes aren't limited to helping you understand how hormonal imbalances can shape your experience of your physical body and the world around you. They can also help you understand how a hormonal imbalance may influence the way *others* experience *you*. This is because your Hormonal Archetype has an organic impact on the way you show up in the world. It influences your behavior, your demeanor, and your energetic expression. Think about the times in your life when you have felt your best: What did that encompass? How did you show up in the world when you felt this way?

Over your lifetime, your Hormonal Archetype will change and overlap due to the changing nature of the body and of our being. You'll find that different characteristics dominate your physical, psychological, and energetic experiences for a time, and then they change. You can move in and out of an archetype. The ancient Greeks referred to "chronos" time—the sequential, *chrono*logical time of calendars and appointments and day-to-day existence—as opposed to "cosmos" time, which is eternal and enduring. In chronos time, you have the power to change the way you act, appear, and engage with the world around you. Your movement through the archetypes can be "chronos," acting in a linear way that relates to aging and body progression. Or it can operate in "cosmos" time, influenced and affected by your actions, the way you think, and how you engage in the world. In other words, these archetypes encompass the whole of your spirit, as well as your specific biology.

All of this means that yes, your archetype (or archetypes) are part of who you are. But they do not define you. The archetypes are actually a framework for understanding that you have the power to change, if you wish to. And this is where your heroine's journey begins.

The Heroine's Journey

The call to begin your journey could arrive in the form of a sudden drop in your estrogen or progesterone levels, bringing symptoms of insomnia, hot flashes, mood swings, irritability, irregular periods, or weight gain. Or your cortisol levels might abruptly surge, causing skin flushing, skin thinning, stretch marks, high blood pressure, or weight gain. You might feel an acute lack of sexual desire and find that the amount of testosterone in your blood has dropped, or you may feel fatigued in a way you never have before and discover that your thyroid hormone levels have fallen off the low end of the chart. Whatever your symptoms or experiences, this call means you are preparing to cross a threshold. You are leaving the ordinary world, where your hormones were operating in sync and at levels that were normal for you, and entering into a new one, where changes in your hormones are causing you significant pain or unease. Perhaps you've gained 10 pounds, and no matter what you do, you can't seem to drop the weight. Perhaps you feel agitated or irritable in ways you never have before. Perhaps you lose weight or begin losing your hair. Perhaps you lose interest in the things that used to bring you joy. Maybe you can't get out of bed. Maybe you can't sleep.

Whatever your experiences, they signal your entry into a new world—the start of your *adventure*. At first, you're bound to feel lost. But before long, guides will appear along your path: Women who have been where you are. Women who share—or have shared—your archetype. Doctors who have the knowledge and experience to help you. These guides can help you navigate the inevitable challenges that await—the physical, emotional, and energetic tests that threaten to pull you into the abyss.

Here your inner heroine will experience both a defeat and a victory. A death and a rebirth. Now your new self emerges, fortified with freshly acquired knowledge, strength, and awareness, and you're ready to find your way home—to walk the road back, navigating your way out of the labyrinth to reenter a world of wellness you thought you'd left forever. Each of the twelve archetypes has a journey all its own. In the moment you recognize your archetype, you know your journey awaits.

Answering the call means leaving the familiar behind. It means seeking out the help you need and educating yourself. It means becoming an advocate for yourself and constantly striving to achieve balance. It means prioritizing and addressing your physical, emotional, and spiritual needs. This is why the heroine's journey is rarely easy. There are bound to be some rough patches. This is why I tell my patients: *Stick with it. Stick with me. Stay on the path and see where it takes you.*

Are you prepared to take this journey? Are you ready to really dig deep? Are you ready to explore the depths of your soul in order to figure out these hormonal imbalances? Are you ready to experience joyful living again?

Hormone Typing

As I listened to the stories of my patients' life experiences, in combination with the symptoms and health issues they were reporting and the data revealed by their hormonal testing, I began to craft a series of standardized questions that would capture these experiences. I built out my archetype framework, incorporating a holistic approach to the needs of the symptom groups prevalent in my practice. I began with estrogen, the quintessential and dominant female hormone, compiling a list of the common physiological, psychological, and emotional effects of higher and lower estrogen levels. I then considered the seven other critical female hormones in the same light (see chapter two for more information on these), ultimately arriving at the twelve archetypes I'll describe in the next chapter.

I ultimately identified 36 questions that led directly to the twelve archetypes. This quiz is fun and can be fascinating, but it is also remarkably accurate at revealing the current state of a woman's hormone profile when compared against the results of actual hormonal testing.

Hormone testing is the best option when you want to be precise, and any of the tests discussed in this book can be more sensitive and more specific than my Hormone-Typing Quiz. But for insightful results, I would recommend combining hormonal testing with the quiz, in conjunction with the treatment of a trusted physician or hormone specialist, before making any significant changes to your lifestyle or health approach. The quiz can also serve as a solid starting point for a discussion with your physician or healthcare specialist before you undergo testing. Additionally, in chapter four of this book, I go into detail about the hormonal profiles of each archetype, allowing you to consider which symptoms, characteristics, and challenges you recognize in your own story. I think you will find these to be an invaluable addition to what your quiz responses reveal.

Finally, it is time to take the online quiz! The quiz questions center on your physical well-being and lifestyle, asking about the functioning of your reproductive system, about your diet, and about your sleep, mood, and energy levels throughout the day. It also asks questions about your life at home, including your relationship with your spouse or partner, and your job satisfaction. Because the quiz has a mathematical component, it isn't as simple as listing the 36 questions here—the analysis needs computing power, so I have included the URL here for you to access the quiz online: **www.tassonemd.com/quiz**. You can also scan the QR code on page 14 of this book to access the quiz.

Whether you now pause for a moment to take the quiz or continue reading, you are about to enter the world of the twelve Hormonal Archetypes. The information in the book up to this point has laid the groundwork for how to approach your discoveries within these archetypes. Each includes a set of physical, psychological, and energetic experiences. As you read through the archetypes, including the one assigned to you via the online quiz, I encourage you to think about how your own health narrative takes shape. How would you describe your heroine's journey up to this point, and where do you ultimately want this journey to lead you?

4

Understanding the Twelve Hormonal Archetypes

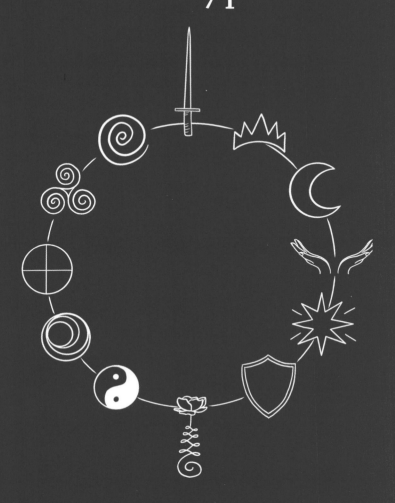

After taking the online assessment (see page 63), you will have gained knowledge and insight into what may be your dominant and secondary archetypes, though, as previously mentioned, these archetypes are fluid and there is overlap between them. This chapter serves to build on the results of the online quiz, and it will invite you to take a closer look at each of the archetypes in detail. Notice where you intersect with these descriptions. I've included a patient story with each archetype, and I think you'll find similarities between more than one of these patient stories and your own story. In this chapter, you will also find a comprehensive symptom chart that includes both physiologic (physical) symptoms and psychological (emotional and mental) signs that correspond to the various archetypes. Keep in mind, however, that while your symptoms are part of your story, they do not tell the whole story. As you read through each of the archetypes, I encourage you to take notes, noticing where you recognize yourself. Think about how you want to own and rewrite your heroine's journey based on the signs and clues you find in these archetypes. Many women are able to identify their archetype(s) by reading the opening descriptions alone, but I recommend that you read each entry in full, approaching this process with a spirit of curiosity. Be sure to stay open to the subtleties of each.

Once you have determined your dominant archetype and possibly some overlapping secondary archetypes as well, you will move on to the SHINES protocols in chapter five, which provide a detailed plan tailored to your archetype. Remember that your hormones are in a constant state of flux, so while you may identify one dominant archetype now, that may change as your body changes throughout your life. What goes on in your body affects your external life, and what takes place in your outside life affects your body. It is all connected, and the archetypes and protocols detailed in this book address your needs as a whole human being. I am confident that you will find yourself on these pages.

The Queen
Estrogen Dominance

"A queen—a queen who bowed to no one, a queen who had faced them all down and triumphed. A queen who owned her body, her life, her destiny, and never apologized for it."

—SARAH J. MAAS

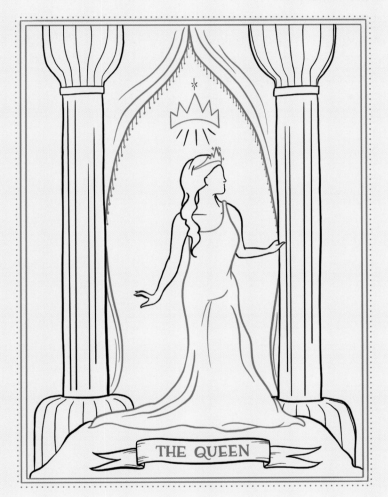

THE QUEEN

noun queen \'kwēn\

a: a woman eminent in rank, power, or attractions.

b: a goddess or a thing personified as female and having supremacy in a specified realm.

In this section, we delve into the Queen archetype. Beginning with one patient's story, we will take a look at the Queen's overarching symptomology and the underlying causes of the hormonal imbalance that characterizes this archetype.

Patient Example

Susan arrived in my office carrying two cell phones. She was speaking on the one that was pinned between her chin and her shoulder and texting furiously on the other. Her thumbs didn't stop moving when she looked at me and mouthed, *I'm so sorry!*

This went on for a few minutes. I had known Susan for years and was accustomed to her grueling work routine. As the head of a large, prestigious real estate firm, she was constantly dealing with some crisis or other. Today was no exception.

"It never stops," she said when she had finally dispensed with the call and stuffed both phones in her purse. "I feel like hell."

Susan was thirty-eight and married with two children, ages ten and twelve. Until recently, she had more or less been able to physically and emotionally keep pace with her busy life at work and at home. But now she was suffering frequent migraines, which were new to her, and her libido had all but disappeared. Initially, she had attributed both to exhaustion. But then other symptoms began to take hold.

During the preceding six to eight months, Susan had gained 10 pounds, despite the fact that she was "eating clean," as she put it—she'd been on a Paleo diet for nearly a year—and working out her usual three early mornings each week. She'd also significantly cut back on her alcohol consumption. While she understood that her metabolism would start to slow down as she aged, the relatively sudden addition of 10 pounds to her five-foot-two, 135-pound frame came as a shock.

These were not the only symptoms Susan was suffering. She also complained of periodic memory lapses she described as "brain fog." While she never forgot "big" things, such as her employees' or clients' names or a major task on her work or home to-do lists, she often couldn't remember where she'd left her car keys or whether she'd taken her vitamins. This didn't trouble her too much, until one day when she forgot to pick up her ten-year-old at school. Then the brain fog seemed a bigger deal. "I feel like I'm living in a fishbowl," she told me. "I'm in the water and looking at the world around me, but it's just not the same. It's not as clear as it used to be."

Susan also complained of certain premenstrual symptoms. For one thing, she reported feeling highly emotionally changeable. "I feel like I'm walking on the edge of a cliff," she said. "Like every little thing is *the* thing that's going to take me over it." Whether it was her husband arriving home late or one of her kids knocking a glass of milk off the table, life's common and relatively small inconveniences were constantly threatening to be the final straw. Susan also noted that her breasts were tender and swollen. She was nearly a full cup size larger, as she typically had been before her menstrual cycles and at the beginning of each of her pregnancies.

Susan was still menstruating regularly, but now her periods were longer than they had been—seven days on average. She was also having some occasional spotting between cycles, which she'd never had before. This was worrying, of course, and also inconvenient. "I always need to be prepared," she told me, "and sometimes I just forget. I'm afraid to wear certain clothes, in case I have one of those days. It's a crappy feeling. I feel like I'm losing control of yet another aspect of my life."

The Queen: Symptomology Summary

Queens who are estrogen dominant tend to present with symptoms like Susan's. Most of the time, they're gaining weight and don't understand why, their periods (and intermittent spotting) tend to be more intense and less predictable, and they suffer intense headaches, as well as what Susan called "brain fog." As in Susan's case, these symptoms taken together contribute to the feeling that they are losing control—of their bodies and, to a degree, of their minds. (For women who have experience with birth control pills, I describe estrogen dominance as being like taking two birth control pills per day.)

Many of the new patients I see have already consulted other physicians about their problems, only to be rebuffed. "My doctor said I needed to calm down," one woman told me. "He said my weight gain was fine. I'd turned forty, after all, so I should get used to it . . . But the weight gain wasn't all. There was much more to it. I was always exhausted and always on edge. Most of all, I know my body, and I knew something wasn't right." The last thing this patient needed to hear was "It's all in your head." And the truth was, it wasn't.

For a Queen, trusting her instinct that *something is not right* and getting the acknowledgment she needs and deserves from the people on whom she relies for counsel and support is the critical first step in her journey. While internal and external acknowledgment are essential to any archetype's progress, these are especially important for a Queen—her body being her domain. Accustomed to garnering the attention and admiration of people around her, she is even more prone to feeling debilitated by her physician's disregard. She may even feel injured by a spouse's or partner's well-intentioned but misguided attempts at support. As one patient described, "When I told my husband I'd gained ten pounds, he told me I looked exactly the same. That I looked fine. I know he was trying to be kind, but I felt like he wasn't listening. Like he didn't believe me when I told him something was *wrong*."

While each woman's experience is unique, you may use the following guide to a Queen's physical, psychological, and emotional symptoms to help determine whether this is your archetype.

Physiological Symptoms

Water retention*	Among Queens, water retention is common and can contribute to symptoms including weight gain, increased blood pressure, and headaches.
Weight gain**	In the short term, a Queen's weight gain may be attributable to water retention. But over time, an estrogen-dominance-driven metabolic imbalance can cause a woman to retain fat, especially around her abdomen and hips; this is driven by the fact that estrogen and insulin work hand in hand in creating an environment around how you utilize glucose in the body.
Cravings***	Queens tend to have cravings. Salty and sugary foods top the list. As one of my patients put it, "I could eat all my kid's Halloween candy." Even if she doesn't normally eat or even crave salty or sugary foods, a Queen is likely to be drawn to both, and may feel less able to resist the urge to raid the pantry, the refrigerator, or anywhere else snacks might be found.

* N. S. Stachenfeld, "Hormonal Changes During Menopause and the Impact on Fluid Regulation, *Reproductive Sciences* 21, no. 5 (2014): 555–61, https://doi.org/10.1177/193 3719113518992.

**A. Gambineri, D. Laudisio, C. Marocco, et al., "Female Infertility: Which Role for Obesity?" *International Journal of Obesity Supplements* 9, no. 1 (2019): 65–72, https://doi .org/10.1038/s41367-019-0009-1.

*** S. Krishnan, R. R. Tryon, W. F. Horn, L. Welch, and N. L. Keim, "Estradiol, SHBG and Leptin Interplay with Food Craving and Intake Across the Menstrual Cycle," *Physiology & Behavior* 165 (2016): 304–12, https://doi.org/10.1016/j.physbeh.2016.08.010.

(continues)

Irregular menstruation	Queens are prone to irregular menstrual cycles. These may occur more frequently (e.g., every two to three weeks) and/or be longer in duration. A Queen's menstrual flow may be heavier than she is accustomed to, and she may also experience spotting between her cycles.
Interference with thyroid hormone*	Estrogen dominance can cause the thyroid gland to become dysfunctional. When estrogen levels become dangerously high, the levels of thyroid binding globulin also become elevated. The latter means you have less active thyroid hormone in your system. If your estrogen levels remain too high for a long period of time, you may begin to experience some hypothyroid-related symptoms—those that characterize the Underdog archetype (see page 156). Among these are cold hands and feet, as well as overarching sluggishness and fatigue
Additional symptoms	Anxiety • Bloating • Breast swelling and tenderness • Decreased libido • Fatigue • Fertility issues • Fibrocystic breasts • Hair loss • Insomnia • Mood swings • Heavy menses • Mid-cycle pain

* P. M. Maki, "Women and Memory," *Menopause* 22, no. 1 (2015): 4–5, https://doi.org/10.1097/GME.0000000000000386.

Psychological and Emotional Symptoms

"Foggy Brain"*	This refers to memory lapses that while relatively minor in terms of their consequences, are nonetheless troubling for the Queen who experiences them. These may manifest as trouble accessing certain details, such as the title of a book you read recently or the name of a person you met, or forgetting an appointment or where you left your keys. An important aspect of foggy brain is that it compounds. The more it happens, the more it is likely to happen—and the more it is likely to cause distress. Sometimes, patients report anxiety around this, fearing they may be suffering a neurological disorder, such as dementia. The anxiety, too, can feed on itself, which can negatively affect mental functioning and contribute to a Queen's sense that she is losing control.
Mood swings, emotional changeability, and feeling out of control**	The Queen who has reached a severe state is likely to experience extreme and unpredictable mood swings. Often, patients describe feeling like they're "tiptoeing along the edge of a cliff" and say they have to bring all their physical, emotional, and psychological energy to bear to keep the winds blowing around them from taking them over it.

* S. Ahmadi, M. R. Eshraghian, M. Hedayati, and H. Pishva, "Relationship Between Estrogen and Body Composition, Energy, and Endocrine Factors in Obese Women with Normal and Low Ree," *Steroids* 130 (2018): 31–35, https://doi.org/10.1016/j.steroids.2017.12.008.

(continues)

**J. K. Warnock, L. J. Cohen, H. Blumenthal, and J. E. Hammond, "Hormone-Related Migraine Headaches and Mood Disorders: Treatment with Estrogen Stabilization," *Pharmacotherapy* 37, no. 1 (2017): 120–28, https://doi.org/10.1002/phar.1876.

*** L. Y. Maeng and M. R. Milad, "Sex Differences in Anxiety Disorders: Interactions Between Fear, Stress, and Gonadal Hormones," *Hormones and Behavior* 76 (2015): 106–17, https://doi.org/10.1016/j.yhbeh.2015.04.002.

Feelings of "bitchiness" and aggression***	Although I take pains to avoid using the term "bitchiness," many of my patients use it to describe themselves. "My kids say I'm mean," a patient will tell me. "My husband says I rule with an iron fist." Whether at home or work, a Queen whose estrogen dominance is making her more emotionally changeable and prone to irritability is likely to present differently to others. Her interactions with family, friends, coworkers, and others may become more emotionally charged, contributing to feelings of alienation and a Queen's tendency to accuse herself of "bitchiness." Of course, any Queen who feels like she's burning the candle at both ends and has little to no capacity to withstand anything going wrong is bound to respond negatively—even aggressively—to inconvenient or disconcerting information or events. "Everyone is afraid to give me any bad news," Susan told me about the other real estate agents at her firm. "They all assume I'm going to explode at them."

When estrogen dominance is transient, causing only temporary physiological or psychological dissonance or discomfort, it may not have lasting or far-reaching effects. Persistent estrogen dominance has been linked to breast cancer, uterine cancer, ovarian cysts, and infertility.[1] It has also been linked to increased blood clotting (including deep vein thrombosis and pulmonary emboli), allergies, autoimmune disorders, and accelerated aging.[2]

When it comes to assessing your symptoms and your overall sense of well-being, trust your instincts. Pay attention to that inner voice that tells you something is *just not right*. Don't leave these symptoms unchecked.

The Queen: Underlying Causes

A number of factors and conditions can give rise to estrogen dominance. In the following pages, we consider the most common internal and external causes of this imbalance, any of which may lie at the heart of the Queen archetype.

CESSATION OF OVULATION

During the first two weeks of a woman's menstrual cycle, she is naturally estrogen dominant. Levels of the hormone rise during this period, peaking just before ovulation. After ovulation, progesterone takes over, balancing out the estrogen to the point where progesterone becomes the dominant hormone during the last two weeks of the cycle.[3]

Beginning in perimenopause, ovulation can become irregular or cease altogether. When this happens, estrogen rises during the first two weeks of the menstrual cycle, then continues to dominate, unopposed by progesterone, since in the absence of ovulation, increased production of progesterone does not occur.

BIRTH CONTROL PILLS, HORMONE REPLACEMENT THERAPY, AND OTHER MEDICATIONS

Birth control pills contain synthetic versions of estrogen and/or progesterone and in most cases prevent pregnancy by preempting ovulation (they also work by disrupting tubal motility and thickening the cervical mucus). When a woman continuously takes birth control pills that contain synthetic estrogen, she runs the risks associated with excess estrogen going unopposed by progesterone, or estrogen dominance. This is particularly true for women whose estrogen levels are already elevated due to perimenopause, polycystic ovarian syndrome (PCOS), or other internal or external factors.

Hormone replacement therapy (HRT) can also drive estrogen dominance. Estrogen-only medications increase levels of estrogen while leaving it unopposed by progesterone. Physicians will often place women who've undergone a hysterectomy solely on estrogen, which puts them in an estrogen-dominant state.

Finally, if you suffer from an autoimmune or inflammatory disorder and are taking an immunosuppressant or steroid-based medication to combat it, you can expect your estrogen levels to rise.

OBESITY

The amount of estrogen a woman produces increases alongside her body fat levels.[4] Women who are obese (those whose body fat exceeds 28 percent) run the greatest risk of body-fat-driven excess estrogen production and, therefore, estrogen dominance.[5] Simply put, fat cells are estrogen-making machines. They are now greatly regarded as another endocrine organ: Not only can they create estrogen, but they can convert excess testosterone to estrogen as well. (For women with PCOS, a condition that also causes the body to create extra testosterone, this means even *more* estrogen.) You can see the horrible cycle: Fat begets more estrogen, and more estrogen can beget more fat.

STRESS

Excessive stress causes levels of cortisol, insulin, and epinephrine to rise.[6] Taken together, these changes can result in the adrenal glands working overtime, running on a hamster wheel of sorts and kicking off the downstream effect of an overarching hormonal imbalance. This broader disruption can lead to a rise in estrogen production.

ENVIRONMENTAL CONTRIBUTORS TO ESTROGEN DOMINANCE

FOOD

Phytoestrogens are naturally occurring plant-based compounds found in beans, seeds, and grains. Because phytoestrogens' chemical structure resembles that of estrogen, these compounds can mimic estrogenic activity and affect both the production and breakdown of estrogen in the body.

A common source of phytoestrogens is soy. It should be noted that many women who are not eating meat because of vegetarian or vegan diets may be eating more soy-related foods. Although various health benefits are associated with soy consumption, including protection against certain types of cancer, menopausal symptoms, heart disease, and osteoporosis, the phytoestrogens contained in soy can pose a danger for women who are estrogen dominant or at risk of becoming so. Part of the phytoestrogen class of isofla-vones, the soy-based extracts genistein, daidzein, and glycitein have known estrogenic effects. Another class of phytoestrogens called coumestans are found in split peas, pinto beans, alfalfa, and clover sprouts, among other foods.

Estrogen is also found in beef and other meat, as well as various dairy products. Exogenous hormones (taken orally, topically, or vaginally— including estrogen and growth hormones) and synthetic, chemical-based compounds with estrogenic effects known as xenoestrogens found in animal feed are largely to blame for this. Many brands have stopped using products that contain estrogen and other hormones, advertising that their meat and dairy products are "hormone-free." But as we'll see in the following section, the pervasiveness of synthetic estrogenic compounds in our environment makes these difficult for meat producers to avoid.

In addition to consuming estrogen in plant- and animal-based foods, your estrogen levels may increase if you are not eating enough fiber. Excess estrogen is expelled via the bowel, so slowing the rate of excretion increases the likelihood that excess estrogen will be reab-sorbed into the system. Eating high levels of refined carbohydrates can compound this problem.

SYNTHETIC ENVIRONMENTAL AGENTS

Xenoestrogens, synthetic compounds that can mimic estrogenic ac-tivity, are found in thousands of man-made products, most notably chemicals and plastics.[7] One of the largest sources of these is a class of chemicals known as organochlorines. Found in pesticides, herbi-cides, and fungicides, as well as in cosmetics products that contain parabens and stearalkonium chloride, organochlorines are also com-monly used in dry-cleaning and plastics manufacturing.

As for plastics, exposure to a compound called PET (polyethyl-ene terephthalate) can contribute to estrogen dominance. A form of polyester, PET is used to make plastic bottles and food containers, as well as certain personal care products. Plastics can also expose you to BPA (bisphenol A), the estrogenic effects of which have been well documented. Widely used in the production of containers for liquids, BPA is released from plastic when heated. This is why environmental health experts warn against microwaving food or liquid in plastic containers.

Birth control pills are another potential and somewhat controversial source of estrogen in the environment. Some scientists have argued that via human excretion or disposal into sewer systems or landfills, birth control pills are leaching synthetic estrogen into soil and waterways. During recent years, countries around the world have considered mandating the removal of the most harmful synthetic estrogens from rivers, lakes, and estuaries.

Personal hygiene products and cosmetics and body products may have chemicals that can have estrogen-like effects on the body.

Lastly, chemicals used in common cleaning products can also have a hormone-like effect on the body and should be avoided for more natural products.

POLYCYSTIC OVARIAN SYNDROME (PCOS)

When a woman has PCOS, tiny cysts on her ovaries and hypothalamic dysfunction prevent her from ovulating. It is only when a woman ovulates that her progesterone production picks up and opposes the estrogen she has produced during the first two weeks of her cycle. Stimulated by hormones from the pituitary gland, these little cysts make large amounts of estrogen and testosterone. This means that women with PCOS are inevitably prone to estrogen and testosterone dominance. The most popular treatment for PCOS is birth control pills, which can intensify estrogen dominance. Oral contraceptives as a treatment for PCOS are not actually treating the issue, but covering it up. They aren't treating the underlying hormonal imbalance, but instead merely shutting off the ovaries and trading bioidentical estrogen dominance for synthetic estrogen dominance.

HEPATIC STRESS

The liver is responsible for breaking down hormones, including estrogen. If it is overtaxed due to illness, alcohol consumption, or medications (including OTC remedies such as Tylenol and Advil), it does this less efficiently, leaving excess estrogen circulating in your system.

The Unbalanced Heroine

Progesterone Deficiency

"And now I may dismiss my heroine to the sleepless couch, which is the true heroine's portion—to a pillow strewed with thorns and wet with tears. And lucky may she think herself, if she get another good night's rest in the course of the next three months."

—JANE AUSTEN

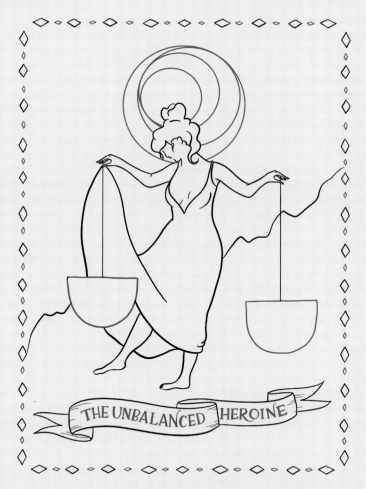

adjective un·bal·anced \ˌən-ˈba-lən(t)st\ noun ˈher-ə-wən\

: a mythological or legendary figure, often of divine descent, endowed with great strength or ability who is not balanced, such as not in equilibrium.

In this section, we consider the archetype of the Unbalanced Heroine, which is characterized by a deficiency of progesterone. Progesterone, produced primarily in the corpus luteum within the ovaries, as well as in smaller quantities in the adrenal glands (and in the placenta during pregnancy), influences a series of vital functions, including sleep, and plays a major role in the menstrual cycle and pregnancy.

During a woman's 28-day menstrual cycle, production of progesterone rises after ovulation (approximately day 14), peaking around day 21. The hormone's primary function is to stabilize the uterine lining (or endometrium) in order to create a supportive environment for a fertilized egg. If a woman does not become pregnant, her progesterone levels begin to fall. By day 28 of her cycle, her uterine lining sheds, and she menstruates. If she does become pregnant, her progesterone levels continue to rise after day 21. The hormone is produced by the corpus luteum (the now transformed lining of the ovulated cyst wall) for roughly ten weeks, until the placenta takes over, leveling off the production of progesterone after the first trimester.

For the Unbalanced Heroine, increases and decreases in progesterone levels do not follow this path. One potential cause of this deviation is that she does not ovulate, a condition known as anovulation. Ovulation is critical to progesterone production, so if ovulation does not occur, over time a progesterone deficiency (and estrogen dominance) will take hold. Ovulation may cease due to a variety of conditions, including excessive stress, extreme weight loss or gain, ovarian dysfunction, and a number of hormonal and/or other chemical imbalances.

An Unbalanced Heroine may continue to ovulate, if irregularly. In these cases, after ovulation, her ovaries do not release sufficient amounts of progesterone to support the growth of the uterine lining. This gives rise to a condition known as luteal phase defect, which is named for the second (or luteal) phase of the menstrual cycle.[8] These Unbalanced Heroines tend to experience severe PMS or premenstrual dysphoric disorder (PMDD). The potentially debilitating symptoms of this disorder include depression and feelings of hopelessness, as well as tension, anxiety, and irritability. Additional symptoms include fatigue, joint and muscle aches, headaches, and interrupted sleep. Luteal phase defect can also cause miscarriage.[9] In the event that an Unbalanced Heroine's egg becomes fertilized following ovulation, her thin endometrial lining may not sustain implantation.

In addition to these primary physiological effects, progesterone can also significantly impact the Unbalanced Heroine's emotional and psychological experiences. Commonly referred to as a calming hormone, progesterone not only helps regulate sleep, but also moderates heightened emotional responses and reduces anxiety. Some studies have shown that progesterone can also intensify a woman's (or a man's) tendency to bond with their offspring.

In this section, we consider two Unbalanced Heroines' stories. We also take a close look at the archetype's causes and symptomology, including those that take hold immediately or more slowly over time.

Patient Examples

ANNA

Anna was nineteen when she first visited me in my office. She was a college sophomore who was struggling with what she called her "freshman 15" and an irregular menstrual cycle. She had not had a regular period in three months. Anna also reported feeling more stressed about her studies than usual, and said she was consistently experiencing a high degree of emotional sensitivity. Her moods were changeable, she explained, and intense. Sometimes, she felt depressed. At other times, she felt extremely irritable. She also reported difficulty sleeping, which left her feeling tired during the day and added to her anxiety about keeping up with her coursework.

Given her collection of symptoms, I suspected a progesterone deficiency, and checked her levels. Although they fell into the "normal" range, her numbers were on the low side during her luteal phase. I assessed that her progesterone levels could account for many of her symptoms, including the changes to her mood, her interrupted menstrual cycle, and her weight gain. Progesterone is also a natural diuretic, I explained to Anna, so some of her "freshman 15" may partially have been due to water retention.

I also checked Anna's estrogen-to-progesterone ratio. In some cases, low progesterone can combine with estrogen dominance. In general, I like to see an estrogen-to-progesterone ratio of 10 to 1. When this reaches 100 to 1, an Unbalanced Heroine may be taking on aspects of the Queen archetype (see page 67), meaning that her progesterone-deficiency-related symptoms are exaggerated *and* she is experiencing the effects of estrogen dominance (the combination of a Queen and an Unbalanced Heroine is the Mother archetype; see page 90). In these cases, Unbalanced Heroines can benefit from a combination of a progesterone-replacement-focused SHINES protocol and one that helps address the symptoms associated with the Queen archetype.

As Anna did, you may find that the Queen archetype overlaps. Where the two archetypes likely overlap, I point this out. Ultimately, a thorough assessment of your symptoms, including your hormone levels, will lead you and your physician or other healthcare provider to precisely determine which imbalance you have.

SUZANNE

At the age of thirty-five, Suzanne had had two miscarriages. She was keen to try to become pregnant again, and she wanted my help to determine whether a hormonal imbalance had caused her to miscarry before.

Suzanne told me each of her miscarriages had occurred during what she estimated to be the first six to eight weeks of her pregnancies. She also reported having struggled with symptoms of PMDD, including severely depressed mood, irritability, and interrupted sleep, and she noted that her periods had become irregular during the past two to three years. Suzanne explained that her cycles had become both shorter and more difficult to predict. This had made it difficult for her to pinpoint when she was ovulating.

When I tested Suzanne's hormone levels, I discovered that her progesterone level was low-normal. Her estrogen-to-progesterone ratios were a little high, though not high enough to warrant her embarking on an estrogen-dominance-related protocol. I recommended that she commence the Unbalanced Heroine's SHINES protocol, including treatment with progesterone during the last two weeks of her cycle (insofar as we were able to predict this). In the event that she became pregnant, her elevated progesterone levels would help sufficiently strengthen the endometrium to support implantation of the fertilized egg. Within ten weeks of conception, her placenta would take over progesterone production, though I recommended that we continue to monitor Suzanne's progesterone levels for the duration of pregnancy.

Suzanne adhered to a SHINES protocol for several months after our initial visit. Before a year had passed, she became pregnant. Her pregnancy was normal, and she delivered a healthy baby at full term.

The Unbalanced Heroine: Symptomology Summary

Unbalanced Heroines tend to present with the following physiological, psychological, and emotional symptoms:

Physiological Symptoms

Breast tenderness and/or fibrocystic breasts • Fibroids	Progesterone blocks the effect of estrogen and will thin out the lining of the uterus. When progesterone is absent, the lining will grow unabated. With endometriosis, a condition in which endometrial-like tissue grows outside the uterus (mostly in the pelvis) without the effects of progesterone, this tissue can cause pain and scarring.
Catamenial migraine[*]	Catamenial migraines occur regularly alongside the menstrual cycle and are particularly prevalent in Unbalanced Heroines. These intense headaches begin on day 1 or 2 of menstruation and can last for 2 to 3 days.

Hot flashes and night sweats[**]	Unbalanced Heroines of any age who have low levels of progesterone and normal levels of estrogen may experience both hot flashes and night sweats.
	
	   Caused by sudden surges in vasodilation, hot flashes are feelings of intense warmth that can spread across the head, neck, and face before extending to the entire body. When these occur during the night, releasing heat and causing perspiration, they are called night sweats.
	
	   Hot flashes typically last between thirty seconds and a few minutes, causing an increase in skin temperature and redness. They may also cause an increase in heart rate, heart palpitations, and dizziness.

Physiological symptoms associated with severe premenstrual syndrome or PMDD[***]	**Fluid retention**, including periodic or longer-term weight gain; swelling of the ankles, hands, and feet; and fullness of the breasts. **Gastrointestinal symptoms**, including abdominal cramps, bloating, constipation, nausea, vomiting, and backache. **Neurological and vascular symptoms**, including headache, dizziness, fainting, increased bruising, and heart palpitations. **Skin conditions**, including acne and aggravation of disorders such as cold sores.

[*] V. Tanos, E. A. Raad, K. E. Berry, and Z. A. Toney, "Review of Migraine Incidence and Management in Obstetrics and Gynaecology," *European Journal of Obstetrics & Gynecology and Reproductive Biology* 240 (2019): 248–55, https://doi.org/10.1016/j.ejogrb.2019.07.021.

[**] J. C. Prior, "Progesterone for Treatment of Symptomatic Menopausal Women," *Climacteric* 21, no. 4 (2018): 358–65, https://doi.org/10.1080/13697137.2018.1472567.

[***] J.-Y. Yen, H.-C. Lin, P.-C. Lin, T.-L. Liu, C.-Y. Long, and C.-H. Ko, "Early- and Late-Luteal-Phase Estrogen and Progesterone Levels of Women with Premenstrual Dysphoric Disorder," *International Journal of Environmental Research and Public Health* 16 (2019): 4352.

(continues)

Psychological and Emotional Symptoms

Irritability • Agitation • Anger • Insomnia • Difficulty concentrating • Depression • Severe fatigue • Anxiety • Confusion • Forgetfulness • Poor self-image • Emotional sensitivity • Crying spells • Moodiness • Interrupted sleep	A progesterone deficiency causes these symptoms because it breaks down into GABA, an amino acid that works as a neurotransmitter in your brain, making you feel more prone to anxiety and insomnia.

The Unbalanced Heroine: Underlying Causes of Symptomology

EMOTIONAL STRESS

One potential underlying cause of the Unbalanced Heroine's symptomology is stress. Intense stress can cause ovulation to cease, which, over time, can result in an extreme progesterone deficiency. This can occur in women of any age.

I have seen stress exert these effects in many of my patients. Around the year 2000, I was working as a military OB/GYN stationed at Fort Sill, an artillery base in Lawton, Oklahoma. There, I worked with hundreds of female soldiers who had entered into combat training. At Fort Sill, their job was to learn how to use various weapons, including mortars and multiple-launch rocket systems (MLRS). This entailed everything from physically firing the weapons to providing tactical support to a ground battalion.

Most of these women were in their twenties and healthy overall. But the stress associated with the psychologically and physically demanding work they were doing day in and day out began to cause them to cease ovulating. This, in turn, caused many of them to suffer from progesterone deficiency, which had an impact on their sleep, moods, and anxiety levels. Given the demanding nature of the circumstances in which they lived and worked—and the larger journey to which they'd been called—supporting these Unbalanced Heroines with a tailored protocol was critically important.

MEDICAL CONDITIONS AND TREATMENTS

Various illnesses and chronic conditions can cause hormonal imbalances that influence progesterone production. Thyroid disease and rheumatoid arthritis are two common examples. Cancer patients who undergo chemotherapy and/or radiation can also suffer damage to the ovaries, which can affect the production of both estrogen and progesterone.

The Mother

Estrogen Dominance and
Progesterone Deficiency

"In a child's eyes, a mother is a goddess. She can be glorious or terrible, benevolent or filled with wrath, but she commands love either way. I am convinced that this is the greatest power in the universe."
—N. K. JEMISIN

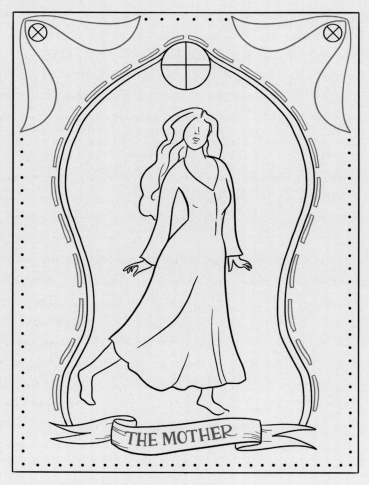

THE MOTHER

noun moth·er \ ˈmə-thər \

a: a female parent.

b (1): a woman in authority; specifically: the superior of a religious community of women.

In this section, we consider the Mother archetype. Characterized by a pair of imbalances—estrogen dominance and progesterone deficiency—the Mother archetype possesses attributes of both the Queen and the Unbalanced Heroine.

Mothers not only run the show as a Queen can, but they also may suffer from a lack of the soothing and caregiving support progesterone provides. Often, Mothers are dedicated to their work, whether this is a busy job outside the home or work within it, and they're also dedicated to their families and larger communities—to their partners, children, parents, friends, and various organizations to which they belong. As such, I've found that Mothers can go for months or even a year or more before addressing their symptoms with me. Accustomed to tending to everyone else first, they do not seek help for their own issues until they are collapsing in bed at seven o'clock each night; their menstrual cycles have either stopped or significantly changed in quality, frequency, or duration; they have gained 15 to 20 pounds; and/or they're fed up with battling the fatigue caused by the fever pitch at which they're operating.

If you have tested into the Mother archetype, I suggest reading this section with an eye to those symptoms that most closely resonate with yours. This will help you determine whether estrogen dominance or progesterone deficiency is the more significant driver of your symptoms. Consider also the potential underlying causes of each of these conditions to help determine how and when your archetype is likely to have taken hold. For additional information on estrogen dominance, you may consult the section on the Queen archetype (page 67). For more on progesterone deficiency, you may refer to the Unbalanced Heroine (page 81).

Patient Example

As soon as Melanie entered my office, she all but collapsed into a chair. "I'm *exhausted!*" she said. "And whatever I do, I *swear* it's only getting worse." Now thirty-five, this stay-at-home mother of two young children had been my patient since she was thirty. And while I was certain some of her fatigue was attributable to her responsibilities at home, I could tell there was more to Melanie's story.

When I asked Melanie about her other symptoms, she systematically listed them out for me. During the past year, she had gained 25 pounds. Now, she told me, she weighed as much as she had at the height of her first pregnancy. "I feel bloated all the time," she told me. "I can't even wear my rings anymore, my fingers are so swollen. I feel like I'm *always* about to get my period." In addition to feeling bloated, Melanie suffered extreme physical and psychological premenstrual symptoms, including terrible cramping, mood swings, and irritability. On top of all this, Melanie's menstrual cycle had become irregular. Sometimes, she would go three months between cycles, often experiencing spotting during this time.

Melanie went on. "Sometimes, I get hot flashes," she said. At one point, these had become so severe, she thought she might be entering menopause early. Melanie also reported suffering intermittently from migraines, which she'd never experienced before, as well as insomnia. "I'm in bed as soon as the kids are," Melanie explained, "but then I'm up in the middle of the night, pacing the floor, waiting for one of them to wake up."

While some of Melanie's symptoms indicated estrogen dominance, the insomnia in particular caused me to think that a progesterone deficiency had also taken hold. I recommended a DUTCH test, which revealed the combination of imbalances: Melanie's estrogen was on the high side of the "normal" range, and her progesterone on the low side. More revealing, perhaps, was the ratio between these figures. Although each fell within "normal" range, Melanie's estrogen-to-progesterone ratio was 1,000 to 1. In a woman whose estrogen and progesterone are in balance, this ratio is roughly 10 to 1. (In women who are estrogen dominant only—i.e., Queens—this ratio is approximately 100 to 1.)

The Mother: Symptomology Summary

The Mother's symptomology combines elements of the Queen's and the Unbalanced Heroine's symptomologies. A Mother is likely to experience some of these symptoms, but not all. As you review them, consider which align most closely with your own. This will help you ascertain the degree to which estrogen dominance and progesterone deficiency have each contributed to the rise of your archetype and the role each is playing in your overall hormonal health.

Physiological Symptoms: Estrogen Dominance	
Water retention	Water retention is common and can contribute to other symptoms, including weight gain, increased blood pressure, and headaches.
Weight gain	In the short term, weight gain may be attributable to water retention. But over time, an estrogen-dominance-driven metabolic imbalance can cause a woman to retain fat, particularly around her abdomen and hips.
Cravings	Cravings for salty and sugary foods are common. Even if she doesn't normally eat or even crave salty or sugary foods, a Mother is likely to be drawn to both, and may feel less able to resist the urge to raid the pantry, the refrigerator, or anywhere else snacks might be found.

(continues)

Irregular menstruation	Mothers are prone to irregular menstrual cycles. These may occur more frequently (e.g., every two to three weeks) and/or be longer in duration. A Mother's menstrual flow may be heavier than she is accustomed to, and she may also experience spotting between her cycles.
Interference with thyroid hormone	Estrogen dominance can cause the thyroid gland to become dysfunctional. When estrogen levels become dangerously high, the levels of thyroid binding globulin also become elevated. The latter means you have less active thyroid hormone in your system. If your estrogen levels remain too high for a long period of time, you may begin to experience some hypothyroid-related symptoms—those that characterize the Underdog archetype (see page 156). Among these are cold hands and feet, as well as overarching sluggishness and fatigue.
Additional symptoms	Breast swelling and tenderness Fibrocystic breasts Hair loss Insomnia Night sweats

Physiological Symptoms: Progesterone Deficiency

Breast tenderness and/or fibrocystic breasts	The reason for the tenderness is the stimulation of the breast tissue and cysts by higher levels of estrogen.
Fibroids	The mostly benign muscular tumors cause pelvic pain, pressure, and increased bleeding.
Catamenial migraine	Catamenial migraines occur regularly alongside the menstrual cycle. These intense headaches begin on day 1 or 2 of menstruation and can last for 2 to 3 days.
Hot flashes and night sweats	Mothers of any age who have low levels of progesterone and high levels of estrogen may experience both hot flashes and night sweats. Caused by sudden surges in vasodilation, hot flashes are feelings of intense warmth that can spread across the head, neck, and face before extending to the entire body. When these occur during the night, releasing heat and causing perspiration, they are called night sweats. Hot flashes typically last between thirty seconds and a few minutes, causing an increase in skin temperature and redness. They may also cause an increase in heart rate, heart palpitations, and dizziness.

(continues)

Physiological symptoms associated with severe premenstrual syndrome or PMDD	**Fluid retention**, including periodic or longer-term weight gain; swelling of the ankles, hands, and feet; and fullness of the breasts. **Gastrointestinal symptoms**, including abdominal cramps, bloating, constipation, nausea, vomiting, and backache. **Neurological and vascular symptoms**, including headache, dizziness, fainting, increased bruising, and heart palpitations. **Skin conditions**, including acne and aggravation of disorders such as cold sores.

Psychological and Emotional Symptoms: Estrogen Dominance

"Foggy brain"	This refers to memory lapses that, while relatively minor in terms of their consequences, are nonetheless disconcerting or troubling for the Mother who experiences them. These may manifest as trouble accessing certain details, such as the title of a book you read recently or the name of a person you met, or forgetting an appointment or where you left your keys. An important aspect of foggy brain is that it compounds. Sometimes, patients report anxiety around this, fearing they may be suffering a neurological disorder, such as dementia.

Mood swings, emotional changeability, and feeling out of control	The Mother who has reached a severe state is likely to experience extreme and unpredictable mood swings, feeling on edge or like she's "just barely holding on." Mothers often describe generalized feelings of loss of control. In fact, in many instances, I've documented "I feel totally crazy" as a patient's chief complaint.
Feelings of "bitchiness" and aggression	Although I take pains to avoid using the term "bitchiness," many of my patients use it to describe themselves. "My kids say I'm mean," a patient will tell me. "My husband says I rule with an iron fist." Whether at home or work, a Mother whose estrogen dominance is making her more emotionally changeable and prone to irritability is likely to present differently to others. Her interactions with family, friends, coworkers, etc., may become more emotionally charged, contributing to feelings of alienation and a Mother's tendency to accuse herself of "bitchiness." Of course, any Mother who is on her last straw, feeling like she's burning the candle at both ends and has little to no capacity to withstand anything going wrong, is bound to respond negatively—and even aggressively—to inconvenient or disconcerting information or events. Here again, we see the importance of how your Hormonal Archetype shapes not only your experience of the world but how the rest of the world experiences you.

(continues)

Psychological and Emotional Symptoms: Progesterone Deficiency	
Psychological and emotional symptoms associated with severe premenstrual syndrome or PMDD	Agitation • Anger • Anxiety • Confusion • Crying spells • Depression • Difficulty concentrating • Emotional sensitivity • Forgetfulness • Insomnia • Interrupted sleep • Irritability • Moodiness • Paranoia • Poor self-image • Severe fatigue

When estrogen dominance is transient, causing only temporary physiological or psychological dissonance or discomfort, it may not have lasting or far-reaching effects. Persistent estrogen dominance has been linked to breast cancer, uterine cancer, ovarian cysts, and infertility. It has also been linked to increased blood clotting (including deep vein thrombosis and pulmonary emboli), allergies, autoimmune disorders, and accelerated aging.

The Mother: Underlying Causes of Symptomology

A common factor in the rise of the Mother archetype is birth control medication. If you are taking a birth control medication that contains synthetic estrogen, it may be contributing to your estrogen dominance and exacerbating the relevant symptoms. Switching to a progestin-only birth control medication may help bring your estrogen and progesterone closer to balance; however, the progesterone is also synthetic, and while birth control pills are okay for birth control, they aren't necessarily fixing estrogen dominance. Synthetic progesterone may not have the same effects as the progesterone produced by your own body or a bioidentical replacement.

CONDITIONS THAT CAN EXACERBATE THE MOTHER'S SYMPTOMS

Certain illnesses and chronic conditions may give rise to the Mother archetype. Thyroid disease and rheumatoid arthritis are both associated with the diminished production of progesterone. Cancer patients who undergo chemotherapy and/or radiation can also suffer damage to the ovaries, which can affect the production of both estrogen and progesterone.

Polycystic ovarian syndrome (PCOS) can also contribute to the rise of the Mother archetype. When a woman ovulates, her progesterone production picks up and opposes the estrogen she has produced during the first two weeks of her cycle. When a woman has PCOS, tiny cysts on her ovaries prevent her from ovulating, which means that women with PCOS are inevitably prone to estrogen dominance. Adding to this, the most popular treatment for the condition is birth control pills, which can intensify the condition and exacerbate symptoms of the Mother archetype.

Underlying Causes of Estrogen Dominance

A number of factors and conditions can give rise to estrogen dominance. In the following pages, we consider the most common internal and external causes of this imbalance, any of which may contribute to the Mother archetype taking hold.

CESSATION OF OVULATION

During the first two weeks of a woman's menstrual cycle, she is naturally estrogen dominant. Levels of the hormone rise during this period, peaking just before ovulation. After ovulation, progesterone takes over, balancing out the estrogen to the point where progesterone becomes the dominant hormone during the last two weeks of the cycle.

Beginning in perimenopause, ovulation can become irregular or cease altogether. When this happens, estrogen rises during the first two weeks of the menstrual cycle, then continues to dominate, un-opposed by progesterone, since in the absence of ovulation, increased production of progesterone does not occur.

OBESITY

The amount of estrogen a woman produces increases alongside her body-fat levels. Women who are obese (whose body fat exceeds 28 percent) run the highest risk of body-fat-driven excess estrogen production and, therefore, estrogen dominance. Simply put, fat cells are estrogen-making machines. They are now greatly regarded as an-other endocrine organ: Not only can they create estrogen, but they can convert excess testosterone to estrogen as well. (For women with PCOS, a condition that also causes the body to create extra testoster-one, this means even *more* estrogen.) You can see the horrible cycle: Fat begets more estrogen, and more estrogen can beget more fat.

STRESS

Excessive stress causes levels of cortisol, insulin, and epinephrine to rise. Taken together, these changes can result in the adrenal glands working overtime, running on a hamster wheel of sorts and kicking off the downstream effect of an overarching hormonal imbalance. This broader disruption can lead to a rise in estrogen production.

ENVIRONMENTAL CONTRIBUTORS TO ESTROGEN DOMINANCE

FOOD

Phytoestrogens are naturally occurring plant-based compounds found in beans, seeds, and grains. Because phytoestrogens' chemical structure resembles that of estrogen, these compounds can mimic estrogenic activity and affect both the production and breakdown of estrogen in the body.

A common source of phytoestrogens is soy. Although various health benefits are associated with soy consumption, including protection against certain types of cancer, menopausal symptoms, heart disease, and osteoporosis, the phytoestrogens contained in soy can pose a danger for women who are estrogen dominant or at risk of becoming so. Part of the phytoestrogen class of isoflavones, the soy-based extracts genistein, daidzein, and glycitein have known estrogenic effects. Another class of phytoestrogens called coumestans are found in split peas, pinto beans, alfalfa, and clover sprouts, among other foods.

Estrogen is also found in beef and other meat, as well as various dairy products. Exogenous hormones (including estrogen and growth hormones) and synthetic, chemical-based compounds with estrogenic effects known as xenoestrogens found in animal feed are largely to blame for this. Many brands have stopped using products that contain estrogen and other hormones, advertising that their meat and dairy products are "hormone-free." But as we'll see in the following section, the pervasiveness of synthetic estrogenic compounds in our environment makes these difficult for meat producers to avoid.

In addition to consuming estrogen in plant- and animal-based foods, your estrogen levels may increase if you are not eating enough fiber. Excess estrogen is expelled via the bowel, so slowing the rate of excretion increases the likelihood that excess estrogen will be reabsorbed into the system. Eating high levels of refined carbohydrates can compound this problem.

As is true with most hormone imbalances, overconsumption of alcohol can cause significant stress and exogenous triggering of hormone receptors. Alcohol consumption over time also stresses the liver and can thus decrease the body's ability to clear hormone metabolites.

SYNTHETIC ENVIRONMENTAL AGENTS

Xenoestrogens, synthetic compounds that can mimic estrogenic activity, are found in thousands of man-made products, most notably chemicals and plastics. One of the largest sources of these is a class of chemicals known as organochlorines. Found in pesticides, herbicides, and fungicides, as well as in cosmetics products that contain parabens and stearalkonium chloride, organochlorines are also commonly used in dry-cleaning and plastics manufacturing.

As for plastics, exposure to a compound called PET (polyethylene terephthalate) can contribute to estrogen dominance. A form of polyester, PET is used to make plastic bottles and food containers, as well as certain personal care products. Plastics can also expose you to BPA (bisphenol A), the estrogenic effects of which have been well documented. Widely used in the production of containers for liquids, BPA is released from plastic when heated. This is why environmental health experts warn against microwaving food or liquid in plastic containers.

Birth control pills are another potential and somewhat controversial source of estrogen in the environment. Some scientists have argued that via human excretion or disposal into sewer systems or landfills, birth control pills are leaching synthetic estrogen into soil and waterways. During recent years, countries around the world have considered mandating the removal of the most harmful synthetic estrogens from rivers, lakes, and estuaries.

HEPATIC STRESS

The liver is responsible for breaking down hormones, including estrogen. If it is overtaxed due to illness, alcohol consumption, or medications (including OTC remedies such as Tylenol and Advil), it does this less efficiently, leaving excess estrogen circulating in your system.

UNDERLYING CAUSES OF PROGESTERONE DEFICIENCY

PSYCHOLOGICAL AND PHYSICAL STRESS

Intense stress can cause ovulation to cease, which, over time, can result in an extreme progesterone deficiency. This can occur in women of any age.

I have seen stress exert these effects in many of my patients. Around the year 2000, I was working as a military OB/GYN stationed at Fort Sill, an artillery base in Lawton, Oklahoma. There, I worked with hundreds of female soldiers who had entered into combat training. At Fort Sill, their job was to learn how to use various weapons, including mortars and multiple-launch rocket systems (MLRS). This entailed everything from physically firing the weapons to providing tactical support to a ground battalion.

Most of these women were in their twenties and healthy overall. But the stress associated with the psychologically and physically demanding work they were doing day in and day out began to cause them to cease ovulating. This, in turn, caused many of them to suffer from progesterone deficiency, which had an impact on their sleep, moods, and anxiety levels. Given the demanding nature of the circumstances in which they lived and worked—and the larger journey to which they'd been called—supporting these Mothers with a tailored protocol was critically important.

The Wisewoman

Estrogen Deficiency

"When a wise woman speaks, smart people listen and learn from her."

—GIFT GUGU MONA

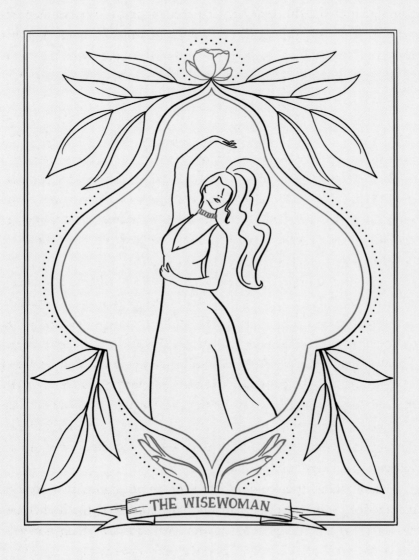

THE WISEWOMAN

noun wise·wom·an \ˈwīz-ˌwu̇-mən\
: a woman versed in charms, conjuring, or fortune-telling.

In this section, we consider the Wisewoman archetype. Characterized by a severe lack or total absence of estrogen (and also of progesterone and most likely testosterone), this archetype largely takes hold in women over the age of fifty who naturally become menopausal. From the time they enter perimenopause, Wisewomen experience a range of physical, psychological, and spiritual symptoms rooted in the cessation of estrogen (and progesterone) production in the body, and the archetype becomes a permanent part of who they are.

Wisewomen may also be younger, however. If a woman has had a total hysterectomy and a bilateral oophorectomy (removal of the ovaries), for example, or is suffering from a condition or taking a medication that severely diminishes or prevents estrogen production, she may become a Wisewoman. If her ovaries have been removed, the archetype will remain permanently. If a medical condition gives rise to the archetype and then resolves, the archetype will be temporary.

Regardless of her age, when a Wisewoman is called to adventure, she is thrown into a world where the formidable and predominant hormonal force behind her physical development and her sexual and reproductive experiences has ceased to exert its impact. This drives some of the most profound physical, psychological, and spiritual changes associated with any of the twelve archetypes. Taken together, these changes represent a new phase in a woman's life. The journey into Wisewomanhood is a rite of passage that is at once natural, normal, and rife with opportunities for enhanced self-awareness and spiritual and emotional growth.

I have treated thousands of Wisewomen during my two decades in practice. Some of these patients have embraced the archetype, challenges and all. Many women who have naturally reached menopause have told me that for them, the archetype symbolizes a welcome, calmer period following decades of life's inevitable trials and tribulations—an earned badge of honor. Other women have resisted entering into this phase. Younger and older women alike have told me they are filled with regret about the losses they perceive it entails.

Regardless of whether a woman embraces or resists her Wise-woman archetype, at the outset of her heroine's journey, she is an acolyte. Again, the shift its onset represents is one of the most fundamentally important and significant changes a woman will ever experience, which is why I counsel my patients to seek out a mentor; I advise the same for those of you reading this book. This mentor may be a woman who has lived through the experience herself, having been in menopause for years. Whether she has managed this with hormone modulation, taken a holistic approach such as SHINES provides, or simply gritted it out (as my ninety-five-year-old grandmother liked to remind me she did), the important thing is that she endured the labyrinth's turmoil, emerging as a more balanced, knowledgeable, and powerful version of herself. Your mentor may also be a physician or other healthcare practitioner who can draw on their experience with other women who have walked the path you're on. Whomever you choose to help guide and support you, the counsel and encouragement of people who have intimate knowledge of what you're going through will be a critical element of support as you make your way along this journey.

I know from experience that finding a mentor can be difficult. During my two decades of working with women during all phases of their physical development, I have come to understand that within both the medical community and society as a whole, we have yet to embrace this phase of a woman's life as the new beginning it is. We have yet to acknowledge the opportunities it opens up, including self-reflection and bringing wisdom to bear as you take better care of your body, mind, and soul than you may have in the past. Finding a guide is worth it, as is mentoring younger women once you've reached the other side.

Although all the archetypes in this book hold opportunities for self-development and transformation, the Wisewoman is uniquely endowed with the potential to make a significant impact on the world around her. Called by the physical changes that take hold within her to reflect on herself, the life she's living, and the sagacity she now possesses, the Wisewoman has the power to educate, influence, and lead.

In this section, we consider one Wisewoman's story. We also take a close look at the archetype's causes and symptomology, including those that take hold immediately or more slowly over time. Finally, we will explore the various aspects of the SHINES protocol through which a Wisewoman becomes an oracle, mapping out her journey toward sustained inner peace and understanding.

Patient Example

At fifty-two years old, Maria had been in what she described as "pre-menopause" for a little more than two years. She had menstruated more or less regularly for most of her life, but when she turned fifty, her cycle became less predictable, and her periods became more infrequent. By the time she was sitting in my office, she hadn't menstruated in six months, the longest such duration for her.

For several months, she'd been waking up in the middle of the night, sweating. She'd also been experiencing hot flashes, which were far more intense than she'd anticipated. "I feel each one start inside my chest," she described. "At first, it's a little ball of heat. But it quickly gets bigger and bigger until it bursts out into my entire body like an atomic bomb." Adding to her physical symptoms, Mary's moods had become markedly changeable. "Yesterday, I cried at a dog food commercial," she said. "And I am always short with my kids. They're teenagers and all, but sometimes, I know I'm overreacting." Mary also admitted she'd tried to remain in denial about her symptoms. "I knew menopause was coming," she said, "but I didn't want to admit it. Now I have no choice. The reality is, I can't sit still at my desk without a fan blowing on me, and my colleagues have caught me turning down the air conditioner so many times, it's turned into a joke."

Mary's symptoms hardly made her feel wise, she told me. Or womanly. She described feeling uneasy in her own skin. "Even my clothes feel wrong," she said. "I feel so awkward and uncomfortable, I'm constantly distracted. It's interfering with my life at home and at work." Mary linked this unease to her general disinterest in sex. Vaginal dryness had also made intercourse uncomfortable, and while she missed intimacy with her partner, she did not feel inclined to reignite it.

The Wisewoman: Symptomology Summary

Women who are estrogen deficient tend to present with symptoms like Mary's, including amenorrhea (the cessation of menstruation), hot flashes, vaginal dryness and irritation, night sweats, insomnia, and emotional instability. But each woman's experience is different. Symptoms appear (or do not) at a unique pace and frequency. This makes tracking your symptoms from the outset critically important.

As with other archetypes, the Wisewoman's journey begins with the realization that a significant shift is underway. Regardless of whether your symptoms arise as a result of age or medical intervention, the journey ahead promises to be a challenging *and* fulfilling one—and one that I hope this book helps you to embark on with a strong sense of self-respect and protectiveness. As I tell my patients, even natural shifts can be difficult to endure, and there is no reason to deny yourself the help that is readily available to support, sustain, and empower you on every level.

Although each Wisewoman's journey is singular, the following pages provide a basic guide to her physical, psychological, and emotional symptoms.

Physiological Symptoms

| Hot flashes and night sweats | Caused by sudden surges in vasodilation, hot flashes are feelings of intense warmth that can spread across the head, neck, and face before extending to the entire body. When these occur during the night, releasing heat and causing perspiration, they are called night sweats.

Hot flashes typically last between thirty seconds and a few minutes, causing an increase in skin temperature and redness. They may also cause an increase in heart rate, heart palpitations, and dizziness.

Estrogen deficiency causes hot flashes in approximately 75 percent of women. The majority of women transitioning into menopause experience them for two years or less. |
|---|---|

(continues)

Vaginal dryness (vaginal atrophy)	Estrogen helps maintain the natural lubrication of the vaginal walls, in addition to maintaining their thickness and elasticity. A drop in estrogen causes both a loss of lubrication and a thinning of the vaginal walls, a condition known as vaginal atrophy. Vaginal atrophy can not only make sexual intercourse painful, it can also cause vaginal irritation and itching; urinary issues, including urgency, burning, and incontinence; and a shortening and tightening of the vaginal canal.[*] Taken together, these symptoms are now known as "genitourinary syndrome of menopause."
Relaxation of the pelvic muscles	Together with vaginal atrophy, this can contribute to urinary incontinence and increase the risk that a woman's uterus, bladder, urethra, or rectum will project into the vagina.[**]

[*] Johns Hopkins Medicine, "Introduction to Menopause," http://www.hopkins medicine.org/healthlibrary/conditions/gynecological_health/introduction_to _menopause_85,P01535.

[**]B. Bleibel and H. Nguyen, "Vaginal Atrophy," in *StatPearls* (Treasure Island, FL: StatPearls Publishing, July 6, 2020).

Insomnia	In addition to the difficulty that night sweats may cause, a naturally or surgically induced progesterone deficiency may contribute to difficulty sleeping. Progesterone upregulates GABA receptors, which can help with sleep and relaxation. Difficulty sleeping can also occur if you are having hot flashes in the middle of the night, as they can be stimulatory and wake you up.
Changes to skin and hair	Estrogen is present in all cells of a woman's body, including the skin. A deficiency causes a loss of plasticity and general health of the skin, giving rise to thinning, wrinkling, and age spots. Some women also experience thinning of the hair on the scalp, in addition to an increase in the growth of facial hair.
Cardiac issues	In addition to the heart palpitations hot flashes may cause, estrogen deficiency may give rise to intermittent dizziness, heart palpitations, and tachycardia, as well as sensations including numbness, prickling, tingling, and increased sensitivity.[*] A lack of estrogen can also decrease the good cholesterol and increase the bad cholesterol, increasing the risk of heart attack.

[*] Johns Hopkins Medicine, "Introduction to Menopause."

(continues)

| Weight gain | In particular, estrogen deficiency can cause abdominal weight gain. This may be in part because fat cells produce estrogen, and with the body attempting to protect itself from the estrogen deprivation of menopause, this is a natural way to protect itself. |

Psychological and Emotional Symptoms

| Mood swings | Several studies have linked fluctuating and decreasing levels of estrogen during perimenopause and menopause with unpredictable shifts in mood. Some physiological symptoms, including insomnia and fatigue, can also contribute to sudden feelings of anger, sadness, nervousness, or even euphoria. |
| Depression | In addition to emotional changeability, estrogen deficiency can also contribute significantly to persistent depression (depressed mood lasting most of the day on most days). A depressed state is most likely caused by a combination of factors relating to menopause, including the generalized stress and anxiety that can accompany the physiological changes taking hold. |

As we discussed earlier in this section, every Wisewoman is at first an acolyte, embarking on one of the most significant heroine's journeys of her life. If you feel concerned or overwhelmed by your physiological or psychological symptoms, know that you're not alone. There are healthcare practitioners and communities of women who can provide guidance and support.

The Wisewoman: Underlying Causes of Symptomology

Estrogen deficiency may arise naturally as a result of menopause, or as a result of surgery or other medical intervention.

MENOPAUSE

Menopause is a natural and inevitable phase of female development that encompasses all the changes a woman experiences shortly before and after she ceases to menstruate. On average, a woman will be in her late thirties when her ovaries begin to produce less estrogen and progesterone (the hormones responsible for initiating and sustaining her menstrual cycle). The finite number of eggs she is born with are released and fall over time, and on average, women enter menopause between the ages of 45 and 55. For some women, the phase naturally commences as early as the age of 40 or as late as the age of 60+. The average age is currently 51.

Approximately 1 percent of women will suffer from a condition known as premature ovarian failure, in which a woman's ovaries fail to produce sufficient estrogen and progesterone to sustain the menstrual cycle before she reaches the age of forty.[10] No single cause of this condition has been identified, though it has been linked to certain genetic factors and autoimmune diseases.

SURGICAL REMOVAL OF THE OVARIES

Women of any age who undergo a total hysterectomy (or bilateral oophorectomy) for medical reasons immediately enter menopause. In these cases, the onset of menopausal symptoms is swift, and the symptoms themselves can be severe. For these Wisewomen, having a mentor to guide them during the acolyte phase of their journey is particularly crucial. Surgical removal of the ovaries is in many cases not life or death and is a very personal decision.

MEDICATIONS

Treatment with some medications may also cause temporary estrogen deficiency. Women who are prescribed medications like Lupron Depot and Orilissa for endometriosis, for example, generally see a decrease or cessation of their menstrual cycle while they are taking the medication and are likely to experience the various physiological, emotional, and spiritual aspects of the Wisewoman archetype within two to four weeks. Chemotherapy and radiation may also temporarily or permanently disrupt or halt menstruation, resulting in the archetype taking hold.

The Workaholic
Cortisol Excess

"I'm a workaholic. Before long I'm traveling on my nervous energy alone. This is incredibly exhausting."

—EVA GABOR

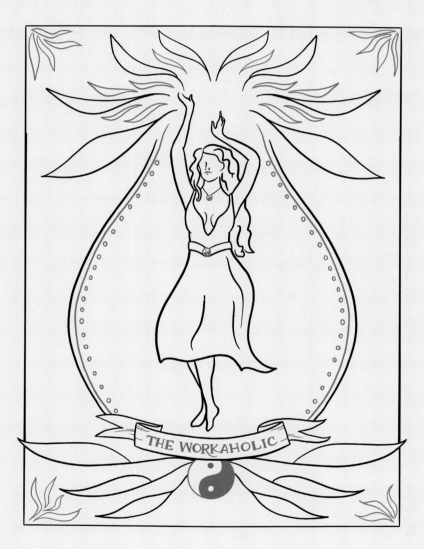

noun work·a·hol·ic \wər-kə-ˈhȯ-lik, -ˈhä-\
: a compulsive worker.

In this section, we consider the Workaholic archetype. Characterized primarily by abnormally high levels of cortisol, this archetype can take hold in women of any age, though it most commonly occurs among women between the ages of thirty and fifty-five.

Before we embark on a larger discussion of the Workaholic archetype, it is important to clarify the role of cortisol in the body and the various potential negative effects of abnormally high levels of this steroid-based hormone over the long term.

First, cortisol is not a sex hormone. Rather, it belongs to the glucocortoid class of hormones. It is made in the adrenal cortex of your adrenal glands, which are located just above your kidneys. Cortisol is the body's primary stress hormone, meaning that it's released as part of the body's response to threatening situations. It also signals the liver to increase glucose production to prepare the body for physical activity and prevents the release of certain substances in the body that cause inflammation. This is why hydrocortisone (the medical version of cortisol) is administered to patients suffering from conditions such as rheumatoid arthritis.

Unlike estrogen, progesterone, and certain other hormones that, while important, are not critical for survival, cortisol is absolutely essential for life. Excessive amounts of the hormone can give rise to a series of physical and physiological difficulties, however, including increased stress and generalized anxiety, troubled sleep, suppressed immunity, abdominal weight gain, headaches, body aches, and gastrointestinal upset. High levels of cortisol can also suppress thyroid function, inhibiting the conversion of thyroxine (T4) to triiodothyronine (T3), the active form of thyroid hormone. Taken together, these symptoms can result in persistent fatigue, particularly when elevated cortisol levels have gone unchecked for an extended period of time.

It is important to note here that when we discuss cortisol excess in the context of the Workaholic archetype (and that of the Chairwoman; see page 182), we are limiting ourselves to a discussion of abnormally high or low levels of the hormone, which the SHINES protocol can help address. We are not discussing the far more serious and potentially life-threatening conditions of Cushing's syndrome (cortisol excess) or Addison's disease (cortisol deficiency), both of which are indeed potentially life-threatening illnesses and require very specific medical intervention.

Patient Example

Wendy entered my office in a flurry of motion. At forty-three years old, she had reached a high point in her career in advertising and was running three boutique branding and PR agencies of her own, one of which was just getting off the ground. And, as Wendy explained to me as she went through her handbag to find each of her phones and turn them off, two of that agency's ten staffers had just walked off the job after she'd confronted them about their lack of effort. "It's always this way," she said. "When I want something done right, I have to do it myself."

Then Wendy told me about the symptoms she'd been experiencing. The worst, she said, was insomnia. She always had trouble falling asleep, and once she did, she remained asleep for only short periods. She assumed this was the cause of her consistent headaches and intermittent feeling that she had *something* to do but couldn't remember what. Would I write her a prescription for Ambien? she wondered.

In addition to the insomnia, Wendy complained about abdominal weight gain that had seemingly come out of nowhere. She was exercising as much as ever, spending all the time she could spare at the gym, and her eating habits hadn't changed. Wendy often skipped breakfast. Lunch was a Pop-Tart at her desk, snacks were popcorn and crackers from the vending machine downstairs. When I asked her about the Pop-Tarts, she explained that she constantly craved sugary foods and snacks. She had always liked sweets, she explained, but recently, she felt like eating little else.

Wendy also relied on coffee to keep her going. When I asked how much coffee she thought she drank each day, she estimated six to eight cups. "When I'm falling asleep at my desk at two in the afternoon, what else am I supposed to do?" she said. Wendy was also taking Excedrin to stave off those headaches she'd mentioned, adding to her daily caffeine intake.

When I asked Wendy about her menstrual cycle, she reported that it was relatively regular, but that she sometimes went a month or two without a period and then experienced an unusually heavy one. "I figured it was the stress," she told me. She also blamed stress for the colds she seemed to keep getting and found hard to kick, and for her decreased interest in sex. "I never have the time or energy anymore," she said.

Listening to Wendy, I was increasingly persuaded that cortisol excess was underlying her symptoms, and that the first step toward balancing out her levels was for her to *slow down*. I had barely begun to explain this when Wendy began to resist. "Oh, no, no, no," she said, when I told her that she needed to cut down on her caffeine intake. I explained that this would not only help her sleep better, but would also help regulate her cortisol levels. But Wendy wasn't having it. Nor was she receptive to my suggestion that she needed to engage in more calming, nonwork activities centering on mindfulness and self-care.

Wendy stayed in the office, however, and seemed to be more and more willing to hear what I had to say as I began to map out the road from cortisol excess to cortisol deficiency. "Picture your life and career in the longer term," I said. "Imagine it as the Boston Marathon. See yourself at the starting line. Are you planning to sprint off? Probably not. But let's say you do. Let's say you sprint for the first mile, the first three miles. Now what? By mile four, you're out of steam. You begin to walk. By mile ten, you're crawling, and you still have sixteen to go. This is the risk of allowing cortisol excess to reach its natural end."

I explained to Wendy that her current "sprint" was causing her adrenal glands to produce more and more and more cortisol to help her keep up her frenetic pace. "Cortisol *does* play a critical role in our lives," I continued. "It can help save us from clear and present dangers. It's how our ancestors outran tigers, after all. But once they'd escaped from their predators, their levels went back down. In our modern, hectic lives, constant stress can keep our cortisol levels high, even when a threat has passed. This is what has you feeling like you're not just burning a candle at both ends but holding a blowtorch to it."

I told Wendy she would not be able to keep going at her current pace for long. Without sleep or proper nutrition, her overworked adrenal glands would hit their maximum production and begin to peter out. By reducing the amount of physical and psychological stress she was experiencing, improving her diet, and supplementing these efforts with appropriate prescription and nonprescription treatments, she could head off the eventual crash of cortisol deficiency. (We take a closer look at cortisol deficiency in the section on the Saboteur archetype; see page 125.)

The Workaholic: Symptomology Summary

As we have discussed, elevated levels of cortisol can cause a series of symptoms, from interrupted sleep (even in the absence of stimulant effects such as those from caffeine) to headaches to dysregulated menstrual cycle and chronic fatigue. This fatigue can be caused in part by the tendency of elevated levels of cortisol to increase catabolism in the body (see page 120).

Cortisol and Catabolism

Catabolism, or "destructive metabolism," is the set of metabolic pathways by which the body breaks down more complex substances, including lipids, nucleic acids, and proteins, into smaller units, including monosaccharides and amino acids. The purpose of catabolism is to provide the energy and components needed for anabolism, or "constructive metabolism," the process in which smaller units are synthesized to build up larger ones. A series of signals controls catabolic processes; the majority of these signals are the molecules that are directly involved in hormones, including cortisol.

In general, when your body is in a resting state, it is in an anabolic or "building" phase. When your cortisol levels are consistently high, however, and you're running yourself ragged, your body can remain in a state in which it's breaking itself down—even when you're resting. In such a state, your body is unlikely to be breaking down fat. It's far more likely to be catabolizing your muscles, ligaments, and bones, in addition to thinning your blood vessels and breaking down the collagen in your skin. This makes the skin less elastic and causes stretch marks to appear.

Adding to this, the more time your body spends in a catabolic state, the hungrier you are likely to be. The more the body catabolizes tissue, the more signals it sends to your brain that you need to consume additional calories. During these phases, the body also tends to store fat. This means that over time, the calories you're consuming are more likely to lead to weight gain and related complications such as hypertension. Increased catabolism can also play a role in a disrupted menstrual cycle, given that it can break down communication among the brain, ovaries, and uterus.

In the following pages, we take a closer look at the physiological, psychological, and emotional symptoms that characterize the Workaholic archetype.

Physiological Symptoms	
Gastroesophageal reflux disease (GERD)	Cortisol is a diuretic. In addition to depleting the body's electrolytes, such as sodium and potassium, it can also stimulate gastric acid secretion, which can cause heartburn and reflux.[*]
Insomnia and restlessness	Cortisol levels that remain high during the day and into the evening can make it difficult to fall asleep and may interrupt sleep throughout the night.[**] When your cortisol fails to drop at bedtime as it's supposed to, it can both make it difficult to fall asleep and continue to exert stimulatory effects throughout the night, leaving you feeling tired in the morning.
Fatigue	In combination with the various other symptoms of cortisol excess, remaining in fight-or-flight mode for extended periods of time can leave the Workaholic feeling exhausted, even upon waking.

[*] A. M. Mistry et al., "Corticosteroids in the Management of Hyponatremia, Hypovolemia, and Vasospasm in Subarachnoid Hemorrhage: A Meta-Analysis," *Cerebrovascular Diseases* 42, no. 3–4 (2016): 263–71, https://doi.org/10.1159/000446251.

[**] I. Vargas et al., "Altered Ultradian Cortisol Rhythmicity as a Potential Neurobiologic Substrate for Chronic Insomnia," *Sleep Medicine Reviews* 41 (2018): 234–43, https://doi.org/10.1016/j.smrv.2018.03.003.

(continues)

Weight gain	Workaholics are particularly prone to gaining weight around the abdomen. Studies have shown that animals in a state of elevated cortisol are predisposed toward obesity.[*]
Immunosuppression	Cortisol has a negative feedback effect on interleukin, a glycoprotein involved in immune responses, thereby interfering with the body's communication with its T-cells. Cortisol is ordinarily anti-inflammatory and contains the immune response, but chronic elevations can lead to the immune system becoming "resistant," an accumulation of stress hormones, and increased production of inflammatory cytokines that further compromise the immune response.[**]
Osteoporosis	Cortisol can reduce bone formation.[***]
Sagging skin and wrinkles	Cortisol breaks down collagen in the skin, causing it to thin and prematurely age. Cortisol also breaks down collagen in the joints, causing stiffness and pain.

* S. D. Hewagalamulage, T. K. Lee, I. J. Clarke, and B. A. Henry, "Stress, Cortisol, and Obesity: A Role for Cortisol Responsiveness in Identifying Individuals Prone to Obesity," *Domestic Animal Endocrinology* 56, suppl. (2016): S112–S120, https://doi.org/10.1016/j.domaniend.2016.03.004.

**A. Vitlic, J. M. Lord, and A. C. Philips, "Stress, Ageing and Their Influence on Functional, Cellular and Molecular Aspects of the Immune System," *Age* 36 (2014): 1169–85.

***A. Krishnan and S. Muthusami, "Hormonal Alterations in PCOS and Its Influence on Bone Metabolism," *Journal of Endocrinology* 232, no. 2 (2017): R99–R113, https://doi.org/10.1530/JOE-16-0405.

Increased wound healing time	Both high levels of stress and elevated cortisol levels have been linked to increased wound healing time.
Headaches	This tends to be a tension or stress (musculoskeletal) headache and is that headache that feels like your head is in a vise. This type of headache can wake you up at night; it's generally painful but definitely not the worst headache of your life, and resolves with therapeutic treatment like sleep, meditation, cold packs, or OTC medications such as ibuprofen, aspirin, or acetaminophen.
Decreased libido	High levels of cortisol can have a negative impact on testosterone levels. Decreased libido may also arise alongside other symptoms, including fatigue.[*]
Cravings	Workaholics commonly crave salty and sugary foods.

* R. Basson, J. I. O'Loughlin, J. Weinberg, A. H. Young, T. Bodnar, and L. A. Brotto, "Dehydroepiandrosterone and Cortisol as Markers of HPA Axis Dysregulation in Women with Low Sexual Desire," *Psychoneuroendocrinology* 104 (2019): 259–68, https://doi.org/10.1016/j.psyneuen.2019.03.001.

(continues)

Psychological and Emotional Symptoms	
Generalized feeling of being overwhelmed	This is not the kind of anxiety that typically requires medication, per se, but a low and ongoing level of anxious feelings that interfere with the way you want to live your life.

The Workaholic may experience any of these symptoms, often in combination with each other. Over time, the lifestyle changes and other modifications recommended by the SHINES protocol may help any of these abate.

The Workaholic: Underlying Causes of Symptomology

Chronic stress is the primary underlying cause of the Workaholic's symptoms. As established, high emotional and physical alertness raises cortisol levels. Once these levels are elevated, cortisol can feed on its own overproduction, keeping your body and mind in fight-or-flight mode and your adrenal glands responding accordingly. Other, although infrequent, causes of excess cortisol are adrenal tumors and other neoplastic issues with the adrenal gland.

The Saboteur
Cortisol Deficiency

"Many of us are tethered to bodies that sabotage us in our struggle to keep from getting fat, or to slim down when we do."
—ROBIN MARANTZ HENIG

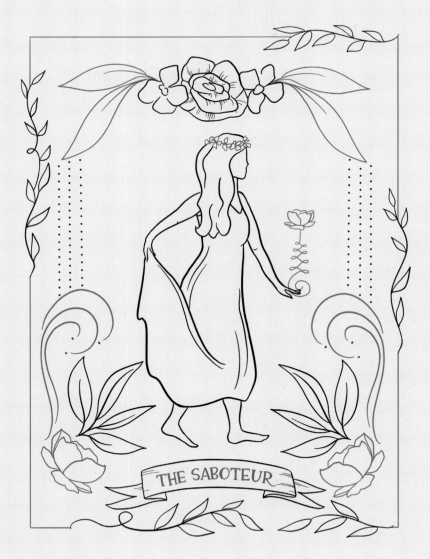

THE SABOTEUR

noun sab·o·teur \ ˌsa-bə-ˈtər, -ˈtu̇r, -ˈtyu̇r \

: a person who destroys or damages something deliberately; a person who performs sabotage.

In this section, we consider the Saboteur. A natural, though not inevitable, outgrowth of the Workaholic archetype, the Saboteur archetype is characterized by symptoms associated with what is known in functional and integrative medicine as adrenal fatigue or adrenal insufficiency. Brought on by long-term physical and/or emotional stress that can drive excessive cortisol production and cause many of the symptoms we discussed in the section on the Workaholic archetype (see page 115), the Saboteur archetype represents the "burnout" phase of cortisol excess.

We can trace the development of the Saboteur through four phases:

During **phase one**, a significant event or events begin to have an impact on your overall emotional and physical functioning. Even "positive" changes in your life can cause stress. Getting married, for example, or taking a new job, or moving to a new city. The stress associated with any of these and/or any "negative" circumstances triggers fight-or-flight responses that drive your adrenal glands to produce additional cortisol and DHEA. If the stress diminishes, your adrenal glands revert to producing normal levels of these hormones. But if the stress persists, your fight-or-flight-response-driven hormone production does, too, and you enter **phase two**.

During this second phase, your cortisol production tends to remain high, while the production of DHEA, estrogen, progesterone, and other hormones begins to drop. Patients who have entered this phase often describe having sufficient energy during the morning hours to prepare themselves for work and/or get their children ready for school, and they tell me they can keep pace with their days until about two or three in the afternoon, when they have to drink a shot of espresso to make it through the rest of the day.

Your body can maintain phase two for only so long. This means that when underlying stress remains unresolved, continuing to inspire the fight-or-flight response, **phase three** begins to take hold. I refer to this as the "resistance phase." During it, your body continues to produce abnormally high levels of cortisol while it also decreases production of other hormones even more significantly than it did during phase two. When this persists, it can lead to what has become known as the "pregnenolone steal."

Pregnenolone, a hormone made from LDL cholesterol primarily in the adrenal glands but also in the ovaries, liver, brain, and skin, is a precursor to progesterone (which can convert to cortisol) and DHEA (which converts to estrogen and testosterone). The "pregnenolone steal" occurs when the body directs pregnenolone away from its natural pathways and increasingly toward the production of cortisol. This results in a further decrease in progesterone and DHEA, which means estrogen and testosterone levels continue to fall as well. The pregnenolone steal as a distinctive physiologic process is not something accepted by the medical industry, and I have included it here for those working with alternative practitioners who may be mentioning it. For the most part it is highly controversial, but it is interesting to discuss.

Finally, the Saboteur will reach **phase four**. This is the point at which the adrenal glands themselves begin to slow down, unable to keep pace with the constant demand that stress creates. Now, with your sex hormones already at very low levels, your cortisol levels also begin to drop. This can leave you feeling permanently fatigued. Or, as my patients often put it, "totally burned out."

Why do I call this archetype the "Saboteur"? There are two major reasons. The first involves the body: The body's physical sabotage of itself gives rise to the archetype. During phases one and two, your body catabolizes muscle and other tissues to supply the body with energy (for details on catabolism, see page 120). During phase three, your body *may* begin to direct pregnenolone toward increased cortisol production, resulting in a decrease in the production of DHEA (and therefore sex hormones) and disrupting overall hormone balance. From the outset, your body races to keep pace with the demands placed on it by various stressors. But ultimately, it compromises itself, leaving you without the physical strength or wherewithal to endure the challenges that gave rise to the archetype in the first place.

The second reason involves the mind: Saboteurs tend to do for others before themselves, and there is a constant pressure to perform, compromising their physical and emotional health in the process. A relatively benign but still telling example comes from a patient of mine who complained that her exhaustion was so acute in part because the demands of work and home simply never stopped. "When I finally collapse in bed at the end of the day," she told me, "I'm so tired, I wonder whether I'll ever be able to get up again. Then I hear my twelve-year-old son calling from across the hall, 'Mom, can I have some ice cream?' My husband says I should ask my son 'Do you have legs?' But I feel guilty telling my son to fetch his own ice cream, so I drag myself out of bed and get it myself."

Adrenal Fatigue and Addison's Disease

"Adrenal fatigue" is a nonmedical diagnosis used by some healthcare practitioners to describe a collection of symptoms that includes fatigue, gastrointestinal disturbances, interrupted sleep, and generalized nervousness or anxiety. Underlying this diagnosis is the assumption that following a prolonged period of stress and the overproduction of stress hormones, the adrenal glands cease to function normally, resulting in a decrease in the levels of stress hormones, sex hormones, and other hormones in the body. Because adrenal fatigue is not a medical diagnosis, there is no official test for it. Your physician can test your cortisol levels, however, using saliva- or urine-based testing. Extremely low levels can help contribute to your intuitive assessment of your archetype. (When possible, I recommend the 24-hour urine-based DUTCH test; see page 54 for more information.) I am going to go on record saying that I am not fond of the tag "adrenal fatigue," because it technically is not a real thing. That said, I do believe there are symptoms and issues that come with having overtaxed adrenal glands, as you will discover in this archetype.

Although some symptoms of adrenal fatigue may overlap with Addison's disease, the two conditions are very different. Addison's disease is a serious, medically diagnosable condition involving adrenal dysfunction resulting from damage to the adrenal gland. Potentially fatal, Addison's disease may be caused by cancer or an infection of the adrenal glands, or autoimmune diseases such as tuberculosis. Sufferers of Addison's disease must consult with a physician, and are generally treated with the prescription anti-inflammatory Cortef or corticosteroids.

Patient Example

Rachel entered my office and slumped into a chair. She appeared exhausted. Forty-two, married, and childless, Rachel was a successful and extremely busy partner at a law firm. Work was more hectic than ever, she told me. She often stayed late at the office, and always took work home with her. "I've been doing this for years," she explained, "but I feel like I can't keep up with it anymore."

When I asked Rachel about her diet, she laughed. "I never have time to cook meals at home, if that's what you're asking. I'm at the mercy of restaurants near the office and the vending machine downstairs." Rachel was also leaning heavily on caffeine to keep pace with her day. But it didn't always have the intended effect. "I used to be able to rely on a shot of espresso at three in the afternoon," she explained, "but that doesn't help at all anymore."

Although she had suffered from interrupted sleep for years, during the few months before our visit, Rachel told me she'd been sleeping like the dead, and she simply could not sleep enough. No amount left her feeling well-rested or energized. Rachel had also gained roughly 10 pounds during these months, mostly in her abdominal area, and sensed that her temper was becoming shorter and shorter. "Where I could handle stress at work and home before," she said, "now everything feels like the straw that's breaking the camel's back." Premenstrual syndrome and her menstrual cycle also seemed to rob her of more physical and emotional energy than they had before. This, she believed, was exacerbating her weight gain and emotional changeability.

Rachel's relationship with her husband had also become strained. The couple had shared little emotional or physical intimacy during the past several months. Rachel assumed this was owing, in part, to her demanding schedule and tiredness. "We're like ships in the night," she said. "Every night."

Rachel had also become more susceptible to illness. Where she had always been the person who managed to avoid coming down with whatever cold or flu was going around, now she was constantly battling respiratory infections that seemed to linger for weeks; one had even turned into pneumonia. It was spring when we met, and for the first time in her life, Rachel was suffering from allergies. Pollen bothered her, she said. And although she had always been able to eat dairy, she'd recently become lactose intolerant. Rachel also complained that her skin felt thin and dry, and that no topical treatments seemed to help.

As I listened to Rachel, it became increasingly clear that she was in the third—if not the fourth—phase of the Workaholic (cortisol excess)/Saboteur (adrenal deficiency) continuum. A recent blood test had confirmed that her levels of iron and thyroid-stimulating hormone (TSH) along with Free T3 and Free T4 were well within normal range. But saliva and urine testing revealed that her levels of cortisol were low, as were her levels of progesterone, estrogen, and testosterone. "I suspect your body has been in fight-or-flight mode for years," I explained. "Now, for the next several months, your work will be about slowing down, eliminating threats and pressures, and tending to your tired system, which has carried you for so long."

The Saboteur: Symptomology Summary

The primary symptoms of the Saboteur archetype mirror those associated with what some healthcare practitioners call adrenal fatigue. Underlying these symptoms are low levels of stress hormones, including cortisol, as well as sex hormones derived from pregnenolone or DHEA, including estrogen, testosterone, and progesterone. Although a series of conditions may contribute to decreased production of any or all these hormones, in the Saboteur's case, the low levels are attributable to the body's efforts to keep pace with long-term physiological and/or psychological stress.

Although Saboteurs' symptoms can vary from woman to woman, most will experience at least some, if not most, of the physiological and psychological symptoms described here.

Physiological Symptoms: Adrenal Insufficiency

Weight gain[*]	Particularly during the early (Workaholic) phases and phase three, elevated cortisol levels can lead to weight gain, typically in the abdominal area.
Fatigue	Saboteurs are likely to experience generalized fatigue on a consistent basis, even with adequate rest. You may find this is particularly the case before and during your menstrual cycle.
Symptoms associated with low blood sugar	Cortisol increases blood sugar. During phase three, when your cortisol levels are higher, you may experience: Cravings for sugary foods Feeling jittery Low body temperature Light-headedness
Immunosuppression[**]	Increased susceptibility to viral and bacterial infections Onset of environmental sensitivities and food allergies
Decreased libido	Increased cortisol production can have a negative impact on testosterone levels. Generalized fatigue may also contribute to this.

* A. M. Chao, A. M. Jastreboff, M. A. White, C. M. Grilo, and R. Sinha, "Stress, Cortisol, and Other Appetite-Related Hormones: Prospective Prediction of 6-Month Changes in Food Cravings and Weight," *Obesity* 25, no. 4 (April 2017): 713–20, https://doi.org/10.1002/oby.21790.

**J. Briegel, *"Cortisol bei kritisch kranken Patienten mit Sepsis: Physiologische Funktionen und therapeutische Implikationen* [Cortisol in Critically Ill Patients with Sepsis— Physiological Functions and Therapeutic Implications]," *Wien Klin Wochenschr* 114, suppl. 1 (2002): 9–19, PMID: 15503552.

Again, the Workaholic and Saboteur archetypes are related. Together, they represent the four major phases of a body's protracted response to long-term stress. Although this section focuses on the Saboteur archetype, if you skipped the section on the Workaholic archetype (page 115), you will likely benefit from reading that as well. It may give you additional insight into the continuum and your experience, and help confirm your identification with the Saboteur archetype.

Psychological and Emotional Symptoms: Cortisol Deficiency	
Low blood pressure	Excess cortisol has been shown to be responsible for elevated blood pressure, and the opposite can also be true.
Muscle and joint pain	Cortisol is a potent anti-inflammatory agent and as such low cortisol can elevate joint and muscle pain.

The Saboteur: Underlying Causes of Symptomology

Ultimately, it is the body's response to prolonged stress that gives rise to the Saboteur archetype. This stress may take a variety of forms, however, and have its root in a combination of physiological and psychological conditions.

EMOTIONAL STRESS

Stress can come in all forms of perceived good and bad changes, which may prompt a fight-or-flight response. Whether it's a marriage or a divorce, a new job or being let go from an old one, life events influence your body's production of stress hormones and sex hormones. Prolonged and chronic stress can create an imbalance that may worsen over time and have negative downstream effects.[11]

DIET

For the Saboteur, diet, and sugar intake in particular, can be a significant source of physical stress. Remember: Humans evolved on a diet that contained no refined sugar, and we still don't require it for survival. It is the "food that nobody needs, but everyone craves," as one group of researchers has put it.[12] During the past two hundred years, a short span in evolutionary terms, Americans' consumption of refined sugar has skyrocketed. According to a recent study, during the early 1800s, the average American consumed roughly 10 grams of refined sugar per day. Today, the average American consumes fifteen times that amount, or roughly 130 pounds of sugar each year.[13] In order to process all that sugar, our bodies produce more cortisol and insulin, putting additional pressure on our pancreas and adrenal glands in the process.

Toxic chemicals found in the air and in food are another aspect of our modern lives that can contribute the Saboteur's symptoms. Chlorine in drinking water, antibiotics in poultry, beef, and other animal products, and pesticides sprayed on fruits and vegetables are all neuroendocrine disruptors. This means they disrupt the communication between your brain and your adrenal glands (as well as the messaging between your brain, your ovaries, and your pituitary gland).

DISEASE AND TRAUMA

Conditions such as asthma, arthritis, diabetes, lupus, Lyme disease, and other chronic illnesses that consistently cause significant physical stress during a long period of time can all contribute to the Saboteur's symptoms. Similarly, athletes who train extensively—whether they're running marathons as an avocation or training for the Olympics—can also keep their adrenals under stress in a way that will see them progress through the four phases of protracted stress response.

Short-term physical trauma can also give rise to the Saboteur archetype. If you have been in a serious car accident, undergone major surgery, or endured several surgeries during a relatively short period, you may also find yourself somewhere along the continuum between excessive cortisol production and adrenal burnout.

The Nun

Testosterone Deficiency

"Be faithful in small things because it is in them that your strength lies."
—MOTHER TERESA

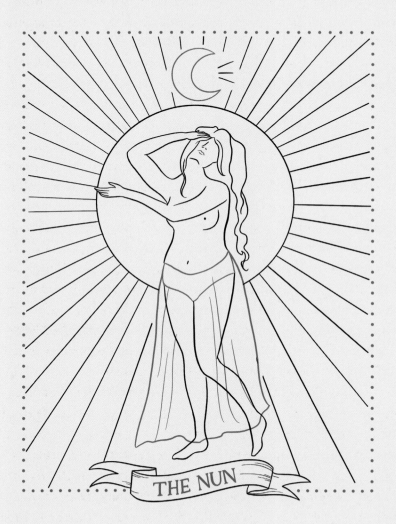

THE NUN

noun nun \ ˈnən \

: a woman belonging to a religious order; *especially*: one under solemn vows of poverty, chastity, and obedience.

In this section, we consider the Nun. The archetype's primary hormonal characteristic is testosterone deficiency.

Produced by the ovaries and adrenal glands, as well as in peripheral tissues (from precursor hormones produced in the ovaries and adrenals), a woman's testosterone generally reaches its highest level during her young adulthood. Production of the hormone decreases over time, falling to roughly 50 percent of its peak by the time she has reached menopause. Although her ovaries will cease to produce estrogen at this point, they will continue to produce smaller amounts of testosterone, as will her adrenal glands. That the hormone continues to play a role in her body's functioning means an imbalance can wreak havoc in various ways. Testosterone is the most often overlooked female hormone imbalance and as of the publication of this book the most common imbalance I see.

Testosterone deficiency can give rise to an array of symptoms, including interrupted sleep, short-term memory dysfunction and/or "foggy brain," weight gain, increased abdominal fat, and diminished physical stamina. Additional symptoms include osteopenia and osteoporosis, male-pattern baldness, mood swings, depression, and anxiety. But perhaps the most commonly cited symptom is diminished libido, or "female sexual interest/arousal disorder," as the *Diagnostic and Statistical Manual of Mental Disorders (DSM-5)* refers to it.[14]

I certainly considered this attribute as I named the Nun archetype. But this choice of "Nun" is less a reflection of decreased sexual desire than of how those women experience the world around them. The array of symptoms associated with testosterone deficiency can leave the Nun feeling generally fatigued and inclined to cloister herself away, avoiding physical and psychological engagement in the world beyond her "walls." While this does not diminish her love for or devotion to the people and causes she cares deeply about, it can close her off from them. As we will see later in this section, the Nun's SHINES protocol speaks directly to this, aiming to support her active and joyful engagement in the world and in her life.

Although a woman's natural testosterone peaks during young adulthood and falls throughout the rest of her life, the Nun archetype can take hold in women of any age. Menopause and menopause-related estrogen dominance can contribute to a testosterone deficiency. But birth control pills can also do this, as can autoimmune disorders such as lupus and rheumatoid arthritis. Among the other potential underlying causes are severe stress and adrenal insufficiency.

A Note on Decreased Libido

In my view, the "problem" of decreased libido in women has been exacerbated by the medical community's focus on men's libido. Within the past twenty years, erectile-dysfunction drugs such as Viagra and Cialis have become enormously popular, generating billions of dollars in revenue each year. Although these drugs contain no testosterone and therefore do not make men more sexually aggressive, per se, they do help improve the strength and stamina of erections and can increase men's general interest in sex. In my clinical experience, when the partners of these men are feeling less drawn to sexual intimacy than they once did, they can end up feeling guilty or inadequate.

The reality is that your libido is likely to be stronger and less strong during different phases of your life. This is inevitable, owing to physiological and psychological conditions alike. At any point, the question is not whether you are feeling more or less interested in sex, but whether your level of interest is *a problem for you*.

Patient Example

Five months after I'd delivered her first child, twenty-eight-year-old Marilyn was concerned that her "pre-baby" energy levels had not returned. Although she'd restarted her workout routine, she found herself unable to exercise at even half the intensity she had before. Marilyn had also recently returned to her hectic job at an advertising agency and was finding it impossible to sustain her old pace. She was less interested in other physical and social activities and reported feeling like her libido was "nonexistent." This worried her, she said, and made her concerned for her relationship with her husband.

I was less surprised by Marilyn's symptoms than she. "You're a *new mom*," I reminded her. "Your body has undergone a massive transformation, and your life has, too. All of this takes a physical and psychological toll and wreaks havoc with your hormones." Marilyn seemed unmoved. I went on. "As for your sex drive, you've transitioned from being a free-loving, sexy wife to having milk leaking out of your breasts while you're up half the night and trying to keep up with the five hundred things you have to do every day. It's not surprising that physical intimacy has taken a back seat." With this, Marilyn seemed to relax.

Although any one of a series of factors may have been the root cause of her fatigue and diminished interest in sex, testing revealed that Marilyn's testosterone levels were, in fact, on the low side of normal. We discussed the impact of her pregnancy and delivery on her hormones, and how factors including stress and her birth control medication were likely contributing to her imbalance. We also discussed how the SHINES protocol could help increase her levels of free testosterone, enabling it to exert its positive impact on her energy and—potentially—her level of sexual desire.

Taken together, the various elements of the SHINES protocol could help alleviate her fatigue and mood-related symptoms, I told Marilyn, improving her physical and emotional stamina and increasing her interest in physical intimacy. Given that testosterone can intensify female sexual arousal, she might also find sex more pleasurable. But we would need to carefully monitor her levels, ensuring that they returned to healthy levels without becoming *too* elevated. "If your testosterone levels were as high as your husband's, you *might* want to have sex with him," I explained, "and you'd almost certainly want to rip his face off."

The Nun: Symptomology Summary

Nuns tend to present with the following physiological, psychological, and emotional symptoms:

Among women who present with the Nun archetype, the most common complaint is decreased sexual desire. Symptoms of testosterone deficiency can vary widely, however. If you are suffering from any of the conditions listed here, consult with your physician and explore the possibility that the Nun archetype has taken hold.

The Nun: Underlying Causes of Symptomology

In women, approximately 50 percent of testosterone is made by the ovaries. The adrenal glands produce the balance. Therefore, a testosterone deficiency can arise when ovarian or adrenal dysfunction takes hold.

HORMONAL CONTRACEPTIVES AND HORMONE REPLACEMENT THERAPY (HRT)

Birth control pills and other forms of hormonal contraceptives prevent pregnancy by interrupting the body's natural hormone production cycle. Containing synthetic estrogen and progestin, these medications generally prevent ovulation. Interrupting the ovaries'

Physiological Symptoms: Testosterone Deficiency

Diminished genital arousal and orgasmic response	Decreased vaginal lubrication may also occur.*
Chronic or acute fatigue	In addition to generalized exhaustion, testosterone deficiency can also contribute to muscle weakness. The fatigue I see with these patients is usually in the later afternoon.
Weight gain	Testosterone deficiency can cause the body to retain fat, particularly around the abdomen.
Interrupted sleep	Testosterone levels follow a bit of a circadian rhythm, so it is thought that low testosterone can contribute to insomnia.
Hair thinning/ hair loss	Testosterone is thought to have an anabolic effect on the hair in those women with testosterone deficiency, and those women can see hair thinning. Care should be exercised, however, as excess testosterone can also be associated with male-pattern hair loss.
Osteoporosis and osteopenia	Similar to low estrogen, low testosterone can cause the body to leach calcium from bones.

* André Guay and Susan R. Davis, "Testosterone Insufficiency in Women: Fact or Fiction," excerpt from *World Journal of Urology* 20 (2002): 106–10, http://www.bumc.bu.edu/sexualmedicine/publications/testosterone-insufficiency-in-women-fact-or-fiction.

(continues)

Psychological and Emotional Symptoms: Testosterone Deficiency	
Decreased sexual desire	This includes a decrease in sexual thoughts, fantasies, and actions.*
Depression and anxiety	While the literature does not support a consistent relationship between testosterone levels and depressive symptoms, most studies do suggest that lower testosterone could contribute to depressive symptoms. This could be due to the fact that testosterone is a modulator of GABA receptors and inhibits 5-HT$_3$ receptors centrally.

* Guay and Davis, "Testosterone Insufficiency in Women: Fact or Fiction."

production of estrogen and progesterone also negatively affects their production of testosterone.

Estrogen replacement therapy can also negatively impact testosterone levels. When your estrogen levels rise, so do your levels of sex hormone binding globulin (SHBG), a protein produced in the liver. SHBG binds to estrogen, dihydrotestosterone, and testosterone, decreasing the bioavailability of each. This means that if you take a birth control pill, the amount of active testosterone in your body may decrease, and research has shown that birth control pills can decrease sex drive.[15]

MENOPAUSE

A woman's testosterone levels begin to drop during her twenties. By the time she reaches menopause, her levels are likely to be half what they were at their peak. Women who experience premenopausal ovarian failure or undergo an oophorectomy (removal of the ovaries) will also suffer an acute reduction in testosterone production.

CHRONIC ILLNESS

Women suffering from autoimmune disorders (particularly those that cause inflammation) such as lupus and rheumatoid arthritis, or thyroid conditions, including Hashimoto's disease, often experience decreased androgen production. Addison's disease and hypopituitarism (the loss of pituitary gland hormone production) can also cause testosterone deficiency.[16]

ADRENAL INSUFFICIENCY

The adrenal glands are responsible for roughly half your total testosterone production, so adrenal fatigue can also contribute to testosterone deficiency. Whether it's stress, disease, or even extreme athletic training that is at the heart of the adrenal "burnout," the glands' diminished functioning can be a significant factor in the Nun archetype taking hold. For more on adrenal fatigue, see the sections on the Workaholic archetype (cortisol excess, page 115) and the Saboteur (cortisol deficiency, page 125).

OBESITY

In a woman who is overweight or obese, the levels of circulating estrogen in her body can increase. As stated earlier, when estrogen levels rise, there is a subsequent increase in the levels of sex hormone binding globulin (SHBG), which then decreases the amount of freely circulating testosterone. Another unfortunate effect of obesity is that you may feel less confident about your body and feel self-conscious with your partner. Unfortunately, the psychological aspects of obesity can also affect sexual function.

The Warrior

Testosterone Excess

"Not many women got to live out the daydream of women—to have a room, even a section of a room, that only gets messed up when she messes it up herself."

—MAXINE HONG KINGSTON

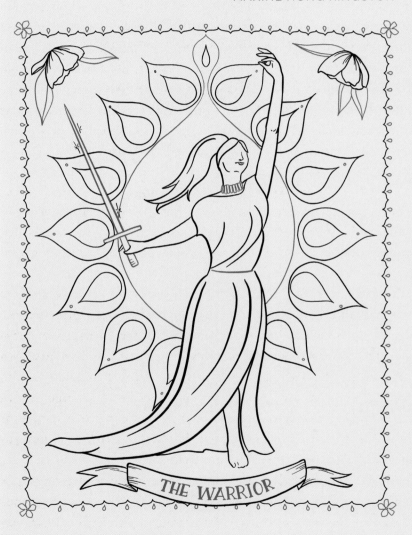

THE WARRIOR

noun war·rior \ ˈwȯr-yər , ˈwȯr-ē-ər , ˈwär-ē—also ˈwär-yər \

: a person engaged or experienced in warfare; *broadly*: a person engaged in some struggle or conflict.

In this section, we consider the Warrior. Characterized by testosterone excess, this archetype can take hold in women of any age during any phase of their physical development, including pregnancy.

Produced by the ovaries and adrenal glands, as well as in peripheral tissues (from precursor hormones produced in the ovaries and adrenals), a woman's testosterone generally reaches its highest level during her young adulthood. Production of the hormone decreases over time, falling to roughly 50 percent of its peak by the time she has reached menopause. Although her ovaries will cease to produce estrogen at this point, they will continue to produce testosterone, as will the adrenal glands. That the hormone continues to play a role in her body's functioning means an imbalance can wreak havoc in various ways.

Although testosterone is typically thought of as a "male" hormone, it plays a significant role in every woman's physical health and overall well-being. It has an impact on your cardiovascular and musculoskeletal health, energy levels, libido, and experience of sexual pleasure.

While a Warrior may experience some of the "positive" effects of testosterone excess, such as improved muscle tone, increased energy, and enhanced libido, she may also experience such undesirable symptoms as acne, excess body hair growth and/or hirsutism (male-pattern hair growth, generally on the face, chest, and/or back), balding near the hair line, clitoromegaly (abnormal enlargement of the clitoris), and deepening of the voice. Some of these symptoms diminish or reverse when a Warrior's hormones are brought into balance. Others persist. Some become permanent.

When I work with a Warrior, our first step is to determine the cause of her testosterone excess. The first and perhaps most obvious of these is that she is taking a testosterone replacement medication or a supplement that is driving up her production of the hormone. Some forms of testosterone replacement therapy and excessive doses of OTC DHEA supplements can cause a woman's testosterone levels to rise too high, too quickly, with deleterious effects. A second, related cause is that she is being exposed to exogenous testosterone without being aware of it. Women whose male partners are using topical testosterone treatments can fall into this category. Polycystic ovarian syndrome (PCOS), a condition in which multiple benign cysts form on a woman's ovaries, is also associated with excess testosterone production, as are ovarian, adrenal, and other types of tumors.

In the following pages, we consider the stories of two Warriors before taking a closer look at the archetype's causes and symptomology. In the next chapter we will go on to explore the various elements of the SHINES protocol that can help a Warrior weather her battle and come to experience ease in victory.

Patient Examples

AMANDA

When Amanda visited me in my office, she appeared to be in good spirits. A pharmaceutical representative whose schedule was always packed, the thirty-eight-year-old mother of two seemed well rested and energized. An avid athlete, she told me she'd been keeping up with her workouts in addition to the rest of her hectic life, and that overall, she didn't feel poorly. She wasn't in any consistent physical pain, she said, and was sleeping relatively well. She hadn't suffered any sort of viral or bacterial infection in some time, but still, she explained, *something* was off.

Amanda's menstrual cycles had become erratic, and she was experiencing some spotting between them. She was also noticing a bit of extra hair growth on her chin. "I figured it was just my genetics," she said, "but lately, I've found myself plucking hairs every day. It may seem like a small thing, but I know my body, and this feels like a sign that something is wrong." Amanda also described some changes to her mood. "I'm not sure anyone would say I have *anger issues*," she said, "but I feel like I'm always on edge. I often sense that I'm heading into attack mode, like I'm ready to jump into a fight . . . It takes a lot of effort to take a few breaths and rein myself in, and I'm beginning to think I'm going to lose it one of these days. I just don't feel like myself."

Listening to Amanda, I began to think that excess testosterone might be driving her symptoms. I tested her total testosterone and found it was *ten times as high* as I would expect to see in a woman her age. When I asked Amanda whether she was taking a testosterone replacement medication, she said no, and I immediately became concerned that a tumor might be the cause of her elevated levels. A vaginal ultrasound revealed no masses on her uterus or ovaries. But before I ordered a CT scan, I wanted to confirm she was not being exposed to exogenous testosterone. "I understand you're not taking testosterone replacement medication yourself," I said, "but what about your husband?"

At that point, Amanda told me her husband was using Andro-Gel, a topical testosterone therapy for men. Each night, she explained, he took a shower and applied the gel to his stomach. He slept with his shirt off, which meant that any time his skin came into contact with Amanda's, the gel spread across her exposed skin. Given that AndroGel was (and is) dosed for men, relatively low levels of the medication could have been responsible for raising Amanda's testosterone levels to several times what they should be.

The first step in bringing Amanda's testosterone levels back into balance was to eliminate her exposure to her husband's AndroGel. The next would be to continue to monitor her testosterone levels to ensure they were restored to a normal level that worked for her. An improvement of her symptoms would tell us we were on track. Although she was grateful we'd identified the root cause of her extremely high level of testosterone, Amanda was also concerned that lowering this would curb her athletic edge. She'd recently started competing in Tough Mudders and wanted to keep dominating in competitions.

I had to admit to Amanda that her athletic performance might suffer a bit. Her overall energy level could also wane, I explained. But the risks of long-term excess testosterone were significant. In addition to her disrupted menstrual cycle, facial hair growth, and quickness to anger, I said, she might experience a host of other symptoms, including increased cholesterol and elevated blood pressure, male-pattern baldness, permanent changes to her voice, and an irreversible mutation of her clitoris.

Within two months, Amanda's testosterone levels were within normal range, if on the high side of normal, and her symptoms had all improved. We also monitored her estrogen, progesterone, and cortisol levels to help ensure she was returning to overall hormonal balance.

How Afraid of Your Husband's or Boyfriend's Testosterone Replacement Medication Do You *Actually* Need to Be?

A good rule of thumb is that a gel- or cream-based medication needs thirty minutes to dry after application. If your partner is using a topical hormone treatment, it's a good idea to avoid direct contact between his skin and yours for at least this long. (At least one of you being clothed can also solve the problem.) While stories like Amanda's are not as rare as you might think, infrequent exposure puts you at very little risk.

When I discuss this with my patients, I recall a story about my stepfather. Many years ago, I was visiting my mother and stepfather in Arizona, and one morning, I heard my stepfather screaming in the shower. I ran upstairs to find him standing in the bathroom, wrapped in a towel, yelling at me to "GET IT OFF! GET IT OFF!" I scanned for a scorpion. But all I found was one of my mother's estrogen patches stuck to his foot. I peeled it off and assured him he wouldn't be growing breasts anytime soon.

The point is: Be cognizant of exposure to exogenous testosterone. But when such exposure is extremely limited, it's very unlikely to cause a problematic excess.

EMILY

This second patient example offers insight into the Warrior whose testosterone excess is being driven by PCOS.

At thirty-three years old, Emily had been married for a few years, and now she and her husband wanted to have a child. They had been trying unsuccessfully for about a year, and now Emily wanted my help. She explained that since she'd stopped taking her birth control pills a year earlier, her periods had been both infrequent and irregular. She assumed this was related to the fact that she hadn't become pregnant, but, she said, she was also suffering from other symptoms that concerned her. She had noticed increased hair growth on her stomach, for example, in addition to some on her chin. She was also losing hair on her head, mostly from the top, near her hairline. "Every time I shower, I can see I'm losing small clumps," she explained. Emily had also gained roughly 20 pounds during the past year, though she hadn't made any significant changes to her diet or exercise routines. Emily was five feet four and 170 pounds, and her weight was high for her height. And when I checked her body mass index (BMI), it was also high: 35. "I'm afraid this is just going to get worse," she said.

Given her symptoms, I suspected Emily was suffering from PCOS, and that her birth control medication had masked it for years. I suspected her PCOS was the underlying cause of not only testosterone excess, but also estrogen excess and progesterone deficiency. This is what sets Warriors with PCOS apart from the rest: Their archetype is multifaceted, incorporating aspects of the Queen (see page 67) and the Unbalanced Heroine (see page 81).

So, how can PCOS help give rise to the Warrior archetype? This has to do with the condition's impact on two hormones that factor significantly into the production of testosterone in women: follicle-stimulating hormone (FSH) and luteinizing hormone (LH). FSH stimulates what are called granulosa cells in the ovaries and ovarian cysts to produce estrogen. LH stimulates ovary- and ovarian-cyst-based theca cells to produce testosterone. In normally functioning females, the FSH-to-LH ratio is roughly 2 to 1. In women who have PCOS, this ratio is flipped to 1 to 3. In the end, women who have PCOS tend to experience increased production of both estrogen *and* testosterone, as well as decreased production of progesterone. Emily's flipped FSH-to-LH ratio added the element of relative imbalance between estrogen and testosterone, which helps account for the symptoms of testosterone excess.

PCOS contributes to increased testosterone production in a second way. In women and men, testosterone helps regulate insulin levels. Women who have PCOS also tend to suffer from insulin resistance and hyperinsulinemia, a condition in which insulin levels in the blood are generally high relative to glucose levels. In women who have PCOS, then, increased testosterone may be part of the body's natural effort to regulate insulin. High insulin also contributes to weight gain by causing the body to store fat. This is why the Warrior with PCOS may have a hard time increasing muscle mass and losing weight, even when she diets and exercises.

As it turned out, Emily was, in fact, suffering from PCOS. Her estrogen and testosterone levels were each well outside "normal" range, and her progesterone levels were far below it. We discussed the impact of testosterone excess and the fact that it was likely causing the growth of hair on her body and face, the loss of hair on her head, and her acne. We also discussed that excess estrogen and a progesterone deficiency were likely combining to cause interrupted sleep, irregular periods, and water retention. "Your birth control medication masked the PCOS for years," I explained. "But now our challenge is to take a multifaceted SHINES approach to help bring your testosterone, estrogen, and progesterone back into balance while we also explore options for treating your PCOS."

The Warrior: Symptomology Summary

Warriors tend to present with the following physiological, psychological, and emotional symptoms:

Physiological Symptoms	
Irregular menstrual cycles or amenorrhea (cessation of menstruation)	This could be due to PCOS.
Hirsutism	Male-pattern body hair growth, particularly on the face, chest, and back. Increased hair growth in the abdominal area is common.

(continues)

Hair loss	This is most likely to occur on the top of the head, near the hairline. In women who have excess testosterone, the hair loss that ensues is most likely male pattern.
Clitoromegaly (enlargement of the clitoris)	It is important to note that this condition can be permanent.
Deepening of the voice	It is important to note that this condition can be permanent.

Psychological and Emotional Symptoms	
Irritability	Some women describe feeling quick to anger and uncharacteristically inclined toward aggression.

An array of circumstances and conditions can give rise to the Warrior archetype. This means that symptoms among Warriors can vary. If you are experiencing X number of these symptoms and/or are aware that you may have been exposed to or experienced one or more of the underlying root causes of testosterone excess, I encourage you to have your levels of testosterone—and other hormones—tested. Excessive testosterone production may trigger or indicate other imbalances.

The Warrior: Underlying Causes of Symptomology

Early in this section, we discussed the three most common causes of testosterone excess in women: intentional or unintentional exposure to testosterone replacement medications or supplements, tumors in the ovaries or adrenals that disrupt the body's natural production of the hormone, and PCOS. There are also other, rarer causes of the condition.

EXPOSURE TO MEDICATIONS OR SUPPLEMENTS

Some of the Warriors I've treated have sought me out after consulting with another physician or hormone expert, and have already started a **testosterone replacement therapy medication** when they come to see me. Many of these women have had testosterone pellets inserted under their skin. This form of testosterone replacement therapy can be dangerous for women because of the way it causes levels of the hormone to spike and quickly drop. Additional dangers of this form of therapy for women are increased risk of deepening voice and an enlarged clitoris, which can be permanent changes.

Available by prescription or over the counter, **DHEA supplements** can also contribute to the Warrior archetype's taking hold. Popular with men and women alike, DHEA supplements are believed to help promote a healthy constitution and longevity, improving bone density and heart health, fighting fatigue, and increasing the production of testosterone (and estrogen). Once DHEA enters into your system, it breaks down into androstenedione, the direct precursor to testosterone.

When I prescribe DHEA for my patients, I recommend doses of between 6.5 and 12.5 mg/day. In women, doses of 25 mg/day and higher can increase their testosterone to levels at which they begin to experience undesirable side effects, including elevated cholesterol. Although DHEA can yield some positive benefits, taking a supplement without a physician's oversight can lead to hormonal imbalances, which, if left unchecked, can have deleterious effects.

TUMORS

In some cases, ovarian tumors, adrenal tumors, or other masses can drive increased testosterone production in women. Diagnosing this requires eliminating potential causes that are more easily recognized and scanning for growths. Even benign tumors that resolve on their own can cause temporary imbalances.

POLYCYSTIC OVARIAN SYNDROME (PCOS)

PCOS can contribute to the Warrior archetype's taking hold by virtue of its impact on two hormones that factor significantly into the production of testosterone in women: FSH and LH. FSH and LH stimulate ovarian granulosis cells and theca cells respectively, triggering these to produce estrogen and testosterone. In normally functioning females, the FSH-to-LH ratio is roughly 2 to 1; in women who have PCOS, this ratio is flipped to 1 to 3. This means that women with PCOS tend to have higher absolute levels of testosterone in addition to an estrogen-testosterone imbalance.

PCOS also contributes to increased testosterone production due to the condition's impact on insulin. Insulin resistance and hyperinsulinemia (a condition in which insulin levels in the blood are generally high relative to glucose levels) are both associated with PCOS. Testosterone helps regulate insulin, which may account for why women with PCOS tend to have elevated testosterone levels. Increased production of the hormone may indicate the body's effort to regulate its insulin.

OTHER ILLNESSES AND CONDITIONS

Cushing's syndrome and Cushing's disease, conditions in which the body suffers chronic exposure to excessive levels of cortisol, can give rise to testosterone excess.

In rare instances, pregnant women may develop masses known as theca lutein cysts on their ovaries.[17] Because these cysts are lined with testosterone-producing theca cells, women who have them are likely to produce excess testosterone. Although many of the symptoms diminish or resolve altogether following pregnancy, some, such as deepening of the voice and clitoromegaly, do not. This condition also poses a risk to the fetus, which may display ambiguous sexual development or, if it is female, clitoromegaly. If you are or become pregnant and experience the symptoms described in this section, I strongly encourage you to consult your physician.

A third condition that can contribute to excess testosterone in women is congenital adrenal hyperplasia (CAH). Often diagnosed during childhood, this condition causes dysfunction of the adrenal glands, which can, in turn, affect the production of cortisol, mineralocorticoids (which regulate sodium and potassium levels), and/or androgens. According to the Mayo Clinic, CAH often results in diminished cortisol levels and an overproduction of testosterone.

If you have not been diagnosed with CAH by adulthood, it is unlikely you will be. If you have been diagnosed with the condition, however, certain elements of the Warrior's SHINES protocol may help alleviate symptoms of testosterone excess.

The Underdog

Hypothyroidism (Low Thyroid)

"Ultimately, 'Cinderella' is the story of the underdog. You root for her in this fairy tale; the girl who has nothing, deserves so much more, and gets it."

—LILY JAMES

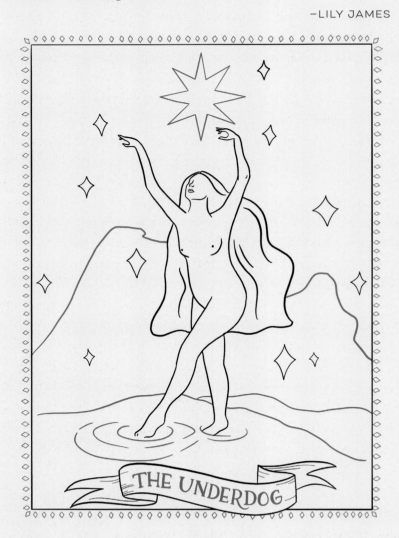

THE UNDERDOG

noun un·der·dog \ ˈən-dər-ˌdȯg \
: a loser or predicted loser in a struggle or contest.

In this section, we consider the Underdog. Characterized by hypothyroidism, or "underactive thyroid," this archetype can arise in women of any age. Women are significantly more likely to develop hypothyroidism than men are—five to eight times more likely, according to the American Thyroid Association—and their chances of doing so increase with age.[18]

Despite the relative prevalence of hypothyroidism, Underdogs can often go undiagnosed. This has to do with standard medical practices around testing for the underactive thyroid. Traditionally, physicians have measured patients' thyroid-stimulating hormone (TSH) levels. Produced by the pituitary gland, high levels of TSH indicate decreased thyroid activity, and lower levels indicate more. But a hypothyroid diagnosis requires that these levels fall outside the "normal" range, which spans from 0.4 to 5 milli-international units per liter (mIU/L). If your level is 3.5, you may fall within the normal range, but this level may be abnormal for *you*. If you've gained 20 pounds during the past year, suffer from chronically low body temperature, and have begun experiencing sporadic short-term memory loss, diminished thyroid activity may well be at the root of your symptoms.

Adding to this, TSH levels can reveal only so much about what the thyroid is *actually* producing. This small, butterfly-shaped gland produces two hormones that, taken together, exert effects on all the body's tissues. Known as T4 (tetraiodothyronine, thyroxine) and T3 (triiodothyronine), these hormones influence a number of the body's vital functions, including metabolism, heart rate, breathing, muscle strength, body temperature, and menstrual cycle.[*]

That thyroid hormones have such varied effects means the Underdog's symptoms can be far-flung. These include weight gain, fatigue, muscle and joint aches, and, in some cases, irregular menstrual

---

[*] The thyroid also produces a hormone called calcitonin, which helps regulate the amount of calcium circulating in the blood.

cycles or amenorrhea (the cessation of menstruation). Where these can be explained by other causes, Underdogs are at an increased risk of going undiagnosed.

T4 (Tetraiodothyronine or Thyroxine) and T3 (Triiodothyronine)

T4 and T3, as they are commonly known, are the two thyroid hormones that drive your metabolic processes, including those associated with digestion, circulation, and even brain activity. They are almost identical in molecular structure, differing by only a single iodine atom.

When triggered by TSH (which is produced by the pituitary gland), the thyroid combines iodine stored in its cells with the amino acid tyrosine to produce both T3 and T4. It does this at a ratio of roughly 20 percent T3 to 80 percent T4. T3 is the more "active" of the two hormones, meaning that it is the form that actually exerts metabolic effects. T4 converts to T3 according to the body's need for it. Conversion occurs when T4 binds to cells in peripheral tissues throughout the body, dropping an iodine atom in the process.

This is why it is so important to test for blood serum levels of TSH, Free T4, *and* Free T3. Even if your TSH levels are within normal range, your thyroid may not be producing sufficient levels of T4 and T3 and/or your conversion of T4 to T3 may be impeded. Any of these conditions may give rise to symptomatic subclinical hypothyroidism.

I named the Underdog for the overarching nature of her experience of herself and her body: Her potential self seems within her reach, but she cannot access it. So many patients have told me they feel like the girl who used to be a star athlete but is now always chosen last when teams pick sides, or who stays home when her friends ask her to come out because she just doesn't have the energy to socialize the way she'd like to. Underdogs can imagine leading the life they want to—and, in some cases, used to—but they don't feel like they have the drive or the energy to access and hold on to it. This is what the SHINES protocol is designed to help the Underdog achieve.

A note about hormone-based interventions for the Underdog: The use of medications to treat hypothyroidism or subclinical hypothyroidism (which is an early, mild form) is a delicate matter. Intervening in the thyroid's functioning in this way can effectively "shut it off" permanently, making an Underdog dependent on medications for the rest of her life. This is why, for the Underdog in particular, both careful diagnosis of hypothyroidism and consideration of alternative approaches are critical.

In the following pages, we consider one Underdog's story and take a closer look at the archetype's causes and symptomology. In the next chapter we will explore the Underdog's SHINES protocol, which I've designed to help restore your access to the strength and vitality residing within you.

Hypothyroidism and Hashimoto's Thyroiditis

Hashimoto's thyroiditis is an autoimmune disorder that involves the degradation and, potentially, destruction of the thyroid gland. This occurs when an overabundance of white blood cells in the thyroid turn from maintaining the health of the tissue to attacking it.

Progressing in five stages (labeled from 0 to 4), the condition initially gives rise to symptomatic—but subclinical—hypothyroidism, which, as we've discussed,

(continues)

can be misdiagnosed. Symptoms of Hashimoto's include those associated with other forms of hypothyroidism such as fatigue, infertility and miscarriage, weight gain or loss, anxiety, and depression, in addition to acid reflux, gut wall dysfunction, food sensitivity, certain nutrient deficiencies, and more.

During the early stages of Hashimoto's, levels of TSH, T3, and T4 are likely to be within "normal" range. It is only in the later stages that these levels may drive a clinical diagnosis. Alternative means of diagnosis are blood serum testing for elevated levels of the thyroid antibodies peroxidase and thyroglobulin (between 90 and 95 percent of Hashimoto's sufferers will have these antibodies) and ultrasound scans that can reveal singular structural features and blood flow patterns in the thyroid tissue.

As with any Underdog who is struggling with subclinical hypothyroidism, early-stage Hashimoto's sufferers can benefit from thyroid medication in addition to lifestyle changes, particularly those involving nutrition. Many of these changes are designed to help bring the immune system into balance, given that Hashimoto's is an autoimmune disorder and not a disease of the thyroid, per se.

As Hashimoto's progresses, prescription thyroid hormone replacement becomes increasingly vital. For some, the need for medication will be lifelong.[19]

Patient Example

When Miranda called to schedule a visit, I could hear the exhaustion in her voice. Thirty-year-old Miranda had been a patient of mine for five years, and I had never heard her sound so tired. She had a two-year-old at home, which was bound to account for some of her fatigue. But my intuition told me that a hormonal imbalance could also be a significant factor. When she told me she was most concerned about her irregular menstrual cycle and some spotting, which she'd never experienced before, I was persuaded that we should test her hormone levels. And by the time Miranda mentioned she was also concerned that she would *never* lose the 20 pounds she'd gained during her pregnancy, I suspected her thyroid hormone levels were off.

Adding to all this, it was summer in Austin when Miranda came in for her consult, and she was wearing a jacket. "I don't need it *outside*," she explained, "but I'm too cold anywhere there's air-conditioning. My coworkers make fun of me for keeping a blanket in my desk drawer, but I don't care. I need it!" Miranda also appeared as exhausted as she'd sounded on the phone, and when I asked about her energy levels, she told me she struggled mightily to get out of bed each morning. Even a healthy breakfast and coffee didn't seem to help. "I'm always sluggish," she said. "Like my body just never kicks into gear. I'm missing work more than I ever have. And I do my best to muster the energy to keep up with my two-year-old, but it's a struggle every single day." Miranda's low energy was also keeping her out of the gym. "I want to lose the baby weight," she explained. "I'm always conscious of what I'm eating, and I do my best to restrict my calorie intake. But I can't even imagine resuming my old workout routine."

More convinced now that Miranda's thyroid hormone levels were likely causing her symptoms, I considered her history. She had never had thyroid surgery or undergone radiation treatments to her neck, two potential causes of hypothyroidism, and she was not taking any medications or supplements that might interfere with the functioning of her pituitary or thyroid glands. For Underdogs, family history is also relevant, so I asked about the women in her family—whether her mother, sisters, or even aunts or grandmothers had ever suffered from a thyroid disorder. As it turned out, Miranda's mother had been treated for thyroid cancer, and her older sister had been diagnosed with underactive thyroid two years earlier.

A physical exam revealed no swelling or nodules on Miranda's thyroid gland. But a blood serum test indicated that her levels of

TSH fell on the high side of the "normal" range. This indicated that her thyroid hormone levels might be low. When I looked at these—and at T3 and T4 in particular—each indeed fell on the low side of the normal range for a woman of Miranda's age.

Here was a case where *symptoms* tipped the balance. For me, the fact that Miranda's TSH, T3, and T4 levels were all within normal range did not mean her thyroid wasn't underactive. Taken together with the extreme fatigue, cold intolerance, irregular menstrual cycles, and persistent excess weight she was experiencing, the levels indicated subclinical hypothyroidism. In other words, Miranda's so-called normal levels were *not normal for her.*

I prescribed Miranda a low-dose thyroid medication, and we discussed how the other aspects of the SHINES protocol could also help address her imbalance. I asked that she return in eight weeks for an evaluation, at which point we would reassess her symptoms and retest her blood serum. My hope was that between taking the medication and making changes in her diet and lifestyle, including introducing a gentle exercise routine, Miranda would experience improved thyroid functioning and a reduction of her symptoms. I also explained that our work would not end there. I told her an Underdog's journey can be a long one, with dependency on thyroid medication sometimes lasting a lifetime. For as long as she was on this medication, I told her, we would need to routinely monitor her blood serum levels of TSH, T3, and T4.

When Miranda entered my office eight weeks later, she appeared visibly refreshed. And she wasn't wearing a jacket. "Life is better," she said. "Getting out of bed is becoming easier, and I haven't had to call in sick to work in a month. Keeping up with my son is less of a struggle, and I've finally lost five pounds . . . I haven't gotten back to the gym yet, but I'm taking walks at lunchtime instead of sneaking out to my car for a nap. I can't say I feel like Wonder Woman yet, but I certainly feel a shift has started—and like things are going to keep getting better."

The Underdog: Symptomology Summary

Given the thyroid hormones' broad reach, the Underdog's symptoms can be far-flung and seemingly unrelated. These symptoms also tend to be somewhat common and attributable to other factors, including diet and exercise, as well as other hormonal imbalances.

Physiological Symptoms: Thyroid Hormone Deficiency[*]	
Weight gain	Low thyroid can contribute to weight gain.
Constipation	Slower gut motility can contribute to constipation.
Fatigue (lack of stamina)	Generalized fatigue throughout the day.
Muscle and joint aches[**]	Not well understood, but thought to be affected by cellular metabolism.
Pitting edema	In front of the lower legs.
Infertility	This can result from irregularities in the menstrual cycle/amenorrhea.
Cold intolerance	Due to period irregularities.

[*] L. Chaker, A. C. Bianco, J. Jonklaas, and R. P. Peeters, "Hypothyroidism," *Lancet* 390, no. 10101 (September 23, 2017): 1550–62, https://doi.org/10.1016/S0140-673 6(17)30703-1.

[**] M. M. Fariduddin and N. Bansal, "Hypothyroid Myopathy," in *StatPearls* (Treasure Island, FL: StatPearls Publishing, 2020). Available from https://www.ncbi.nlm.nih.gov /books/NBK519513/.

(continues)

Psychological and Emotional Symptoms	
Depression*	The link to depression is real but it may not resolve with thyroid supplementation, because, as we know, depression is multifaceted.
Memory issues**	Typically described in the clinic as a "brain fog."

* T. Zhao, X. M. Zhao, and Z. Y. Shan, "Subclinical Hypothyroidism and Depression: A Meta Analysis," *Translational Psychiatry* 8, no. 1 (October 30, 2018): 239, https://doi.org /10.1038/s41398-018-0283-7. PMID: 30375372; PMCID: PMC6207556.

** A. Chaalal, R. Poirier, D. Blum, S. Laroche, and V. Enderlin, "Thyroid Hormone Supplementation Restores Spatial Memory, Hipppocampal Markers of Neuroinflammation, Plasticity-Related Signaling Molecules, and <beta>-Amyloid Peptide Load in Hypothyroid Rats," *Molecular Neurobiology* 56, no. 1 (January 2019): 722–35, https://doi.org /10.1007/s12035-018-1111-z. Epub 2018 May 23. PMID: 29796989.

The Underdog: Underlying Causes of Symptomology

AUTOIMMUNE DISORDERS

Hypothyroidism can arise as a result of an autoimmune disorder. Whether the disorder initially targets the thyroid in particular, as is the case with Hashimoto's thyroiditis, or attacks other organ tissues, an imbalance in the body's defenses may be at the root of the Underdog archetype. Conditions such as rheumatoid arthritis, lupus, and fibromyalgia may also negatively affect thyroid function (as mentioned above, Hashimoto's is an autoimmune disorder).

THYROID CANCER

Thyroid cancer patients who undergo surgery to remove their thyroid (thyroidectomy) will inevitably and permanently suffer from hypothyroidism and will rely on medication to replace the hormones produced by the thyroid. Women who undergo a partial thyroidectomy are likely to suffer a degree of hypothyroidism, depending on the extent of the surgery. In these cases, blood serum testing is required to determine the level of functionality in the portion of the gland that remains. I recommend consistent ongoing monitoring of TSH, T3, and T4 levels, particularly in patients who have been prescribed hormone replacement medication.

Radiation treatment for thyroid cancer or other types of cancer can also damage the thyroid, diminishing its functionality. Damage to the pituitary gland that reduces its ability to produce TSH also negatively affects the production of thyroid hormone.

GRAVES' DISEASE

An autoimmune disorder that causes the overproduction of thyroid hormones (hyperthyroidism), Graves' disease may be treated with radiation therapy, radioactive iodine therapy, or the partial or complete removal of the thyroid, any of which may give rise to hypothyroidism.

VIRUSES

The presence of certain viruses in the bloodstream (even if they are dormant) are associated with hypothyroidism. These include the Epstein-Barr virus (EBV), which causes mononucleosis (also known as "glandular fever" and the "kissing disease") and the mumps virus. A 2015 study found evidence of EBV in 62.5 percent of patients suffering from Graves' disease and 80.7 percent of patients diagnosed with Hashimoto's thyroiditis.[20]

Researchers have also linked a number of enteroviruses to hypothyroidism. Named for their transmission route through the intestine, enteroviruses give rise to a range of infections, from a relatively mild summer cold to pericarditis/myocarditis to hand, foot, and mouth disease in children.

OTHER DISEASES

A handful of other relatively rare disorders can directly damage the thyroid and diminish its functioning. One is hemochromatosis, a genetic disorder that causes the body to store too much iron. Excess amounts of the mineral in the thyroid can damage it directly. Hemochromatosis can also result in dangerously high levels of iron in the pituitary, damaging it and influencing its production of TSH.[21]

A condition called amyloidosis results in the deposit of excessive amounts of amyloid—a protein produced in bone marrow—in the tissues of various organs. Amyloid deposits in the thyroid can give rise to what are called amyloid goiters. In some cases, these impede thyroid function significantly enough to cause hypothyroidism.[22] Sarcoidosis, which causes the development of small bunches of inflammatory cells called granulomas in various parts of the body, can result in deposits of these cells in the thyroid gland, causing fibrosis and impairing the gland's functioning.[23]

MEDICATIONS

Some medications may also cause or contribute to the onset of hypothyroidism. Among these are the antiarrhythmic drug amiodarone, as well as interferon, which is commonly used to treat patients who have cancer or hepatitis C. Lithium, which is used to treat psychological and physiological disorders including hyperthyroidism, decreases production of T4 and disrupts the conversion of T4 to T3, the more active form of thyroid hormone.

IODINE IMBALANCE

The thyroid gland needs iodine to produce tetraiodothyronine (thyroxine, or T4). The thyroid stores iodine and combines this with an amino acid called tyrosine to make T4. In peripheral tissues, T4 binds with thyroid hormone receptors, dropping an iodine atom to become the more active form of the hormone, triiodothyronine (T3).

While sufficient amounts of this essential (exogenously produced) nutrient are critically important for healthy thyroid function, an overabundance of iodine in the bloodstream can damage the gland. Keeping your iodine in balance is therefore one of the key elements to maintaining healthy thyroid function.

ENVIRONMENTAL TOXINS

DIOXINS

Dioxins are one group of environmental toxins that can contribute to hypothyroidism. Created by industrial processes such as chemical manufacturing and the burning of hazardous waste, as well as the burning of coal and oil for energy, dioxins are also commonly found in car and truck exhaust, the smoke from cigarettes and wood-burning fires, and pesticides. Dioxins can disrupt various aspects of the body's functioning, including reproduction, and contribute to various hormonal imbalances. In the case of hypothyroidism, research indicates that increased exposure to dioxins can result in lower levels of TSH and T4. According to one study, women were more at risk for this than men.[24]

According to the EPA, dioxins are found in water, air, and soil all over the earth. But the vast majority of human exposure results from the consumption of contaminated animal-derived food products, including meat, dairy, and seafood. (Plants tend not to absorb dioxins. Washing fruits and vegetables generally suffices to remove any dioxin-containing pesticides.)[25] Dioxins are stored in the fatty tissues of humans and animals, where they may continue to exert effects for a number of years. To mitigate or reduce your exposure to dioxins, the National Institutes of Health (NIH) recommends avoiding ingesting excessive amounts of animal fats. Choose meat and fish that is naturally lean and/or remove the skin, in addition to consuming only low-fat or nonfat milk and only limited amounts of butter.[26]

POLYCHLORINATED BIPHENYLS (PCBs)

A series of synthetic chemicals used in the production of certain types of electrical and heavy equipment, oil-based paints, plastics, and insulation, PCBs have been linked to a series of health issues, including adverse effects on thyroid function. Research indicates that PCBs may influence thyroid function in a variety of ways, including by binding with TSH receptors and/or thyroid transport proteins, which limits the amount of circulating T4. PCBs may also have a negative impact on the enzymes necessary for converting T4 to T3 and/or raise the levels of thyroid antibodies.[27]

Although US chemical manufacturers were banned from creating and marketing PCBs in 1979, the compounds are still present in a variety of industrial and consumer products that remain in use. Leaks into the air and soil can occur as a result of illegal dumping, poor maintenance of hazardous-waste sites, and the dumping of PCB-containing objects into landfills that are not properly equipped to contain hazardous waste.[28]

METALS

Exposure to metals such as lead, mercury, cadmium, and aluminum has also been linked to hypothyroidism. Whether naturally occurring or released into air, soil, and water as a result of various industrial processes, these compounds can be hard to avoid. In the United States, environmental lead pollution has resulted from mining operations, for example, and the metal is also contained in (older) paint and certain (generally inexpensive) consumer products. Certain seafood can contain high levels of mercury, and aluminum is found in such common household items as deodorant and cookware. Cadmium is also released into the environment as a result of various industrial processes, but in America, dangerous levels of exposure are linked only to cigarettes and e-cigarettes.

Toxic metals may enter the bloodstream via respiration, digestion, or even simple contact with the skin. Exposure to some heavy metals is inevitable, but reducing exposure can help minimize the likelihood that heavy metals will contribute to hypothyroidism.

While all metals may adversely affect thyroid function, their mechanisms of action can vary. Studies have shown that cadmium reduces the secretion of thyroglobulin, the protein responsible for transporting thyroid hormones throughout the bloodstream, while lead, mercury, and aluminum are all associated with decreased iodine uptake and disruptions of the T4-to-T3 conversion process.[29] Mercury also binds to selenium, a mineral that plays an indirect role in the synthesis of thyroid hormones by virtue of its presence in iodothyronine deiodinases, the proteins responsible for converting T4 to T3.[30]

COMMON HOUSEHOLD PRODUCT ADDITIVES

Another group of toxins that can contribute to hypothyroidism are flame retardants known as polybrominated diphenyl ethers

(PBDEs). Commonly contained in consumer products such as computers, televisions, and furniture, PBDEs can impede the function of thyroid-hormone-binding proteins. These can also disrupt estrogen activity, which some researchers believe may exacerbate postmenopausal women's susceptibility to impaired thyroid function.[31]

Chemicals such as bisphenol A (BPA) and phthalates, which are (or have been) used in plastics, flooring, and some personal care products, can contribute to diminished thyroid function by blocking T3 from binding at receptor sites. In 2012, the Federal Drug Administration (FDA) banned BPA from baby bottles and other drinking cups meant for children. While some states have taken this ban further, there is no federal law prohibiting the manufacture, sale, or use of BPA.

GQ/11 PROTEIN ANTAGONISTS

Gq/11 is a cell protein that desensitizes the thyroid to TSH and blocks the action of T3 within cells. Elevated levels of Gq/11 can therefore contribute to hypothyroidism. Aluminum, silica dust (found in cigarettes as well as rock, soil, and granite), and beryllium (used in the manufacture of missiles, aircrafts, and cell phones) all activate the Gq/11 protein. Fluoride also upregulates Gq/11, in addition to impeding iodine uptake.[32]

The Overachiever

Hyperthyroidism (Excess Thyroid)

"I'm this overachiever type, I'll just work and work, and I'll just do it over and over and over again."

–VENUS WILLIAMS

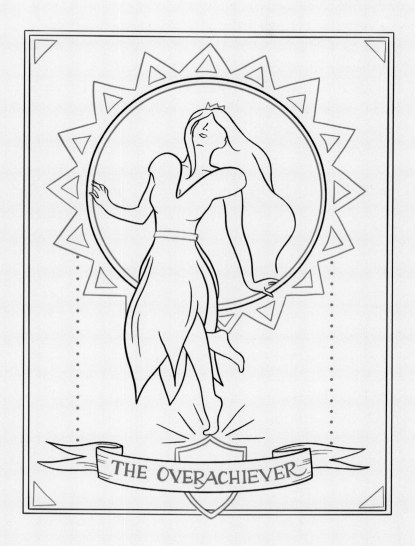

THE OVERACHIEVER

noun over·achiev·er \ ˌō-vər-ə-ˈchē-vər \

: one who achieves success over and above the standard or expected level, especially at an early age.

In this section, we take a close look at the Overachiever archetype. Characterized by an overactive thyroid or overt hyperthyroidism, this archetype can take hold in a woman of any age. Potentially rooted in any of a series of underlying conditions, including autoimmune disorders, nodular growths, viral infection, and pregnancy, hyperthyroidism involves damage to the thyroid and will almost inevitably progress to hypothyroidism if left untreated. Women are at higher risk of hyperthyroidism than men—five to eight times higher, according to research by the American Thyroid Association—and the risk of certain thyroid disorders increases with age.

In Overachievers, the small, butterfly-shaped thyroid gland at the base of the front of the neck produces excess amounts of the thyroid hormones T4 (tetraiodothyronine or thyroxine), T3 (triiodothyronine).[33] Together, these hormones are responsible for regulating a wide range of vital processes in the body, including metabolism, heart rate, breathing, muscle strength, body temperature, and menstrual cycle. As such, excess amounts can cause such varied symptoms as unexplained weight loss, atrial fibrillation (irregular heartbeat), compromised respiration, tremors, gastrointestinal distress, irregular menstrual cycles or amenorrhea (cessation of menstruation), elevated body temperature, excessive sweating, and anxiety.

As much as hyperthyroidism may seem like a "problem you'd love to have," given that weight loss is one of its primary symptoms, the risks that accompany this condition are very serious. For example, hyperthyroidism signals that either the pituitary gland, which produces thyroid-stimulating hormone (TSH), or the thyroid itself has come under attack, either by a growth (or growths) or the body's own immune system. In either case, a prompt diagnosis will be essential to a positive outcome. In the case of the thyroid, determining whether and how it is possible to stem an assault is critical. Damage caused by viruses, antibodies, or tumors can be permanent and give rise to potentially lifelong hypothyroidism.

Adding to this, hyperthyroidism causes extreme stress on all the body's tissues, including muscle and bone. When your metabolism is increased to such a rate that your body is burning through all the calories you consume, it turns to catabolizing your tissues for fuel and nutrients necessary for sustaining bodily functions (see page 120 for more on catabolism). If your heart needs calcium to sustain its increased rate, and you're not consuming enough of the mineral to keep pace with its demands, your body is likely to pull calcium from your bones. If you need 2,000 calories per day to maintain your weight and your body is burning 5,000 calories per day, you not only need 2.5 times as many calories, but 2.5 times as much protein and various essential vitamins and minerals. This is how Overachievers quickly run into deficits that lead to the breakdown of various tissues.

While weight loss may—initially—be a welcome change, the longer it persists, the longer the thyroid remains in danger of permanent injury or burnout. This is the progression of Hashimoto's thyroiditis, for example, an autoimmune condition in which thyroid antibodies attack the gland's healthy tissue. The early stages of Hashimoto's thyroiditis are characterized by hyperthyroidism, which transforms into hypothyroidism as the thyroid tissue degrades. In some cases, this deterioration is irreversible.

Graves' Disease

The leading cause of hyperthyroidism in the United States,[34] Graves' disease is an autoimmune disorder that results in the production of antibodies called thyrotropin receptor antibodies (TRAb) or thyroid-stimulating immunoglobulins (TSI). These antibodies bind with thyroid-stimulating hormone (TSH) receptors

(continues)

on thyroid cells, prompting them to produce and release excess amounts of T4 and T3.

Graves' disease is associated not only with hyperthyroidism, but also with protruding eyes (Graves' opthalmopathy) and the thickening and discoloration of skin, generally on the lower legs and feet (Graves' dermopathy). The presence of these symptoms often indicates that Graves' is the underlying cause of hyperthyroidism, though confirmation of the diagnosis requires testing for one or more of the following: levels of TSH, T4, and T3, TSI, thyroidal blood flow, and the gland's iodine uptake rate. (In mild cases, a patient may test negative for TSI.) A family history of Graves', other thyroid disorders, or autoimmune conditions such as type 1 diabetes, rheumatoid arthritis, or pernicious anemia increases the likelihood of a positive diagnosis.[35]

Treatment for Graves' generally involves antithyroid medications. In some cases, these are prescribed for extended periods (longer than two years). While remission is possible, in extreme and persistent instances of Graves' disease, treatment with surgery or radioactive iodine may be necessary. Either of these may inflict irreparable damage on the thyroid gland and permanently limit its activity.

According to the American Thyroid Association, Graves' disease is seven to eight times as common in women as in men.[36] If you are experiencing symptoms of hyperthyroidism and have some of the risk factors listed above, I recommend consulting with your healthcare practitioner to determine whether a test for Graves' is advisable.

Thyroid Storm

Extreme thyrotoxicosis (the presence of excessive levels of thyroid hormone in the body), also known as "thyroid storm," represents the most extreme end of the spectrum of hyperthyroidism disorder. This condition can be fatal.

Involving the compromised functioning of major organs, including the heart, lungs, liver, and brain, thyroid storm escalates suddenly and requires immediate and significant medical intervention to resolve. Among the common symptoms are fever, profuse sweating, labored respiration, tachyarrhythmia (resting heart rate exceeding 100 beats per minute), delirium or psychosis, jaundice (caused by underlying liver dysfunction), abdominal pain, nausea, vomiting, and diarrhea.[37]

While thyroid storm is a risk for any Overachiever, proper diagnosis and management of your hyperthyroidism is the best protection against it.

Patient Example

When Melinda entered my office, I was struck by how different she looked from when I'd seen her just six weeks before. A new mother, Melinda had been concerned about losing the 30 pounds she'd gained during her pregnancy. But now, just three months after giving birth, she already appeared very thin. Worryingly so, in my view.

At thirty-two years old, Melinda had no history of serious illness. Her pregnancy and delivery had both been free of complications, and her baby was healthy. Melinda was struggling, however. "I'm anxious all the time," she explained. "I'm moody and irritable, and I can't sleep. The baby is sleeping, but I'm not. I'm pacing the floor all night instead." Melinda was also experiencing what she referred to as hot flashes, and complained of feeling uncomfortably warm much of the time. When I asked about her apparent weight loss, Melinda said she was happy she seemed to be losing her baby weight despite "eating like a fiend," but lately, she'd been having trouble producing enough milk to breastfeed. "I'm worried it will only get worse," she said.

When Melinda stepped on the scale, we discovered she was down to 120 pounds, 20 pounds below her pre-pregnancy weight. "I've lost more than I thought," she said. Melinda was also slightly tachycardic, with a resting heart rate of 105. Her body temperature was normal, though her limbs were warm to the touch. Her skin was also dry. When I asked Melinda whether her menstrual cycles had resumed since the birth of her baby, she told me they had not. By now, I suspected she was suffering from hyperthyroidism, and I asked about her family history. Some years before, Melinda told me, her mother had suffered some difficulties with her thyroid and had had a nodule removed.

When I examined Melinda, I felt no nodules on her thyroid, though it felt slightly enlarged. When I ordered blood serum tests of Melinda's thyroid-stimulating hormone (TSH) and her circulating levels of T4 and T3, I discovered that her TSH was extremely low, while her thyroid hormones were each above normal. An additional test for antithyroid antibodies came back positive for antithyroid peroxidase (anti-TPO) and anti-thyroglobulin (anti-Tg), both of which are associated with Hashimoto's thyroiditis. Taken together, these results indicated that Melinda was very likely in the early stages of Hashimoto's, suffering an autoimmune attack on her thyroid, which was releasing excessive amounts of T4 and T3 into her system as a result.

The Overachiever: Symptomology Summary

The fact that your thyroid hormones have such varied and far-reaching impact means the symptoms of hyperthyroidism can also be far-flung. While unexplained weight loss is a primary and defining symptom of the Overachiever archetype, hyperthyroidism can also give rise to a series of other physiological and psychological conditions, the particular quality or nature of which can reveal the underlying cause of your thyroid's overactivity.

To determine whether the Overachiever is your archetype, I recommend taking the Hormone-Typing Quiz (see page 63) in addition to considering the physiological and psychological symptoms described here. If you are experiencing several of these, I recommend consulting your healthcare practitioner to determine whether testing your blood serum for TSH, T4, T3, and/or antithyroid antibody levels is warranted.

The Overachiever: Underlying Causes of Symptomology

GRAVES' DISEASE

Graves' disease is the most common cause of hyperthyroidism. A hereditary autoimmune disease also known as toxic diffused goiter, Graves' may occur in people of any age, but is seven to eight more times more likely to occur in women than in men and generally takes hold between the ages of thirty and fifty. As discussed earlier in this section, Graves' is characterized by the body's production of antithyroid antibodies called thyrotropin receptor antibodies (TRAb) or thyroid-stimulating immunoglobulins (TSI), which bind with thyrotropin or TSH receptors on thyroid cells, prompting them to produce and release excess amounts of T4 and T3.

Women suffering from certain other autoimmune disorders, including rheumatoid arthritis, lupus, Addison's disease, and type 1 diabetes, are also more likely to develop Graves'.[38] Recent studies have also linked the disease to infection by a bacteria called *Yersinia*

Physiological Symptoms: Hyperthyroidism

Sudden, unexplained weight loss	Increased appetite is likely. Weight loss occurs even with increased calorie consumption.
Muscle weakness and general fatigue	This is a condition called thyrotoxic myopathy.
Heat intolerance	Excessive sweating may also occur.
Enlarged thyroid (goiter) or thyroid nodule	An enlarged thyroid (also known as a goiter) manifests as a swelling near the base of the front of the neck. A nodule (or nodules) may or may not be detectable by touch. When a nodule produces excess T4, it is called toxic adenoma. When multiple nodules do this, it is called multinodular goiter.
Cardiac issues	These may include tachycardia (rapid resting heart rate), arrhythmia, and heart palpitations.
Tremors	Generally, tremors occur in the fingers and hands.

Dry, thinning skin	Graves' disease can also cause a skin condition called Graves' dermopathy, a thickening and reddening of the skin along the shins and tops of the feet. Painless white patches of skin called vitiligo are also associated with certain types of hyperthyroidism.
Gastrointestinal irregularities	These include increased frequency of bowel movements.

Psychological and Emotional Symptoms: Hyperthyroidism*

Nervousness, generalized anxiety	This is a generalized feeling of being overstimulated as thyroid hormone increases heart rate.
Irritability	As with anxiety, this irritability comes from the feeling of overstimulation.
Panic attacks	The end result of tachycardia or racing heart can cause one to overtly stress and bring on a panic attack.

* M. Mazza, P. Bria, C. Taranto, L. Janiri, and S. Mazza, "Mood, Hormones and Quality of Life," *Clinical Therapeutics* 159, no. 2 (March–April 2008): 105–9, PMID: 18464769.

enterocolitica, which is similar in molecular structure to the thyroid's TSH receptors. The theory is that the same antibodies the body creates to combat the bacterial infection also attack TSH receptors, causing them to produce and release excessive levels of thyroid hormone into the system.[39]

THYROIDITIS

Referring to inflammation of the thyroid, this condition may arise due to a variety of factors. The root cause of some types of thyroiditis may remain a mystery, while others, such as Hashimoto's thyroiditis, can be linked to specific antithyroid antibodies attacking healthy thyroid tissue. This leads to its dysfunction and degradation, and, ultimately, to hypothyroidism. (For more on Hashimoto's thyroiditis, see the Underdog, page 156.) If left untreated, thyroiditis generally results in hypothyroidism, in some cases, permanently.

A few types of thyroiditis fall into the category of "resolving" or "subacute" thyroiditis. This is a self-limited condition associated with transient hyperthyroidism, hypothyroidism, or both. Types of resolving thyroiditis include subacute granulomatous thyroiditis (also known as "painful" thyroiditis or de Quervain's thyroiditis), an autoimmune condition that can be caused by a viral infection, and postpartum thyroiditis, which tends to arise in women with underlying autoimmune conditions, which become increasingly severe following pregnancy and childbirth. Treatment for subacute thyroiditis will vary depending on the severity and duration of symptoms as well as other physiological factors.

NODULES

Thyroid nodules are irregular (and most often benign) growths of thyroid tissue. Their origin is often unknown. They tend to be linked to hereditary factors, and as with other thyroid disorders, they are more common in women than in men. Nodules may be diagnosed during the course of a physical exam and/or with an ultrasound. (Biopsies are required to confirm that nodules are not malignant.)

Nodules may cause no symptoms at all. But in some cases, the tissue inside them may produce and release excess T4 and T3, giving rise to hyperthyroidism. In these cases, the nodules may be treated with alcohol ablation, which causes them to produce less thyroid hormone, or the thyroid itself may be treated with radioactive iodine, which causes it to shrink and produce less T4 and T3. In either case, it is critically important to consistently monitor a nodule or nodules for changes in size and characteristics.

TOXIC MULTINODULAR GOITER (PLUMMER DISEASE)

Toxic multinodular goiter (also known as Plummer disease) is a condition characterized by readily apparent enlargement of the thyroid gland caused by firm thyroid nodules that function independently of TSH and produce and release excess T3 and T4. The condition can also cause such serious symptoms as obstructed breathing and cardiac stress. It occurs mostly in older adults, and is five to ten times more likely to occur in women than in men.[40] Although it has been linked to iodine deficiency, its origins are otherwise unknown. Toxic multinodular goiter may be treated with antithyroid medications, radioactive iodine, or surgery.

The Chairwoman
Estrogen Dominance and Cortisol Excess

"If there is no seat at the table, bring your own chair."

—NINA TASSLER

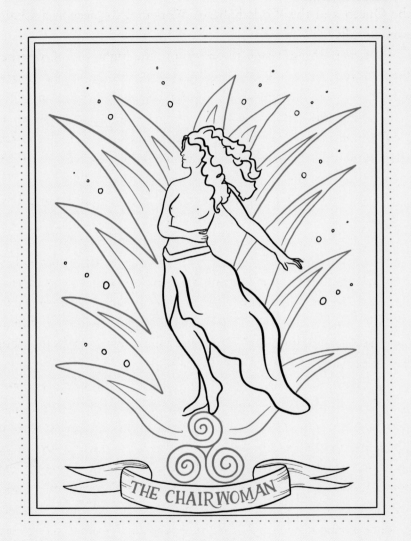

THE CHAIRWOMAN

noun chair·wom·an \ˈcher-ˌwu̇-mən \
: a woman who serves as the presiding officer of a meeting, organization, committee, or event.

In this section, we consider the Chairwoman archetype. Characterized by a pair of imbalances—estrogen dominance and cortisol excess—the Chairwoman archetype possesses attributes of both the Queen and the Workaholic. A Workaholic-Queen is a Chairwoman/CEO.

Always pushing herself to perform at the highest level, whether she's at work or at home, the Chairwoman is known for taking charge. The people around her admire her competence and confidence alike, and they tend to follow her lead. At the same time, the Chairwoman resists delegating the various tasks for which she has taken responsibility, pressuring herself to handle whatever challenges threaten to disrupt her personal and professional worlds.

Fueled by the dual forces of estrogen dominance and cortisol excess, the Chairwoman is often both driven and run ragged. Among the common symptoms of this archetype are lethargy, weight gain, hypertension, and, for those who are premenopausal, menstrual irregularities. Quickness to anger and general changeability of mood also tend to plague the Chairwoman and can cause her to feel particularly lonely at the top. Despite her reluctance to lean on others, the Chairwoman often needs the logistical and emotional support of the people closest to her.

The Chairwoman archetype can take hold in a woman of any age. Typically, however, this occurs when a woman who is suffering from estrogen dominance is also plagued by long-term stress that drives cortisol overproduction. For example, if a woman for whom polycystic ovarian syndrome (PCOS) has given rise to estrogen dominance is also forced to deal with taxing circumstances (even ones that involve positive life changes) that stimulate her cortisol production and keep it high, for a time, the Chairwoman will be her archetype. When either of these imbalances resolves, her archetype shifts: If her cortisol levels recede while her estrogen dominance persists, she becomes a Queen (see page 67). If her estrogen dominance resolves while her cortisol levels remain elevated, she becomes a

Workaholic (see page 115). This means that as a Chairwoman strives to achieve balance, her journey will likely intersect with one or more of the other archetypes'.

If you have tested into the Chairwoman archetype, this means that both estrogen dominance and cortisol excess are exerting physiological, psychological, and emotional effects. But one of these imbalances may play a more significant role in your symptomology than the other. I recommend keeping this in mind as you read this section, noting which aspects of the Chairwoman's experience most closely align with yours. This may have an impact on the goals and specific measures of your personal SHINES protocol.

For additional information on estrogen dominance, you may consult the section on the Queen archetype (page 67). For more on cortisol excess, you may refer to the section on the Workaholic archetype (page 115).

Cortisol Excess: Cushing's Syndrome and Cushing's Disease

Cushing's syndrome and Cushing's disease are both characterized by prolonged elevated cortisol levels in the body. Cushing's syndrome is a condition in which the adrenal glands produce too much cortisol. Cushing's disease is a condition in which the pituitary gland produces excessive amounts of ACTH, a hormone that stimulates the adrenal glands to produce cortisol. Among the symptoms the two conditions have in common are weight gain, hypertension, impaired short-term memory, fatty deposits around the neck, ruddiness of the face, excess body hair growth, and balding.

A Chairwoman's cortisol levels do not rise to the point that would justify a diagnosis of Cushing's syndrome or Cushing's disease. If you suspect you may be suffering from either of these conditions, I strongly encourage you to consult a physician. These illnesses require specific medical intervention and, if left untreated, can be fatal.

Patient Example

I could hear Samantha in the hall outside my office. "But if the accounts are not set up, *no one* will be paid on Thursday," she said. "And if no one is paid on Thursday, there will be *hell* to pay." At forty-two, Samantha was CEO of a relatively large software company and was constantly juggling the demands of its clients and employees. "*Of course* I'll have to handle it," she barked at whoever was on the other end of the line. "As though I have nothing else to do." When I opened the door and invited her inside, Samantha held up the index finger on her free hand, telling me to hold on. "Email me the name and number of the bank rep and I'll call when I'm finished here," she said, hanging up the phone and shoving it into her bulging computer bag. "Honestly," she said as she threw the bag under a chair and collapsed into it, "I'm surrounded by idiots. That place would completely fall apart without me."

Two minutes into our conversation, Samantha was leaning forward in her chair, wringing her hands and anxiously bouncing her knee. Her heel tapped against the floor as she spoke. "I'm here because I can't sleep," she said. "And because I think I'm heavier than I've ever been. I've gained about twenty pounds in the last several months, and even starving myself doesn't seem to make a difference." I nodded, and she went on. "Oh, and my sex drive is nonexistent. I feel so tired and so heavy," she explained. "I'm absolutely never in the mood."

When I asked about any irregularities in her menstrual cycle, Samantha reported that it had become less predictable. Her periods were heavier than usual and sometimes occurred more frequently than every four weeks. She'd also experienced some spotting between cycles. Samantha's blood pressure was slightly elevated, and although she reported no pain, she noted that her legs were often swollen at the end of the day.

As for her weight gain, Samantha insisted she hadn't changed her diet or exercise habits. But the reality was, neither of these was ideal to begin with. And with a hormonal imbalance likely wreaking some havoc on her metabolism, her calorie consumption and expenditure were having a more pronounced effect. Often eating on the go, Samantha was in the habit of picking up breakfast at Starbucks and eating whatever sandwiches and snacks the company's local caterer delivered to the office for lunch. Dinner was generally take-out, and while she tried to find healthy options, few of these featured lean proteins or fresh vegetables. Once devoted to a workout routine, she had given this up, too, sacrificing it in order to meet the relentless demands of her job.

By now, I'd begun to suspect Samantha was suffering from both estrogen dominance and cortisol excess. I asked her about her life at work and home. "At work, I'm surrounded by men," she said. She'd only recently been appointed CEO and was still establishing herself as the leader of her executive team and the larger organization. "I feel like they're constantly judging me, constantly sizing me up," she said. "So, God knows, I can't tell them I'm tired. I also can't tell them I have to take a call from my kids' school about how one of them continually shows up with his homework half-finished or from one of their coaches about how they're not performing in practice. The guys on my team don't take those calls." Samantha said that on top of feeling exhausted, she also felt bad about not having more time for her family, including her husband, from whom she was feeling increasingly distant. "As much as I've always wanted to maintain control of our household, I've also wished he'd step up and help," she said. "Now that I feel like I'm running out of gas, I need him to."

The Chairwoman: Symptomology Summary

The Chairwoman's symptomology combines elements of the Queen's and the Workaholic's.

The majority of the Chairwomen I've treated have presented with symptoms of estrogen dominance that mirror Samantha's, including unexplained weight gain, irregular menstrual cycles and intermittent spotting, intense headaches, and, in a percentage of cases, a sporadic inability to focus that some patients have described as "brain fog." Similar to a Queen, a Chairwoman's symptoms of estrogen dominance can, when taken together, make them feel like they're losing control of their bodies and their minds. (For women who have experience with birth control pills, I describe estrogen dominance as taking two birth control pills per day.)

A Chairwoman's cortisol-excess-related symptoms can be as significant as those arising from her estrogen dominance. Among the most common are interrupted sleep (even in the absence of stimulant effects such as those from caffeine), headaches, irregular and painful menstruation or amenorrhea (cessation of menstruation), and chronic fatigue. This fatigue can be caused in part by the tendency of elevated levels of cortisol to increase catabolism in the body (see page 120 for more on catabolism).

In the following pages, we take a closer look at the symptoms of estrogen dominance and cortisol excess that a Chairwoman is most likely to experience. As you review these, consider which symptoms align most closely with your own. This will help you ascertain the degree to which estrogen dominance and cortisol excess have contributed to the rise of your archetype and the role each imbalance is playing in your overall hormonal health.

Physiological Symptoms: Estrogen Dominance

Water retention	Water retention is common and can contribute to other symptoms, including weight gain, increased blood pressure, and headaches.
Weight gain	In the short term, weight gain may be attributable to water retention. But over time, an estrogen-dominance-driven metabolic imbalance can cause a woman to retain fat, particularly around her abdomen and hips.
Cravings	Cravings for salty and sugary foods are common. Even if she doesn't normally eat or even crave salty or sugary foods, a Chairwoman is likely to be drawn to both, and may feel less able to resist the urge to raid the pantry, the refrigerator, or anywhere else snacks might be found.
Irregular menstruation	Chairwomen are prone to irregular menstrual cycles. These may occur more frequently (e.g., every two to three weeks) and/or be longer in duration. A Chairwoman's menstrual flow may be heavier than she is accustomed to, and she may also experience spotting between her cycles.

Interference with thyroid hormone	Estrogen dominance can cause the thyroid gland to become dysfunctional. When estrogen levels become dangerously high, the levels of thyroid binding globulin also become elevated. The latter means you have less active thyroid hormone in your system. If your estrogen levels remain too high for a long period of time, you may begin to experience some hypothyroid-related symptoms—those that characterize the Underdog archetype (see page 156). Among these are cold hands and feet, as well as overarching sluggishness and fatigue.
Additional symptoms	Breast swelling and tenderness Fibrocystic breasts Hair loss Insomnia Night sweats

Physiological Symptoms: Cortisol Excess

Gastroesophageal reflux disease (GERD)	Cortisol is a diuretic. In addition to depleting the body's electrolytes, such as sodium and potassium, it can also stimulate gastric acid secretion, which can cause heartburn and reflux.

(continues)

Insomnia and restlessness	Cortisol levels that remain high during the day and into the evening can make it difficult to fall asleep and may interrupt sleep throughout the night. When your cortisol fails to drop at bedtime as it's supposed to, it can both make it difficult to fall asleep and continue to exert stimulatory effects throughout the night, leaving you feeling tired in the morning.
Fatigue	In combination with the various other symptoms of cortisol excess, remaining in fight-or-flight mode for extended periods of time can leave the Chairwoman feeling exhausted, even upon waking.
Immunosuppression	Cortisol has a negative feedback effect on interleukin, a glycoprotein involved in immune responses, thereby interfering with the body's communication with its T-cells. Cortisol is ordinarily anti-inflammatory and contains the immune response, but chronic elevations can lead to the immune system becoming "resistant," an accumulation of stress hormones, and increased production of inflammatory cytokines that further compromise the immune response.

Osteoporosis	Cortisol can reduce bone formation.
Sagging skin and wrinkles	Cortisol breaks down collagen in the skin, causing it to thin and prematurely age. Cortisol also breaks down collagen contained in the joints, causing stiffness and pain.
Increased wound healing time	Both high levels of stress and elevated cortisol levels have been linked to increased wound healing time.
Decreased libido	High levels of cortisol can have a negative impact on testosterone levels. Decreased libido may also arise alongside other symptoms, including fatigue.

(continues)

Psychological and Emotional Symptoms: Estrogen Dominance

"Foggy brain"	This refers to memory lapses that, while relatively minor in terms of their consequences, are nonetheless disconcerting for the Chairwoman who experiences them. These may manifest as trouble accessing certain details, such as the title of a book you read recently or the name of a person you met, or forgetting an appointment or where you left your keys.
	An important aspect of foggy brain is that it compounds. The more it happens, the more it is likely to happen—and the more it is likely to cause distress. Sometimes, patients report anxiety around this, fearing they may be suffering a neurological disorder, such as dementia. The anxiety, too, can feed on itself, which can negatively affect mental functioning and contribute to a Chairwoman's overarching sense that she is losing control.

Mood swings, emotional changeability, and feeling out of control	The Chairwoman who has reached a severe state is likely to experience extreme and unpredictable mood swings. Often, patients describe feeling like they're "tiptoeing along the edge of a cliff" and say they have to bring all their physical, emotional, and psychological energy to bear to keep the winds blowing around them from taking them over it.
	Chairwomen often describe generalized feelings of loss of control. In fact, in many instances, I've documented "I feel totally crazy" as a patient's chief complaint.
Feelings of "bitchiness" and aggression	Although I take pains to avoid using the term "bitchiness," many of my patients use it to describe themselves.
	Whether at home or work, a Chairwoman whose estrogen dominance is making her more emotionally changeable and prone to irritability is likely to present differently to others. Her interactions with family, friends, coworkers, etc., may become more emotionally charged, contributing to feelings of alienation and a Chairwoman's tendency to accuse herself of "bitchiness."
	Of course, any Chairwoman who is on her last straw, feeling like she's burning the candle at both ends and has little to no capacity to withstand anything going wrong, is bound to respond negatively—and even aggressively—to inconvenient or disconcerting information or events.
	Here again, we see the importance of how your Hormonal Archetype shapes not only your experience of the world, but how the rest of the world experiences you.

While short-term estrogen dominance may cause only temporary physiological or psychological dissonance or discomfort, persistent estrogen dominance has been linked to breast cancer, uterine cancer, ovarian cysts, and infertility. It has also been linked to increased blood clotting (including deep vein thrombosis and pulmonary emboli), allergies, autoimmune disorders, and accelerated aging.

As for cortisol excess, remaining in a state of high emotional and physical alert can keep the Chairwoman's cortisol levels high. Once your levels are elevated, cortisol feeds on its own overproduction, keeping your body and mind in fight-or-flight mode and your adrenal glands responding accordingly.

The Chairwoman: Underlying Causes of Symptomology

Although estrogen dominance and cortisol excess may occur independently of one another and have distinct underlying causes, when these imbalances take hold simultaneously, giving rise to the Chairwoman archetype, stress is nearly always a common contributing factor. Adding to this, each of the Chairwoman's imbalances can exacerbate the other, powering a feedback loop that can make the archetype even more entrenched.

UNDERLYING CAUSES OF ESTROGEN DOMINANCE

A number of factors and conditions can give rise to estrogen dominance. In the following pages, we consider its most common internal and external causes, any of which may contribute to this aspect of the Chairwoman archetype's taking hold.

POLYCYSTIC OVARIAN SYNDROME (PCOS)

When left untreated, PCOS causes estrogen dominance. As we've discussed at various points in this book, when a woman ovulates, her progesterone production picks up and opposes the estrogen she has produced during the first two weeks of her cycle. When a woman has PCOS, tiny cysts on her ovaries prevent her from ovulating, which means her elevated estrogen goes unopposed, and she becomes estrogen dominant.

Birth control medications are the most popular treatment for PCOS. Unfortunately, some of these can actually exacerbate the symptoms of estrogen dominance.

CESSATION OF OVULATION

During the first two weeks of a woman's menstrual cycle, she is naturally estrogen dominant. Levels of the hormone rise during this period, peaking just before ovulation. After ovulation, progesterone takes over, balancing out the estrogen to the point where progesterone becomes the dominant hormone during the last two weeks of the cycle.

Beginning in perimenopause, ovulation can become irregular or cease altogether. When this happens, estrogen rises during the first two weeks of the menstrual cycle, then continues to dominate, unopposed by progesterone, since in the absence of ovulation, increased production of progesterone does not occur.

OBESITY

The amount of estrogen a woman produces increases alongside her body-fat levels. Women who are obese (whose body fat exceeds 28 percent) run the highest risk of body-fat-driven excess estrogen production and, therefore, estrogen dominance. Simply put, fat cells are estrogen-making machines. They are now greatly regarded as another endocrine organ: Not only can they create estrogen, but they can convert excess testosterone to estrogen as well. (For women with PCOS, a condition that also causes the body to create extra testosterone, this means even *more* estrogen.) You can see the horrible cycle: Fat begets more estrogen, and more estrogen can beget more fat.

ENVIRONMENTAL CONTRIBUTORS TO ESTROGEN DOMINANCE

FOOD

Phytoestrogens are naturally occurring plant-based compounds found in beans, seeds, and grains. Because phytoestrogens' chemical structure resembles that of estrogen, these compounds can mimic estrogenic activity and affect both the production and breakdown of estrogen in the body.

A common source of phytoestrogens is soy. Although various health benefits are associated with soy consumption, including protection against certain types of cancer, menopausal symptoms, heart disease, and osteoporosis, the phytoestrogens contained in soy can pose a danger for women who are estrogen dominant or at risk of becoming so. Part of the phytoestrogen class of isoflavones, the soy-based extracts genistein, daidzein, and glycitein have known estrogenic effects. Another class of phytoestrogens called coumestans are found in split peas, pinto beans, alfalfa, and clover sprouts, among other foods.

Estrogen is also found in beef and other meat, as well as various dairy products. Exogenous hormones (including estrogen and growth hormones) and synthetic, chemical-based compounds with estrogenic effects known as xenoestrogens found in animal feed are largely to blame for this. Many brands have stopped using products that contain estrogen and other hormones, advertising that their meat and dairy products are "hormone-free." But as we'll see in the following section, the pervasiveness of synthetic estrogenic compounds in our environment makes these difficult for meat producers to avoid.

In addition to consuming estrogen in plant- and animal-based foods, your estrogen levels may increase if you are not eating enough fiber. Excess estrogen is expelled via the bowel, so slowing the rate of excretion increases the likelihood that excess estrogen will be reabsorbed into the system. Eating high levels of refined carbohydrates can compound this problem.

SYNTHETIC ENVIRONMENTAL AGENTS

Xenoestrogens, synthetic compounds that can mimic estrogenic activity, are found in thousands of man-made products, most notably chemicals and plastics. One of the largest sources of these is a class of chemicals known as organochlorines. Found in pesticides, herbicides, and fungicides, as well as in cosmetics products that contain parabens and stearalkonium chloride, organochlorines are also commonly used in dry-cleaning and plastics manufacturing.

As for plastics, exposure to a compound called PET (polyethylene terephthalate) can contribute to estrogen dominance. A form of polyester, PET is used to make plastic bottles and food containers, as well as certain personal care products. Plastics can also expose you to BPA (bisphenol A), the estrogenic effects of which have been well documented. Widely used in the production of containers for liquids, BPA is released from plastic when heated. This is why environmental health experts warn against microwaving food or liquid in plastic containers.

Birth control pills are another potential and somewhat controversial source of estrogen in the environment. Some scientists have argued that via human excretion or disposal into sewer systems or landfills, birth control pills are leaching synthetic estrogen into soil and waterways. During recent years, countries around the world have considered mandating the removal of the most harmful synthetic estrogens from rivers, lakes, and estuaries.

HEPATIC STRESS

The liver is responsible for breaking down hormones, including estrogen. If it is overtaxed due to illness, alcohol consumption, or medications (including OTC remedies such as Tylenol and Advil), it does this less efficiently, leaving excess estrogen circulating in your system.

UNDERLYING CAUSES OF CORTISOL EXCESS

The primary underlying cause of the Chairwoman's cortisol excess is chronic stress. Remaining in a persistent state of heightened emotional and physical alert can keep your cortisol levels elevated as the hormone feeds on its own overproduction. Excess cortisol can also have downstream effects on other hormones, including estrogen. This can exacerbate the Chairwoman's estrogen dominance, in some instances, for prolonged periods.

The Chairwoman's cortisol excess does not rise to the level found in women diagnosed with Cushing's syndrome or Cushing's disease (see page 184). These are far more serious and potentially life-threatening conditions that require specific medical intervention.

The Philosopher

Estrogen and Testosterone Deficiency

"How wonderful it is that nobody need wait a single moment before starting to improve the world."
—ANNE FRANK

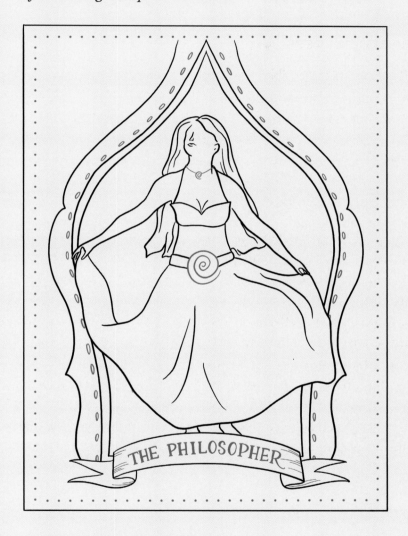

THE PHILOSOPHER

noun phi·los·o·pher \ fə-ˈlä-s(ə-)fər \

a: a person who seeks wisdom or enlightenment: scholar, thinker.

2a: a person whose philosophical perspective makes meeting trouble with equanimity easier.

In this section, we consider the Philosopher archetype. Characterized by a pair of imbalances—estrogen deficiency and low testosterone—the Philosopher possesses attributes of the Wisewoman and the Nun.

Although the Philosopher archetype can take hold in a woman of any age, it most commonly arises in women over the age of forty-five for whom either menopause or perimenopause has caused estrogen (and progesterone) deficiency, and whose production of other hormones, including testosterone and DHEA, has also slowed. The Philosopher archetype can take hold in younger women, however, for whom a total hysterectomy, bilateral oophorectomy (removal of the ovaries), medication, illness, or chronic adrenal insufficiency has terminated or disrupted their production of estrogen, progesterone, testosterone, and other hormones. In the vast majority of cases, the Philosopher archetype is obtained permanently, requiring a lifelong commitment to a SHINES protocol that helps maintain balance.

Each of the deficiencies that characterizes the Philosopher archetype is associated with a set of physiological, psychological, and emotional symptoms. Some of these symptoms correlate to one deficiency or the other. Hot flashes (and night sweats), thinning of the skin, and increased risk of cardiac disease are all associated with estrogen deficiency, for example, while muscle degradation and diminished sexual desire and arousal are both linked to low testosterone.

Several of these symptoms overlap, however, including fatigue, weight gain (particularly around the abdomen), osteoporosis and osteopenia, hair thinning and loss, and mood changeability. Adding to this, other symptoms the Philosopher is likely to experience can contribute to or exacerbate the intensity of others. Estrogen deficiency can cause vaginal atrophy (dryness), for example, which can make sex unpleasant, or even painful. When the Philosopher also experiences the decreased sexual desire and diminished arousal associated with low testosterone, she may be more likely to lose interest in physical intimacy altogether. Similarly, the fatigue correlated with estrogen deficiency may combine with the muscle degradation associated with low testosterone to make it even more difficult for the Philosopher to engage in even mild physical exercise, which, as we will discuss later in this section, is important for the Philosopher's bone, muscle, and joint health.

Whatever a Philosopher's age, her symptoms tend to be significant—life-altering, even—and inspire self-reflection. As we discuss at various points in this section, this archetype's journey involves coming to terms with what this reflection reveals and culminates in embracing the life she has led and looking forward to the life she has yet to live. So many of the Philosophers I've treated have hit their "second peak," as I describe it, and come into their own in a way they hadn't been able to when they were younger. As they've embarked on their journeys toward overall health hormonal balance, committing to their physical, emotional, and spiritual health, Philosophers have started new careers, returned to school, developed new hobbies, skills, and interests. They've asked themselves the "big" existential questions, such as "Who am I?" and "What is it that I really want?" and "How can I live my best life?"—questions they likely asked themselves when they were twenty-five but are now in a very different position to answer, and their responses have led to empowering self-discovery. As one patient described, she felt as though she'd heard a song playing her whole life, and now she was finally dancing to it.

In addition to being in a position to take stock of her life and leverage her wisdom to chart a new course, a Philosopher is also ready to share what she has learned with others. As we discuss in the SHINES portion of chapter five, sharing her thoughts, feelings, experiences, discoveries, and advice with others can be an important aspect of the Philosopher's journey toward balance and enhanced overall well-being.

If you have tested into the Philosopher archetype, this means that both estrogen deficiency and low testosterone are exerting physiological, psychological, and emotional effects. But one of these imbalances may play a more significant role in your symptomology than the other. I recommend keeping this in mind as you read this section, noting which aspects of the Philosopher's experience most closely align with yours. This may have an impact on the goals and specific measures of your personal SHINES protocol.

For additional information on estrogen deficiency, you may consult the section on the Wisewoman archetype (page 104). For more on low testosterone, you may refer to the section on the Nun archetype (page 136).

Patient Example

When Callie called to make an appointment to see me, she described her chief complaint as "menopausal misery." Now fifty-two, she had stopped menstruating two years earlier and struggled with symptoms including hot flashes, mood swings, and insomnia since. Lately, she explained, other difficulties had started to arise. She was tired all the time, she said. She was finding it increasingly difficult to endure her long days at work, and during the evenings and weekends, she felt inclined distance herself from her spouse, sequestering herself so that she could rest and recover from her week. Averse to emotional or physical intimacy with her spouse, Callie was also less interested in socializing with friends than she had been. She did not always enjoy her time on her own, however. "All I want is peace and quiet," she said, "but as soon as I have it, I tend to feel lonely, and the silence becomes a lot to bear."

When I asked what she meant about the silence, Callie explained that her youngest child had left for college four years earlier, and since then, Callie had begun to wonder what would be next for her. When she sat still, she explained, questions about what she had done with her life and what she might do with it now always loomed large. "I feel freedom and pressure at once," she said, "and that's pretty much where it ends. I'm so exhausted, I just don't have the energy to engage with these big questions." This left her feeling depressed, sometimes even hopeless. "I'm only fifty-two, and sometimes, I feel like my life is over," Callie said. "I don't know what I want anymore, or what will drive me to get out of bed each day. I feel like I want my life back, but at the same time, I'm not sure what I want it to look like."

Soon, I suspected Callie was suffering from both estrogen deficiency and low testosterone, and that her generalized lack of passion for her life and feelings of exhaustion at answering the significant questions about what would make her truly happy and what she wanted to do with the rest of her life were rooted in both. "Do I sound crazy to you?" Callie asked. "Because sometimes, I do to me." I told her that to me, she didn't sound crazy at all. As she and I took a closer look at the Philosopher archetype, Callie visibly relaxed. "So it's not just me," she said, and I assured her that no, it was not "just her" at all.

The Chairwoman: Symptomology Summary

In the following pages, we take a closer look at the symptoms of the Wisewoman (estrogen deficiency) and Nun (low testosterone) archetypes that a Philosopher is most likely to experience. As you review these symptoms, consider which align most closely with your own. This will help you ascertain the degree to which each imbalance has contributed to the rise of your archetype and the role it is playing in your overall hormonal health.

Physiological Symptoms: Estrogen Deficiency

Hot flashes and night sweats	Caused by sudden surges in vasodilation, hot flashes are feelings of intense warmth that can spread across the head, neck, and face before extending to the entire body. When these occur during the night, they are called night sweats. Hot flashes typically last between thirty seconds and a few minutes, causing an increase in skin temperature and redness. They may also cause an increase in heart rate, heart palpitations, and dizziness. Estrogen deficiency causes hot flashes in approximately 75 percent of women.
Vaginal dryness (vaginal atrophy)	Estrogen helps maintain the natural lubrication of the vaginal walls, in addition to maintaining their thickness and elasticity. Vaginal atrophy can not only make sexual intercourse painful, but can also cause vaginal irritation and itching; urinary issues, including urgency, burning, and incontinence; and a shortening and tightening of the vaginal canal.[*] Taken together, these symptoms are now known as "genitourinary syndrome of menopause."

[*] B. Bleibel and H. Nguyen, "Vaginal Atrophy," in *StatPearls* (Treasure Island, FL: StatPearls Publishing, July 6, 2020).

Relaxation of the pelvic muscles	Together with vaginal atrophy, this can contribute to urinary incontinence and increase the risk that a woman's uterus, bladder, urethra, or rectum will project into the vagina.
Insomnia	In addition to the difficulty that night sweats may cause, a naturally or medically induced progesterone deficiency may contribute to difficulty sleeping.
Changes to skin and hair	Estrogen is present in all cells of a woman's body, including the skin. A deficiency causes a loss of plasticity and general health of the skin, giving rise to thinning, wrinkling, and age spots. Some women experience hair thinning or loss. In some cases, this combines with an increase in facial hair growth.
Cardiac issues	In addition to the heart palpitations hot flashes may cause, estrogen deficiency may give rise to intermittent dizziness, heart palpitations, and tachycardia, as well as sensations including numbness, prickling, tingling, and increased sensitivity.* Philosophers may also be at increased risk of cardiac arrest.
Weight gain	In particular, estrogen deficiency can cause abdominal weight gain.

* Johns Hopkins Medicine, "Introduction to Menopause," accessed May 1, 2017, http://www.hopkinsmedicine.org/healthlibrary/conditions/gynecological_health/introduction_to_menopause_85,P01535/.

(continues)

Psychological and Emotional Symptoms: Estrogen Deficiency

Mood Swings	Several studies have linked fluctuating and decreasing levels of estrogen during perimenopause and menopause with unpredictable shifts in mood. Some physiological symptoms, including insomnia and fatigue, can also contribute to sudden feelings of anger, sadness, nervousness, or even euphoria.
Depression	In addition to emotional changeability, estrogen deficiency can also contribute significantly to persistent depression (depressed mood lasting most of the day on most days). A depressed state is most likely caused by a combination of factors relating to menopause, including the generalized stress and anxiety that can accompany the physiological changes taking hold.

Physiological Symptoms: Testosterone Deficiency

Diminished genital arousal and orgasmic response	Decreased vaginal lubrication may also occur.*
Chronic or acute fatigue	In addition to generalized exhaustion, testosterone deficiency can also contribute to muscle weakness.
Weight gain	Testosterone deficiency can cause the body to retain fat, particularly around the abdomen.

Interrupted sleep	Testosterone levels follow a bit of a circadian rhythm, so it is thought that low testosterone can contribute to insomnia.
Hair thinning/hair loss	Studies have shown that women with low androgens who use low-dose testosterone will have an increase in hair growth. Testosterone is thought to have an anabolic effect on the hair in those women with testosterone deficiency. Care should be exercised, however, as excess testosterone can also be associated with male-pattern hair loss.
Osteoporosis and osteopenia	Similarly to low estrogen, low testosterone can cause the body to leach calcium from bones.

* A. Guay and S. R. Davis, "Testosterone Insufficiency in Women: Fact or Fiction," excerpt from *World Journal of Urology* 20 (2002): 106–10.

Psychological and Emotional Symptoms: Testosterone Deficiency

Decreased sexual desire	This includes a decrease in sexual thoughts, fantasies, and actions.*

* Guay and Davis, "Testosterone Insufficiency in Women: Fact or Fiction."

The Philosopher: Underlying Causes of Symptomology

For the Philosopher, estrogen deficiency and low testosterone may arise together or independently of each other, depending on the root cause of each. In women, the ovaries produce the majority of the body's estrogen. While the hormone is also produced by the adrenal glands and in fat cells, changes in ovarian function generally underlie a Philosopher's estrogen deficiency.

Roughly half of a woman's testosterone is also produced by the ovaries, which means the same changes in ovarian function that give rise to a Philosopher's estrogen deficiency may also be the root cause of her low testosterone. During perimenopause and menopause, for example, changes in ovarian function generally cause the low levels of each hormone. However, testosterone is also produced by the adrenal glands and peripheral tissues, which means a testosterone deficiency may occur when adrenal dysfunction takes hold.

In the following pages, we look at the most common causes of estrogen deficiency and low testosterone, including those that tend to lead to the diminished production of both hormones.

MENOPAUSE AND PRIMARY OVARIAN INSUFFICIENCY

Menopause is a natural and inevitable phase of female development that encompasses all the changes a woman experiences shortly before and after she ceases to menstruate. On average, a woman will be in her late thirties when her ovaries begin to produce less estrogen, progesterone, and testosterone. Also on average, women enter menopause between the ages of 45 and 55. For some women, the phase naturally commences as early as the age of 40 or as late as the age of 60+. By this time, a woman's estrogen production is likely to have dropped to very low levels, and she may expect her testosterone level to be half what it was at its peak.

Approximately 1 percent of women will suffer from a condition known as premature ovarian failure, in which a woman's ovaries fail to produce sufficient estrogen and progesterone to sustain the menstrual cycle before she reaches the age of forty. No single cause of this condition has been identified, though it has been linked to certain genetic factors and autoimmune diseases. Primary ovarian insufficiency can also negatively affect testosterone production.

SURGICAL REMOVAL OF THE OVARIES

Women of any age who undergo a total hysterectomy (or bilateral oophorectomy) for medical reasons immediately enter menopause. In these cases, both estrogen and testosterone production fall, and the onset of menopausal symptoms is swift. The symptoms themselves can be severe.

MEDICATIONS

In women of any age, treatment with some medications may cause a temporary decrease in the production of estrogen and testosterone. Women who are prescribed Lupron Depot for endometriosis, for example, generally see a decrease or cessation of their menstrual cycle while they are taking the medication and are likely to experience the various physiological, emotional, and spiritual aspects of the Philosopher archetype within two to four weeks. Chemotherapy and radiation may also temporarily or permanently disrupt or halt menstruation, influencing the production of estrogen and testosterone by the ovaries and even the adrenals glands.

Birth control pills and other forms of hormonal contraceptives that disrupt production of estrogen and progesterone by the ovaries also negatively affect testosterone levels. Estrogen replacement therapy can also negatively impact testosterone levels. When your estrogen levels rise, so do your levels of sex hormone binding globulin

(SHBG), a protein produced in the liver. SHBG binds to estrogen, dihydrotestosterone, and testosterone, decreasing the bioavailability of each.

CHRONIC ILLNESS

Women suffering from autoimmune disorders (particularly those that cause inflammation) such as lupus and rheumatoid arthritis, or thyroid conditions, including Hashimoto's disease, often experience decreased androgen production. Addison's disease and hypopituitarism (the loss of pituitary gland hormone production) can also contribute to or exacerbate estrogen and testosterone deficiencies.

ADRENAL INSUFFICIENCY

Adrenal fatigue can contribute to estrogen and testosterone deficiencies. Whether it's stress, disease, or even extreme athletic training that is at the heart of adrenal "burnout," the glands' diminished functioning can be a significant factor in the Philosopher archetype taking hold. When chronic stress causes the adrenals to produce more cortisol and DHEA at the expense of producing sex hormones, estrogen and testosterone levels fall. This is particularly significant for Philosophers who are perimenopausal or menopausal, given that the adrenal glands are critical to the postmenopausal production of estrogen and testosterone.

The SHINES
Protocol, with
Recommendations
for Each Archetype

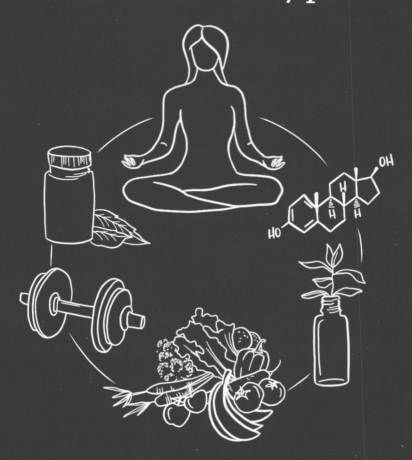

When it comes to holistic hormone health, there is no such thing as a quick fix. Wellness requires work. This is why I consistently remind my patients that the journey toward hormone health is about owning your story and taking charge of it. It is about examining your symptoms and physical issues, but also considering your innate and learned personal characteristics, and the influences—conscious and subconscious—of your life experiences. It's about thoroughly examining how these influences shape your engagement with the world, its impact on you, and your impact on it.

That is where the SHINES protocol comes in, which I have developed as a multifaceted approach to hormone health. SHINES combines medical and nonmedical modalities into a comprehensive program that you can tailor to suit your specific needs through the guidance of your archetype. I developed this approach through more than twenty years as a practitioner of integrative medicine, working daily with women to improve their physical health and help them achieve spiritual, emotional, and energetic balance.

The SHINES protocol is made up of six modalities—spiritual practice, hormone modulation, infoceuticals, nutrition, exercise, and supplements—all of which work individually and together to support the optimal functionality of body and mind. As you imagine your hormones as gears in a watch, it's useful to conceive of these six elements as interconnected and working in concert to promote overall wellness.

Spiritual Practice

A spiritual practice is one that inspires introspection, stillness, and inner peace. It need not be religious, though it can be. Contemplative prayer can have centering, healing effects. Meditation—guided or unguided—can also be a helpful restorative practice, as can acupuncture. The archetype-specific spiritual practices are designed to address specific challenges for that archetype, helping you achieve a solitary and peaceful state, a sense of centering and steadiness.

Hormone Modulation

Hormone modulation—or "biohacking," as many healthcare practitioners now refer to it—is the practice of increasing or decreasing certain hormone levels by taking prescription oral, transdermal, or suppository medications. Whether hormonal modulation is right for your archetype depends on the severity of the underlying imbalance and the potential related effects of intervention. Ongoing monitoring by a physician will also help determine appropriate dosing and duration of treatment.

A note on nonprescription hormonal supplements: While there are some over-the-counter (OTC) hormone modulation therapies available, including DHEA, progesterone, and pregnenolone-based options, I recommend that any biohacking be supervised by a physician.

Infoceuticals and Essential Oils

Infoceuticals as used in these protocols are the energetic aspects of healing utilizing such methods as essential oils, acupuncture, and other modalities, like Reiki. These also include Energetic Integrators (EI), which are remedies composed of filtered water and plant-derived microminerals that have been imprinted with bioinformation that directly pinpoints and helps resolve distortions in your body's energetic fields. Energetic Integrators

1 through 12 (EI1–EI12), discussed in this book, are designed to target blockages or disruptions of energetic fields caused by physical, emotional, environmental, or chemical toxins and exacerbated by an archetype's specific symptomology. In addition to these, I offer my favorite essential oils for each archetype, which complement the energetic challenges of that particular archetype.

Nutrition

The majority of Americans are terrible at eating well. It's hard, and we avoid it. (I know this from personal experience. A dream of mine is to have a show on the Food Network, where I drive from state to state in search of the country's best hamburger.) But eating well for your archetype can have a significant positive impact on your hormonal balance. Yes, it's hard. But it's worth it. For each of the twelve archetypes, there are foods to seek out and others to avoid, as well as preparation techniques to embrace and others to steer clear of. In some cases, traditionally "healthy" foods turn out to be undesirable, and "less healthy" foods turn out to be not so bad for you. In each case, the focus is on the impact certain foods can have on hormonal imbalances and/or on their problematic downstream effects.

Exercise

Like nutrition, exercise is an important contributor to our overall health, one we tend to avoid. But we don't have much of a choice. In our advanced technological age, few of us are manual laborers. Almost none of us grow, harvest, or hunt for our food, which means getting nutrition doesn't necessitate exercise, either. Add our super-busy schedules to the mix, and it becomes even clearer why so many of us avoid exercise. Exercise figures prominently into the SHINES protocols for each archetype. Activities of various types and levels of intensity can positively influence different archetypes, improving strength, balance, and circulation, as well as mental clarity.

Supplements

Dietary supplements play an important role in the SHINES approach and across the board. They can helpfully augment an archetype-based diet and prescription hormone modulation therapy (where this is necessary). I encourage my patients to incorporate these supplements into their broader strategy for hormonal balance. The suggestions for each archetype have been carefully selected for your consideration. There are so many supplements out on the market where claims exceed or outpace the underlying research, sending patients on a wild-goose chase or putting them at risk of exacerbating the symptoms of the imbalances they're trying to resolve.

Each archetype features a SHINES protocol, and I encourage you to review each of the modalities to see how they could complement and contribute to your unique health story. The protocols are not mere means to an end, the solution to a specific problem or symptom that is driving you crazy. Each one is a means to a *beginning*. Write your new health story.

SHINES Protocol: How Do You Soothe a Queen?

For a Queen, the SHINES protocol is all about inspiring a calm sense of power and control. It is about restoring her physical, emotional, and spiritual strength, helping her to channel her native power and energy into finding joyful, healthy balance.

SPIRITUAL PRACTICE

If you are a Queen, your spiritual practice is a method for reclaiming control of your internal kingdom. It's a means of slowing down your rapid thoughts, calming your emotionality and reactivity, and coming back to center in a way that leaves you feeling more in control of the internal world that has felt so outside your control for so long.

To engage in an effective spiritual practice requires expending energy taking care of yourself rather than anyone (or everyone) else. It requires being present with yourself and honest about your needs, fears, and desires. It also requires being as gentle with yourself as you can be, as well as being present in the now, temporarily closing out your awareness of any stress-inducing external circumstances and focusing exclusively on bringing a sense of order to your internal realm.

It may be that you do this for just one moment at a time. Let's face it: It is a challenge for a Queen to carve out extended periods of time for calm, centering reflection away from the world that demands so much from her. But that demand need not be a barrier to engaging in soothing spiritual exercises. These don't have to take hours, or even tens of minutes, each day.

In the following pages, we'll look closely at different spiritual practices that can help pacify a Queen, including practices that require little time but soothe you effectively, nonetheless.

YOGA

For its physical and mental-focus requirements alike, yoga can be an excellent spiritual practice for a Queen. Of all the types of yoga to choose from, the best options are those that are the gentlest and most restorative. Many yoga studios and gyms now offer classes in a variety of styles. But if you cannot find a good class that also suits your schedule, I recommend trying online classes. At Glo.com (previously YogaGlo.com), for example, you can find thousands of classes in different styles for practitioners of all levels. For a relatively modest monthly fee, you have instant access to classes that are five minutes to two hours in length. Even for a busy Queen, technology has made getting to yoga class easy.

TAI CHI

This can be a difficult practice to embark upon because it requires a continual commitment of time and energy. But for a Queen, the benefits of tai chi can be significant. Similar to yoga in its physicality and effectiveness at connecting body and mind, tai chi is all about flow. For a Queen for whom things are not flowing—whose brain fog and reactivity have her feeling constantly on edge—tai chi can physically impose an ease that leaves you feeling more centered, confident, and calmly in control of your actions and emotional responses.

GUIDED MEDITATION

I recommend any kind of meditation for a Queen, but if you're resistant to sitting still in total silence, I recommend guided meditation. With a variety of options available online, you can listen to a guided meditation on your phone wherever you are, for whatever period of time you wish or have available. Psychologist, author, and meditation teacher Tara Brach offers a series of free guided meditations on her website, TaraBrach.com, as does the Chopra Center at Chopra .com.

Walking meditation can also be an effective pacifying practice for a Queen. When I talk about this with patients, I often discuss my own experience with this type of meditation. When I lived in Arizona, I liked to take walks in the desert near my home. It was not barren, but filled with dry wash that crackled beneath my feet. I listened so intently to this sound that I became lost in it. These walks were one of the few things that helped me empty my mind of the day's various goings-on. They became my centering meditations.

You may also consider coming up with a mantra for a walking meditation. With each step, I suggest repeating a line that resonates and also conjures a feeling of calm and assurance in peaceful control over your inner kingdom. Try "I feel powerful," repeating this over and over with each step, for as long as your walk lasts.

If this concept appeals to you, I recommend James Endredy's book *Earthwalks for Body and Spirit*. In it, he teaches you how to lead yourself on different kinds of meditation walks, such as "Walks of Attention," "Walks to Connect to the Power of the Earth," and "Walks in Silence."

THE "PERFECT DAY" EXERCISE

This is an exercise I often do with patients, especially those who present with the Queen archetype. It's pretty straightforward: Map out your perfect day, from the moment you wake up until you fall asleep at night, imagining it in as much detail as possible. Where would you be? What you would be doing (or not doing)? Who (if anyone) would be with you?

If you're married, your perfect day needn't include your spouse, though it could. If you have children, the same rule applies. The "perfect day" I'm asking you to describe is about YOU and about *one* perfect day—not the rest of your life. Often, the exercise can reveal what's lacking in your life, and what you need to incorporate into it in order to take better care of yourself. If you're a Queen on the go, chances are you've neglected yourself in your mad dash to tend to your responsibilities at home and/or at work.

The overarching purpose of the exercise is to help clarify what brings *you* joy and help you bring more of it into your life. You may never actually live this perfect day, but with my patients, I've found that the more we discuss it, the closer they're able to draw to it. "Let's try for eighty percent of the way there," I tell them.

One of my patients told me she imagined herself alone, in a cabin in the mountains, drinking a cup of coffee and reading in bed. She said she felt a little bad that she wanted to spend her perfect day alone, without her spouse or children, but I reminded her that the exercise was about what could be missing in her life, what having more of might help bring her inner Queen into a more balanced and contented state. When she told her husband about the exercise, he said, "So, you need some quiet time? The kids and I can give you that." And they did. For her, an important window had opened. The validation of her needs was important, as was the time itself. Each brought her some of the ease her body and mind had craved.

SPIRITUAL PRACTICE—EVEN WHEN YOU'RE PRESSED FOR TIME

Again, your spiritual exercises needn't take up exorbitant amounts of time. Perhaps your walking meditation consists of counting your steps as you walk from your car to your office door, focusing on your breathing. Perhaps your yoga practice is lying fully still on the floor in Savasana (Corpse Pose) for one to two minutes. Completely letting go of your body in this way and focusing exclusively on your breath for even a few moments can impose order on your internal whirring chaos and edginess. Over time, repeating these short exercises can extend their impact.

Another spiritual practice I recommend to busy Queens is the "Xpill," the brainchild of author and leadership guru Robbe Richman. Neither a medication nor a supplement, Xpill is, strictly speaking, a placebo—a purple capsule containing only brown rice protein and no active ingredients. Its inventor describes it as the means of manifesting your intentions to create the life you want to live. "On its own," Richman describes, "[Xpill] cannot heal, fix, or alter you in any way. And yet, the moment you take it your whole life can change."[1]

While the idea that ingesting a little rice protein could help you manifest significant changes in your life may seem outlandish, fans of the Xpill claim that it can inspire a sense of inner peace, equilibrium, and power that puts these within your grasp. As Jack Canfield, coauthor of *Chicken Soup for the Soul, How to Get from Where You Are to Where You Want to Be*, and other books, described his experience with the Xpill, "I have a real sense of standing in my purpose, my strength, my enoughness, my love." I've tried Xpills myself, often on mornings of days I've been heading into surgery. I will think of Robbie Richman's mantra: "With this Xpill, I'm calling on my higher self to generate the best possible outcomes—to help my patients achieve not only optimal physical health, but their greatest dreams and desires."[2]

Whatever your goals may be—to be gentler to yourself today, or to carve out an hour or two for a long walk or an extended session of restorative yoga—when you take a moment to deliberately articulate an intention and, well, "take it," you may feel a sense of increased control and power over your internal and external realms alike.

HORMONE MODULATION

The second aspect of the SHINES method is medically treating your hormonal imbalance when necessary. If you're not taking any hormone medications, this may involve introducing something new. If you are taking one or more of these, however, the work for you and your physician is to figure out what you need to change or eliminate in order to help bring your estrogen levels back within *your normal* range.

ARE YOU TAKING TOO MUCH ESTROGEN?

If you are taking birth control pills or an oral or transdermal HRT medication such as Premarin or Prempro, it's always a possibility that you're simply introducing too much estrogen into your system. This is why I remind patients that it's imperative that we monitor their levels consistently and appropriately at every stage of treatment—before, during, and after the administration of hormone medications.

For one thing, every woman responds differently to these medications. Your rate of absorption will vary, depending on the method of administration, your tissue's permeability, and your overall sensitivity to the medication's active ingredients. For another thing, your hormone levels are influenced by an array of internal and external factors, and subject to constant change.

Sometimes, patients increase their dosages on their own, without their physician's input or consent. Feeling little or no change, they add an extra transdermal patch to the one they're already wearing or take an extra half a pill each morning. This could be dangerous. You should only increase or decrease the amount of a medication you're taking with a physician's consent and consistent ongoing monitoring.

Women who have PCOS are at particular risk when it comes to medication-driven or -enhanced estrogen dominance. A woman with PCOS is likely to be naturally estrogen dominant because she does not ovulate, and her estrogen production goes unopposed by progesterone. To make matters worse, the most popular medical treatment for her condition is birth control pills. Although she may expect the birth control pills to induce her period eventually, she's at risk of becoming significantly estrogen dominant in the meantime.

WHEN TOO MUCH MEDICATION IS NOT THE PROBLEM

If you're estrogen dominant but not taking any hormonal medications, you and your physician may consider introducing a medication that counteracts your estrogen's impact. I suggest starting with progesterone, the number one blocker of estrogen, and consider all the options available, including tablets, gels, suppositories, and injectables.

If you and your physician decide that a progesterone medication is right for you, make sure he or she closely monitors your progesterone and estrogen levels. Changes normally require between one and three weeks to take hold, so it's best to test them at this point and then every several weeks after that. In time, given that other aspects of the SHINES method are likely to influence your levels and diminish the impact of your estrogen dominance, the role of the medication may shift or be entirely diminished.

HORMONE MEDICATION IS NOT THE ONLY ANSWER

Although hormone medications can play an important role in the SHINES protocol, it's critical to remember that for a Queen, the journey from estrogen dominance to balance requires uncovering the root cause of the imbalance, laying bare its numerous effects, and carefully considering the physiological, psychological, and spiritual modalities that will serve you best. Temporarily offsetting or masking estrogen dominance with medication—whether that's birth control pills or progesterone—can never take you as far along your journey toward holistic hormone health as a truly multifaceted approach.

INFOCEUTICALS

Energetic Integrators (EI) 2, 8, and 10 are those best suited to help correct distortions in a Queen's disrupted energy fields.

EI2 helps to restore and balance energy flow through your chest meridian. It interacts with your lungs and heart, affecting the way energy flows between your heart's right and left chambers and acting as a pacemaker of sorts.

Importantly, the energetic balance within your chest meridian strongly correlates to our most emotional experiences. Whether it's love or grief, anything that breaks your heart has the potential to disrupt your estrogen balance. EI2 bioenergetically influences estradiol and estrone, the strongest and weakest of the three forms of estrogen, as well as pregnenolone, the upstream hormone that can be converted into a series of others.

EI8 helps regulate energetic fields within the liver meridian. It bioenergetically influences those parts of the body that deal with endogenous body waste and exogenous environmental toxins, and, like EI2, EI8 also bioenergetically influences estrogen (in addition to prolactin and adrenaline). Exposure to exogenous estrogens contained in food and consumer products can contribute to or exacerbate estrogen dominance. This can also stress the liver, diminishing its ability to break down estrogen. Clearing energetic disruptions along this meridian can help regulate this process.

EI10 operates along the circulation/pericardium meridian. It is a central integrator for the neuroendocrine and circulatory systems, and it is linked to respiration and digestion. As we'll dig into in more detail in our discussion of nutrition for a Queen, a healthy gut can play a critical role in managing estrogen dominance (and overall hormonal balance more generally).

EI10 is also linked to the biological processes of the ovaries. It bioenergetically influences the hypothalamus, which plays a critical role in controlling the ovaries' hormone production. Nerve cells in the hypothalamus release gonadotrophin-releasing hormone, sending messages to the pituitary gland to produce luteinizing hormone (LH) and follicle-stimulating hormone (FSH). These are carried via the bloodstream to the ovaries, where they drive the menstrual cycle.

Given this integrator's influence over the ovaries and the menstrual cycle, it appears in the SHINES protocol for all the archetypes for whom menstrual irregularities or cessation of menstruation play a major role. It can also help bioenergetically regulate premenstrual or menopause-related emotional swings or mood disorders.

EI10 also energetically influences the adrenal cortex, which is responsible for producing corticosteroids and melanocyte-stimulating hormone, and the adrenal medulla, which produces hormones that help you manage physical and emotional stress, including epinephrine (adrenaline) and norepinephrine (noradrenaline).

As with energetic aspects of medicine, healing can be found in energetic blocks within the body. These can be potentially addressed through practices like acupuncture. Keep in mind, I have included the energetic aspects of healing because they are essential for some. You may not find this to be of value, whereas another woman might. In the context of being whole and open-minded, I have included this. There is evidence that acupuncture can alter hormone levels.[3]

ESSENTIAL OILS

Essential oils that improve detoxification pathways and help the liver and gut maximize the detoxification process may potentially help correct or pacify the Queen. The following oils may aid in the detoxification process:

Celery seed	Orange
Chamomile	Rosemary
Lemon	

Essential oils have become commonplace in many households across the world. I do not endorse one oil over another with respect to companies as long as the oil is sustainable and ethically manufactured. I prefer oils to be diffused, but as my friend Dr. Mariza Snyder discusses, they can be applied topically or even ingested when mixed with water. This should be done under the careful supervision of a competent practitioner because essential oils can cause severe complications if not used correctly.

NUTRITION

When it comes to using nutrition to soothe a Queen, the overarching objective is to reduce her total estrogen levels. This involves embracing certain foods and avoiding others.

For a Queen, in nutrition—as in all her life's realms—it's all about taking control. Whether this means spending the time and energy required to shop for the proteins, fruits, and vegetables best suited to her needs and preparing her own meals or enlisting the help of a service such as HelloFresh, which can deliver customized, low-carb options to her door, the key task for a Queen is to preside over this important aspect of her journey toward balance and overall well-being.

FOODS TO EMBRACE

Fiber

Gastrointestinal health is a critical aspect of managing estrogen dominance and hormonal imbalances more generally, and for a Queen, incorporating fiber into her diet is key. In addition to helping maintain digestive regularity and keeping excess estrogen from being reabsorbed into the system, a healthy gut can increase your antioxidant levels. This can help get rid of some of the free radicals that estrogen produces.

I recommend a Queen try to consume at least 25 mg of fiber each day. Within limits, more can be beneficial. Cruciferous vegetables such as broccoli, cabbage, celery, and kale are a great source, as are whole grains and oats, and seeds such as flax and sunflower. Beans, berries, and fruits such as apples and pears contain helpful amounts of fiber, as do nuts such as almonds, pecans, and walnuts.

If you find high-fiber foods unappealing, you may try a supplement. I always recommend trying to get the recommended daily amount from food first. But if you cannot get to 25 mg any other way, I certainly recommend incorporating a supplement into your diet.

When it comes to fiber, I do offer up two notes of caution. The first is that you need to slowly increase the amount of fiber in your diet. Adding too much too quickly can cause your body to produce excess gas, which can lead to mild to severe stomach pain. The second is that cruciferous vegetables can contain phytoestrogens. Some of these, such as lignan, are relatively weak. But they have estrogenic effects nonetheless, so I recommend keeping your consumption of cruciferous vegetables to one serving every other day.

Cruciferous Vegetables

In addition to providing fiber, cruciferous vegetables such as broccoli, Brussels sprouts, cabbage, kale, mustard greens, and turnips contain a compound called indole-3-carbinol (I3C). In recent years, researchers have become interested in I3C as a possible preventive of breast, cervical, endometrial, and colorectal cancers. Studies have also indicated that the compound impedes estrogen receptor cell proliferation in breast tissue.

When you consume cruciferous vegetables, your body naturally produces another compound called diindolylmethane (DIM), which research has shown can help break down estrogen and convert it to its healthy metabolites. DIM has also been shown to have a weak estrogenic effect. This means that it can bind to estrogen receptors, blocking stronger forms of estrogen and thwarting their potentially carcinogenic impact. DIM may also help ease symptoms associated with a Queen's estrogen dominance, including those that mimic premenstrual dysphoric disorder (PMDD), and breast swelling and tenderness. It is also associated with weight loss.

Antioxidant-Containing Fruits and Vegetables

Vegetables rich in antioxidants, including vitamins A, C, and E and beta-carotene, as well as minerals such as copper, zinc, and selenium, can yield significant benefits for the Queen. These unrefined carbohydrates are also a healthy source of fiber, which can help diminish estrogen dominance by aiding the excretion of excess estrogen via the bowel. I recommend seeking out colorful—and different-colored—fruits and vegetables. Good choices for the Queen include:

Bell peppers (yellow, orange, and red)
Broccoli
Brussels sprouts
Cantaloupe
Carrots
Eggplant (including the skin)
Sweet potatoes
Butternut squash

Lean Protein

In addition to helping improve your body composition (by reducing your body fat percentage), a diet high in lean protein has the added benefit of increasing the amount of the amino acids lysine and threonine in the body. These both help the body metabolize estrogen and support liver function. Good sources of lean protein for the Queen include:

Fish, including salmon and tuna
Lean meats, including ground beef and pork loin
Eggs
Low-fat or nonfat dairy products, including milk, yogurt, and cottage cheese
Beans and lentils
Nuts and nut butters
Seeds

Sulfur

Foods that contain sulfur can help detoxify the liver, improving its ability to get rid of toxins from medications, pesticides, and other external sources. This can make its workload lighter and strengthen its ability to break down estrogen. Foods containing sulfur compounds include onions, garlic, and egg yolks. Lemons and limes also contain sulfur. For a Queen, I recommend drinking a glass of water that contains the juice from half a lemon or lime each morning.

Improving the "Good"-to-"Bad" Estrogen-Metabolite Ratio

In addition to a Queen's overall estrogen levels, it's also critical to consider her estrogen metabolites and endeavor to ensure that her diet is designed to maximize her ratio of "good" estrogen metabolites to "bad" ones.

As we discussed in chapter two, the body breaks down estrogen into different metabolites, the most common being 2-hydroxyestrone, 4-hydroxyestrone and 16α-hydroxyestrone. The former is commonly known as "good estrogen," meaning that it does not stimulate cells to divide, which may damage DNA and cause cancer. This good estrogen may also latch on to estrogen cell receptors, exhibiting a blocking action that prevents "bad" estrogen from taking hold and exerting its effects.

This "bad" estrogen is purported to have significant estrogenic activity, and may be linked to breast cancer and other types of cancer. (Studies have shown that women who have a low ratio of 2-hydroxyestrone to 16α-hydroxyestrone have an elevated risk of breast cancer.) Also important, however, there are benefits associated with safer levels of 16α-hydroxyestrone, including helping to prevent osteoporosis.

In order to improve her "good"-to-"bad" estrogen ratio, a Queen should incorporate foods high in S-adenosyl-L-methionine, commonly known as SAMe. She should also look for foods that contain vitamins B2, B6, and B12, as well as methylated folic acid (5-methyltetrahydrofolate) and trimethylglycine.

Omega-3 fatty acids, such as those found in cold-water fish, have been shown to promote the 2-hydroxyestrone pathway over the 16α-hydroxyestrone pathway. The opposite has also been shown to be true: Diets low in omega-3 fats are associated with higher incidence of the 16α-hydroxyestrone pathway.

FOODS TO AVOID

Carbohydrates

A Queen would be wise to minimize her intake of carbohydrates or avoid them altogether. If you're eating a diet rich in carbohydrates, your glucose (blood sugar) levels are going to be higher. When this happens, your body responds by telling the pancreas to increase insulin production. Insulin helps your body store calories as fat, which raises both your weight and your body mass index (BMI). Obesity can drive or exacerbate estrogen dominance, given that fat cells will aromatize excess testosterone into estrogen. Fat cells also hold on to excess estrogen in your system.

If your diet is higher in proteins and healthy fats (such as olive oil, flaxseed oil, and coconut oil) and lower in carbohydrates, your insulin levels will decrease, improving your estrogen metabolism. For a Queen, the best sources of carbohydrates are vegetables and fruits with a low glycemic index. Avoiding processed foods can also make a significant difference. As I tell my patients, I'm a firm believer that if you can grow it, pick it, or kill it, that food is probably a healthy choice for you to eat. Foods that come in a box or a bag should never be your first choice, and if the ingredient list on the packaging contains words you can't pronounce, you're better off avoiding it. It's that simple.

Alcohol

The impact of alcohol on the liver means alcohol interferes with the body's ability to break down estrogen, which can increase a woman's (or man's) overall estrogen levels. For a Queen, I recommend either eliminating alcohol from your diet altogether, or limiting your intake to one glass of red wine per day. If you're in the market for a red wine, Sardinian and Spanish wines happen to be richer in antioxidants than most and, when consumed in moderation, can actually help remove excess estrogen.

Exogenous Estrogens and Phytoestrogens

I recommend the Queens avoid exogenous estrogens, such as those found in beef, poultry, and dairy products, as well as in plastics and certain cosmetics. Make sure to seek out hormone-free foods and limit your exposure to plastics containing BPA and/or other known endocrine disruptors.

Queens should also avoid consuming phytoestrogens, such as those contained in soy. Although there are positive health benefits associated with soy, you will want to make sure you limit your intake of soy products (whether fermented or not) to relatively small amounts. For a Queen, I recommend no more than 25 grams of fermented soy-derived foods per day. If you enjoy soy milk, I recommend switching to almond or rice milk.[4]

EXERCISE

When it comes to exercise, a Queen's goal is to lose fat and gain muscle. Again, higher levels of body fat can drive or exacerbate estrogen dominance. Increasing muscle mass also helps the body burn more calories (meaning fat) at rest.

For the Queen, any kind of exercise is better than none at all. A yearlong study found that women who engaged in three hours of moderate exercise per week had significantly lower levels of circulating estrogens than women who limited their activity to stretching alone. Specifically, women who averaged 171 minutes of moderate exercise spread across five workout sessions per week saw their estrogen levels drop within five months.[5] The researchers discovered that these women experienced increases in their levels of sex hormone binding globulin (SHBG), the blood-borne protein that binds circulating estrogen and makes it inactive.

What does a session of moderate exercise look like? You should aim to reach 60 to 75 percent of your maximum heart rate for 45 minutes. Per the Mayo Clinic, maximum heart rate is 220 minus your age. So, for example, a woman who is thirty-nine has a maximum heart rate of 181. For her, moderate exercise would involve keeping her heart rate between 108 and 135.

Again, any exercise at all is better than none, and a Queen should feel empowered to do whatever works for her. When I counsel a Queen, I never recommend that she obsessively track her steps every day, because chances are, she's already on the move. Yes, you want to get your heart rate up. But not because of stress, and not in a way that causes more stress. We want you to get your heart rate up because you're actually moving your body in a way that feels good, that works, and that gives you the empowering sense that you're doing something you want to do for yourself.

If you're looking for an easy way to kick-start an exercise program, there are a number of iPhone and Android apps you might try. One I like for a Queen is called The Walking. Another is Couch to 5K. These apps and others like them have the capability to guide users through interval-style training, telling you when to speed up, slow down, and speed up again, so that you raise your heart rate and maintain elevated levels for certain periods of time. You can customize these apps, including choosing the music you work out to.

Start where you are. Consult your physician to discuss what options might work well for you, operate with what time you have, and see where it all takes you.

RALLY THE TROOPS

A final note on exercise for a Queen: Secure the support you need from your partner or spouse, your children, your friends, and even your colleagues. Yes, an exercise program can be a solitary endeavor. But having the emotional and logistical support of your kingdom can help you reach new heights of physical wellness, psychological well-being, and energetic equilibrium.

SUPPLEMENTS

I recommend the following supplements for a Queen, but as with any aspect of the SHINES protocol that has a physiological impact, I strongly encourage you to consult your physician before taking any of these. Although they are unlikely to have as dramatic an impact as a prescription medication, they *can* have significant effects. But once you and your physician have determined they pose no health risk, feel free to try any from this list.

VITEX (CHASTEBERRY)

Vitex agnus-castus, commonly known as chasteberry or vitex, is an herbal supplement that has been used for thousands of years by cultures around the globe to help maintain a healthy balance of estrogen and progesterone. Studies have shown that vitex can inhibit the secretion of follicle-stimulating hormone (FSH) by the pituitary gland, which leads to a decrease in estrogen production by the ovaries. Vitex has also been shown to stimulate the secretion of luteinizing hormone (LH), which triggers the formulation of a corpus luteum and increases progesterone production.

For the Queen, I recommend a dose of 900 to 1,000 mg each morning.

I do share a few **warnings** about vitex with patients. First, although vitex may begin working in as few as ten days, studies show that women taking the supplement may need to wait for up to six months to experience it benefits. Second, although there are few significant side effects associated with vitex, some of my patients have reported nausea, gastrointestinal upset, skin reactions, and headaches. Women who suffer from menstrual depression or PMDD have also reported an exacerbation of these symptoms. **Vitex is not recommended for women who are pregnant or breastfeeding.**

MACA

An herb grown in Peru, maca has long been used to promote hormone balance (in men and women) as well as reproductive and menstrual health. Each of the thirteen differently colored varieties of maca exerts distinct effects, and many maca-based supplements combine different varieties of the herb. Some of these can raise estrogen levels, which is why it's critical to use a supplement that contains the right types of maca in the right ratios to address your estrogen dominance.

The particular maca supplement I recommend for a Queen is Femmenessence MacaHarmony, a 100 percent organic and vegan mixture of sustainably farmed maca that has been shown to have a balancing effect on women's levels of estrogen, progesterone, and other hormones. I recommend taking the supplement as directed on the label: two 500 mg tablets daily, taken away from meals. Take the first dose in the morning, before breakfast, and the second dose in the early evening, ideally 30 minutes before you normally experience an energy low. Consider taking half the recommended amount for two weeks, then gradually increasing to the standard amount.

Two notes of **caution** with regard to MacaHarmony: First, I recommend that a Queen take this supplement for two to three months and then take a week off. This can help upregulate your estrogen receptors and enhance the supplement's benefits. Second, Maca-Harmony can amplify the effects of caffeine. So while a Queen is always wise to limit or avoid caffeine, taking extra caution around caffeine when taking this supplement is a good idea.

INDOLE-3-CARBONYL (I3C) AND DIINDOLYLMETHANE (DIM)

Earlier in this chapter, we discussed the benefits associated with I3C, a compound found in cruciferous vegetables, and DIM, a compound the body produces when it breaks down I3C. In recent years, researchers have become interested in I3C as a possible preventive of breast, cervical, endometrial, and colorectal cancers. DIM has been shown to bind to estrogen receptors, blocking stronger forms of estrogen in ways that can limit or weaken their carcinogenic impact. This compound has also been shown to ease symptoms of PMDD, including breast swelling and tenderness, and is associated with weight loss.

For a Queen who doesn't like or can't tolerate some of the plant sources of I3C or DIM, a variety of supplements are available. If you choose to begin taking one of these, I recommend 15 mg/day to start. Over time, as your estrogen levels shift and your symptoms change, you may discuss increasing or decreasing your dose with your physician.

There are some side effects associated with I3C and DIM supplements, including skin rashes, abdominal pain, nausea, and an increase in liver enzymes. DIM may be slightly easier on your digestive system than I3C, because I3C is the unstable precursor to DIM and needs to be activated in the stomach before your body can convert it to DIM.

BOOK RECOMMENDATIONS FOR QUEENS

Ori Hofmeklar and Rick Osborn, *The Anti-Estrogenic Diet* (Berkeley, CA: North Atlantic Books, 2007)

Michael Lam, MD, MPH, *Estrogen Dominance* (Loma Linda, CA: Adrenal Institute Press, 2012)

Mache Seibel, MD, *The Estrogen Window: The Breakthrough Guide to Being Healthy, Energized, and Hormonally Balanced—Through Perimenopause, Menopause, and Beyond* (New York: Rodale Books, 2016)

QUEENS

Marie Antoinette (November 2, 1755–October 16, 1793), *last queen of France and Navarre before the French Revolution.* Marie Antoinette is an example of a Queen who was out of control; not only was she "off with their heads," but she eventually lost her own because she couldn't reign in a comfortable manner. Obviously, for you, losing your head means something completely different, but I still want you to be able to control your emotions in the way you wish, to be that benevolent queen and rule with a mighty but fair hand.

Cersei Lannister, *fictional character in the fantasy-novel series* A Song of Ice and Fire *by American author George R. R. Martin and its television adaptation,* Game of Thrones; *queen of the Seven Kingdoms of Westeros and wife of King Robert Baratheon.* If you're one of the ten people in their country who didn't see *Game of Thrones*, you would want to know that Cersei was another Queen who didn't surround herself with fair and just ministers, and who unfortunately succumbed to the intensity that the Queen archetype can convey.

Queen Victoria (Alexandrina Victoria; May 24, 1819–January 22, 1901)*, queen of the United Kingdom of Great Britain and Ireland from June 20, 1837, until her death; from May 1, 1876, she adopted the additional title of empress of India.* Victoria became queen with the passing of her uncle in 1837, and to keep herself grounded, she would write at least 2,500 words a day in her journal, exemplifying a wonderful spiritual practice. She was small in stature but grand in her presence as a Queen. She wasn't particularly well-liked in the beginning of her reign, but she learned how to balance the stately life with being a strong woman, and later on in her life, her subjects loved her.

SHINES Protocol: How Do You Support an Unbalanced Heroine?

For the Unbalanced Heroine, the primary question is: Will you answer the call? Taking the first step along your journey can be difficult. But facing and moving through any fear or resistance you might feel is all part of restoring and aligning your powers. Whether your initial overriding challenge is amenorrhea (cessation of menstruation), insomnia, anxiety, miscarriage, progesterone-deficiency-related PCOS, or another condition, facing it head on and moving forward is the first, critical step toward reclaiming your access to your heroine's inner strength.

This is not something you need to—or should—do on your own, however. Every hero or heroine needs a sidekick. Batman had Robin, Luke Skywalker had C-3PO and R2-D2, and Dorothy had the Tin Man, the Lion, and the Scarecrow. All these characters got through their journeys with the help of their support structures. Your physician can play a role here, as can other healers. Partners and friends can also make significant contributions.

A 2009 study published in the journal *Hormones and Behavior* concluded that interpersonal closeness increased salivary progesterone levels, a change associated with greater affiliation motivation over time.[6] This suggests that finding a sidekick can help an Unbalanced Heroine on every level—physically, emotionally, and psychologically. Although the journey is yours alone to take, and reaching its end ultimately relies on your strength and resiliency, a sidekick can offer practical knowledge and emotional reinforcement that can help guide you along your path and prop you up when your energy wanes.

SPIRITUAL PRACTICE

HEART COHERENCE: THE EMWAVE DEVICE

Based on research into the heart's effects on the brain, HeartMath's emWave technology provides real-time biofeedback data that helps you achieve "heart coherence," a state in which stress and anxiety may diminish, and overall cognitive functioning may improve. For the Unbalanced Heroine, whose emotions may be changeable and who may tend to experience stress and anxiety, an emWave device can provide significant relief in discrete instances and over time.

The emWave device tracks your heart rhythms and directs you to pace your breathing so the signals your heart sends to your brain are less erratic and disordered. The more stable and ordered these signals become, the better and clearer your cognitive functioning is likely to be. According to HeartMath researchers, using an emWave device can also help reinforce positive feelings and emotional stability, affecting how you perceive the world around you and the way you think, feel, and perform within it.[7] You may feel like this is not much of a spiritual practice; however, this little device can teach you basic meditation-type skills and structured breathing that will open the doors to potentially profound experiences.

Also, the spiritual practice for the Unbalanced Heroine is to find something that is your holy grail. What is it that you have been pursuing? What is your quest? I will often recommend a journal where you can write down your desires and dreams. Getting these down on paper is the beginning of your journey.

HORMONE MODULATION

For the Unbalanced Heroine, hormonal modulation is a fairly straightforward matter: treatment with progesterone. The hormone comes in several forms: capsules, creams, sublingual tablets, and suppositories. Which form of medication is likely to work best depends on the individual. For example, although capsules have the highest absorption rate, they contain peanut oil, so they are inappropriate for any woman with a nut allergy. Suppositories are most commonly used during the first ten to twelve weeks of pregnancy to help prevent miscarriage. Sublingual tablets and creams can both reliably deliver the progesterone you need, but in these formats, it can be difficult to determine the optimal dose.

Whichever progesterone medication your physician prescribes, it is important to note that it will have been created in a laboratory. This is true even of medications marketed as "natural," including the popular Prometrium capsules and Crinone suppositories. "Natural" in this case refers to the medications having been created from diosgenin, a chemical harvested from either yams or soy.

If you and your physician determine that progesterone therapy is right for you, the form of the medication that will work best for you will depend on a series of factors, including your likely physiological response to it as well as the type of progesterone deficiency you're suffering from.

For an Unbalanced Heroine who has progesterone deficiencies during the second half of her menstrual cycle, I recommend taking 10 to 14 days' worth of treatment beginning on roughly day 14 of her cycles. This means that on or around day 25, her progesterone peak will be ended, and menstruation will commence within a few days. I always recommend taking progesterone medication around bedtime, given its potential for making you tired. As for specific dosing of any form of the medication, this will depend on a patient's body mass. Someone who has a higher body mass index (BMI) is likely to need a higher dose than someone whose BMI is lower due to the number of fat cells present in the body.

In most cases, women notice an improvement in their symptoms within one menstrual cycle. But I always encourage patients to continue the medication we choose for at least three months. In my experience, the vast majority of patients feel markedly better by this time. In many cases, they feel better than they have in years.

SIDE EFFECTS OF PROGESTERONE MEDICATIONS

The most prevalent side effect of progesterone replacement therapy is fatigue. Progesterone stimulates the sleep center in the brain by upregulating GABA receptors, which is why I advise patients to take their medication as close as possible to bedtime. Progesterone replacement therapy can also cause an increase in appetite as well as acne, given its slight androgenic component (keep in mind that synthetic progestins have horrible side effects and androgenic components, whereas natural progesterone is actually an antiandrogen). Breast discomfort is also possible, as is some spotting between menstrual cycles. Some patients report headaches and mild depressive symptoms.

A few alternative medicine people in the social media space claim progesterone is completely safe. No medication is completely safe, and existing medical conditions can put a patient at risk of additional side effects from progesterone. If you have a personal or family history of breast cancer, for example, progesterone therapy can pose a danger if that cancer has a progesterone-receptor-positive status. Just as some types of breast cancer are estrogen-receptor positive, others are progesterone-receptor positive. If you or someone in your family has experienced the latter, be sure to discuss this with your prescribing physician. Liver diseases, including hepatitis and cirrhosis, can also put you at increased risk for negative side effects. Hormones are processed by the liver. If yours is already taxed by one of these illnesses or another condition, consult with your physician and weigh the risks associated with stressing it further. A final condition that may put you at risk of experiencing negative side effects is severe depression. Given the tendency of progesterone therapy to make you feel lethargic, it can worsen depressive symptoms. Again, consulting with your prescriber and having a plan in place for careful monitoring is key.

A Note on Over-the-Counter
Progesterone Creams

While some progesterone replacement creams are available over the counter, several studies have confirmed that they may not contain the amounts of progesterone they claim to on the label. Also, progesterone creams labeled as "cosmetic" do not require FDA approval before they come to market, and there is no limit on the amount of the hormone they can contain. Most of these OTC creams have such a minimal amount of hormone they have no physiological effect and actually cost more than a prescription.

INFOCEUTICALS

For the Unbalanced Heroine, the two most important Energetic Integrators (EI) are EI2 and EI10.

EI2 helps to balance out the effects of pregnenolone, a naturally occurring steroid hormone that is a precursor of others, including progesterone. Given that pregnenolone has downstream effects on a series of hormones, it exerts a subtle influence on your entire emotional makeup.

EI2 operates along the lung meridian. At first blush, it may seem that the lungs have little to do with the endocrine system. But as teachers of yoga and meditation have long taught us, the breath can play a highly influential role in emotional health and balance. EI2 also bioenergetically influences the heart. While technically the center of the circulatory system, the heart is also a nucleus of emotion and a seat of your personal identity. For the Unbalanced Heroine on a quest to come into her own, EI2 can help regulate the energy around conflicts between the head and the heart.

EI10 appears in the SHINES protocol for each archetype in

which menstrual irregularities play a major role. Operating along the circulation/pericardium meridian, it is a critical integrator for the neuroendocrine and circulatory systems and plays a major role in overall hormone balance.

EI10 bioenergetically influences the hypothalamus, which helps control the ovaries' hormone production. (Nerve cells in the hypothalamus send messages to the pituitary gland, telling it to produce LH and FSH, which are carried via the bloodstream to the ovaries, where they help regulate the menstrual cycle.) This integrator also bioenergetically influences manifestations of PMS and/or PMDD, including mood swings, irritability, and depressive symptoms.

ESSENTIAL OILS

When you have low circulating levels of progesterone, you can try these essential oils to help bring those levels back up. These will also help with calmness and serenity, thus blocking the deleterious effects of estrogen dominance:

Bergamot	Eucalyptus
Cinnamon bark	Frankincense
Clove bud	Peppermint

In the vein of relaxation and stress reduction, there are also self-care techniques like massage and acupuncture that help to reduce stress and potentially bring the ovulation signals back in line. If massage and acupuncture are going to be used, please remember that it may take more than one session to experience results, and these sessions should be thought of as something you deserve. You are doing this for yourself. I am also a fan of craniosacral therapy for progesterone deficiency to help realign the pituitary gland. Developed by osteopathic physician John Upledger, it is a hands-on technique that uses gentle pressure to realign energetically tensions deep within the body. The theory of this being that overt stressors misalign the brain and spine, thus causing dysfunction, and this gentle hands-on approach brings these imbalances back into proper alignment.

Progesterone and Diosgenin

As we discuss at various points in this book, some progesterone replacement medications are made (in a laboratory environment) from a chemical contained in wild yams called diosgenin. Although various cultures use the roots of wild yams as a natural remedy for reproductive health issues, the human body cannot convert diosgenin into progesterone on its own. This means that neither eating wild yams (the majority of the species are inedible) nor applying a wild yam cream can increase your progesterone levels.

When considering your progesterone replacement options, be sure to check the label. Only those creams containing "USP bioidentical progesterone" may actually support or boost your levels.

NUTRITION

For the Unbalanced Heroine, the role of nutrition is to help boost progesterone production. There are no foods that contain progesterone, per se, so supporting the body's systems in ways that may help the body sustain its existing progesterone levels is ultimately the goal.

FOODS TO EMBRACE

Fiber

Again, estrogen and progesterone work in unison, and with your higher estrogen levels, progesterone may be less effective. By increasing the levels of fiber in your gastrointestinal tract, you can effectively lower your estrogen levels, which can, in turn, make your circulating progesterone levels more effective.

Zinc

This mineral is essential for the production of follicle-stimulating hormone (FSH), which can help you ovulate and thus increase your progesterone levels. Food sources of zinc include beef, nuts, seafood, and pumpkin/squash seeds.

Vitamin B6

This vitamin is found in fish, turkey, dried fruit, and sunflower seeds.

Vitamin C

This vitamin associated with citrus fruits has been shown to boost progesterone by up to 77 percent.

Foods Containing Magnesium

Sufficient amounts of magnesium in your system will help prevent stress-induced inflammation, which in turn supports the healthy functioning of the pituitary gland. This produces LH and FSH, which are carried via the bloodstream to the ovaries, where they drive ovulation and the production of progesterone.

For the Unbalanced Heroine, I recommend an intake of between 400 and 800 mg of magnesium per day. Particularly good food sources include:

Dark leafy greens (spinach and chard)
Nuts (almonds and cashews)
Seeds (pumpkin)
Dark chocolate
Yogurt and kefir
Avocados

Bananas

Figs

Fatty fish, including halibut, mackerel, and salmon

Foods Containing Vitamin C

Research has shown that vitamin C can increase both endometrial thickness and progesterone serum levels during the luteal phase. A 2003 study found that women who ingested 750 mg of vitamin C per day experienced both increased progesterone levels and higher rates of pregnancy.[8]

Although vitamin C can have these supportive effects, it is important not to ingest excessive amounts. Taking more than 1,000 mg/day can cause the cervical mucus to become drier, making it more difficult for sperm to travel from the upper vaginal tract to the uterus.

Good food sources of vitamin C include:

Citrus fruits, particularly oranges and grapefruit

Kale

Red peppers (green peppers contain less vitamin C, but are also a good source)

Brussels sprouts

Broccoli

Tropical fruits, including kiwi and guava

Strawberries

Foods Containing Vitamin B6

Research has shown that vitamin B6 can help decrease estrogen dominance and increase progesterone levels, helping to both ameliorate symptoms of PMS and/or PMDD and decrease the likelihood of miscarriage.[9] Vitamin B6 can also help offset the symptoms of nausea and vomiting during pregnancy.

For the Unbalanced Heroine, I recommend a vitamin B6 intake of 10 mg/day. Good food sources of vitamin B6 include:

Chickpeas and pinto beans
Tuna and salmon
Turkey and chicken breast
Sunflower and sesame seeds
Pistachios
Prunes

Foods That Contain Zinc

For the Unbalanced Heroine, maintaining healthy levels of zinc is particularly important. Similarly to magnesium, zinc helps support the functioning of the pituitary gland, which, as we've seen, secretes FSH and LH, the hormones that trigger ovulation and have the downstream effect of reduced progesterone production. Adding to this, studies have shown that inadequate zinc levels can contribute to symptoms of PMS and/or PMDD.[10]

For the Unbalanced Heroine, I recommend 15 to 25 mg of zinc per day. Good food sources of zinc include:

Oysters and shrimp
Red meats, including lamb and beef
Pumpkin, flax, and watermelon seeds
Cashews and peanuts
Wheat germ

Vitamin E

Research into the effects of vitamin E on women diagnosed with luteal phase defect has shown that it can increase progesterone production by the corpus luteum by improving blood flow to the ovaries. According to a 2009 study, 600 mg of vitamin E administered three times daily significantly increased serum concentrations of progesterone by virtue of its impact on the healthy functioning of the corpus luteum.[11]

For the Unbalanced Heroine, I recommend 400 IU of vitamin E per day. Good food sources of vitamin E include:

Sunflower seeds
Almonds
Safflower and palm oils
Asparagus
Red peppers
Avocado
Spinach
Sweet potato

Fiber

Excess hormones have a tendency to build up in the digestive tract. This is true of estrogen, which is excreted via the bowel. When excess estrogen remains in the bowel for extended periods (in the case of constipation, for example), it can be reabsorbed, contributing to estrogen dominance. For the Unbalanced Heroine, estrogen dominance can exacerbate the symptoms of low progesterone.

Adding to this, progesterone itself is a smooth muscle relaxant. The intestines are encased in layers of smooth muscle, which means when women increase their progesterone levels, they are subject to constipation. Pregnant women are particularly prone to this, given their increased levels of the hormone. For the Unbalanced Heroine, maintaining enough fiber in their diet to facilitate normal bowel transit is an important element of their overarching SHINES approach.

Seed Cycling

Seed cycling is a process by which you can help support your body's natural hormone-balancing processes. Although any of the archetypes discussed in this book may benefit from seed cycling, those whose symptomology is rooted in estrogen or progesterone excess or deficiency are most likely to benefit.

Seed cycling involves introducing different seeds into your diet at different points during your menstrual cycle. Among the seeds you can use are pumpkin, sunflower, and sesame. The cycling process works as follows: During days 1 to 14 of your cycle, called the follicular phase, you consume 1 tablespoon of flaxseeds and 1 tablespoon of hulled pumpkin seeds. Flaxseeds contain lignans that bind excess estrogen in the body and help to eliminate it. This can be particularly helpful for the Unbalanced Heroine suffering from the effects of estrogen dominance. Pumpkin seeds are utilized for their essential fatty acids and zinc. Zinc helps support progesterone production via a downstream effect that begins in the pituitary gland.

During days 15 to 28, or the luteal phase, you change the type of seeds you are consuming to 1 tablespoon of sesame seeds and 1 tablespoon of hulled sunflower seeds. The lignans in sesame seeds also help to balance out estrogen levels, though less potently than those in flaxseeds. Sunflower seeds are utilized for their selenium content, which can help support liver function and overall hormone balance as your cycle comes to a close.

One important note about seed cycling: Your body can't digest the seeds on its own. Grinding or crushing the seeds and adding them to a soup, a smoothie, or a serving of yogurt is the best way to access their essential, benefit-yielding ingredients. Take care not to grind them for too long—overheating the seeds can cause

(continues)

their natural oils to become rancid. You may also choose to add some oils to the seed-cycling process. This, too, can enhance its benefits. During the follicular phase, I recommend 1.5 to 2 g of fish oil per day. During the luteal phase, I recommend switching to primrose oil in the same amount.

EXERCISE

At every turn of your journey, it's important to tend to your body and remain as physically fit as possible. The type of exercise you choose to help you maintain your muscular strength, flexibility, joint health, and cardiovascular fitness is less important than simply finding one (or more). Discovering what best suits your physical, emotional, *and* logistical needs is the critical first step to developing an exercise plan that will give your body and mind the strength they need to endure the trials you'll face. Suffice it to say, just getting your body moving can be half the battle, so don't judge yourself—just get out there and do something.

PILATES

For any Unbalanced Heroine, I recommend practices that can help strengthen your core (I mean, what type of hero/heroine doesn't need a strong core to swing that sword?), the muscles of your abdominal area, hips, and lower back. In particular, I recommend Pilates. Named for its German inventor, Joseph Pilates (whose father was a prize-winning gymnast and mother was a naturopath), Pilates involves performing a series of resistance exercises that emphasize body alignment, muscle stretching and strengthening, balance, and coordination.

Pilates is low-impact and may or may not involve the use of specialized apparatus. It may also be modified for individual practitioners according to their goals, abilities, and physical improvement over time. If you are interested in giving Pilates a try, you may consider trying a mat-based workout first. You may find a series of these workouts, varying in length and practitioner experience level, online at www.pilatesanytime.com.

AIKIDO

Aikido is another practice I often recommend for Unbalanced Heroines. A Japanese method of self-defense, aikido has its root in three words: *ai*, meaning "joining," *ki*, meaning "spirit," and *do*, meaning "the way." Translated into English, *aikido* means "the way of joining the spirit," and it is this element as much as any physical one that makes it a fortifying practice for the Unbalanced Heroine. Aikido training focuses on flexibility and endurance. Although students of aikido may build muscle mass, the emphasis is less on this than on overall body control and balance.

Aikido utilizes methods of *nonresistance* rather than offensive attacks to fell opponents. Although the art involves learning a series of locks, holds, and throws, the *first* thing a new student of aikido learns is how to *fall* correctly. This is an invaluable skill for anyone embarking on a journey during which they're likely to encounter obstacles, large or small, that threaten their progress.

Above all else, aikido emphasizes the importance of developing the ability to relax the mind and body in even the most stressful or dangerous situations, so that you can act from a place of calm confidence—exactly what the Unbalanced Heroine must always strive to do. As aikido's founder, Morihei Ueshiba, is quoted as saying, "In Aikido, we never attack. An attack is proof that one is out of control. Never run away from any kind of challenge, but do not try to suppress or control an opponent unnaturally. Let attackers come any way they like and then blend with them. Never chase after opponents. Redirect each attack and get firmly behind it."[12]

Another important characteristic of aikido is that the practice relies on two people—the *uke*, the student who is learning to receive or absorb an attack, and the *nage*, the teacher or person who administers the technique being taught. In aikido training, the uke and nage are regarded not as separate entities, but as two parts of a whole, each of which has an equally important role to play. Thus, in aikido, the importance of a sidekick arises again. Since aikido is not an art anyone can learn on their own, the practice can help the Unbalanced Heroine learn to forge sustaining relationships with trusted cohorts.

WALKING

Paralleling the quintessential heroine's journey (which initially takes you away from home but ultimately leads a new, enlightened version of you back to where you began), walking provides the Unbalanced Heroine with significant opportunities for physical and spiritual healing and growth. In addition to the physical changes it can help bring about, including improved bone and muscle strength, balance, coordination, and blood pressure, walking requires that you remain mindful of your surroundings and your progress. This is a skill that can serve you well as you make your larger journey.

An important note about walking is that you do not need to have excessive amounts of time—or energy—to do it. Even when you're feeling sluggish, and a trip to the gym or the dojo is just too much, a twenty-minute walk can yield worthwhile benefits. As answering the call is the critical first step for the Unbalanced Heroine, walking can become an easily accessible first step. Leaving your house to take time for yourself, devoting the time and energy you can to paying attention to what's going on in your body and mind, and allowing yourself to transform in the small physical and spiritual ways, *is* answering the heroine's call to adventure.

A second important note about walking is that your sidekick can join you. In his book *Earthwalks for Body and Spirit*, writer James Endredy describes a walk for two or more participants. This is how it works: One person (your trusted partner) takes the lead, handing you a rope to hold on to as they lead you blindfolded along a relatively unobstructed path. As Endredy describes the potential impact of this exercise:

> As you follow this practice, two forces will become apparent to you. The first is the force of your rational mind holding you back from embracing the mystery, trying to remain in control as you pursue the "risky" activity of walking blindfolded. The other force is your other self who craves the excitement of breaking free from this physical and rational world and yearns to express itself. . . . We do not often enough give our other side a chance to emerge—make the most of this time and let go of your rational mind. There will be plenty of time after the walk is over for it to take over again.[13]

Although Endredy emphasizes the potential for freedom from your rational mind in this particular context, any walk can provide this for you. Any walk during which you engage in mindful contemplation of your surroundings and your immediate and larger journey can yield physical, emotional, and spiritual benefits that can support you along the road to balance and overall well-being.

SUPPLEMENTS

Apart from hormone modulation therapy, certain vitamin and mineral supplements can help support progesterone production and ameliorate some of the physical and psychological symptoms that characterize the Unbalanced Heroine archetype.

MAGNESIUM

Again, magnesium helps reduce stress-induced inflammation. This, in turn, supports the healthy functioning of the pituitary gland and the production of LH and FSH, the hormones that drive ovulation and the production of progesterone.

For the Unbalanced Heroine, I recommend an intake of between 400 and 800 mg of magnesium per day, in the form of magnesium glycinate.

VITAMIN C

Vitamin C can increase both endometrial thickness and progesterone serum levels during the luteal phase. For the Unbalanced Heroine, I recommend a supplement of between 250 and 500 mg per day.

Although vitamin C is water-soluble and the body excretes excess amounts via urine, taking megadoses of the vitamin can cause gastrointestinal distress, headaches, insomnia, and kidney stones. Taking more than 1,000 mg/day can also cause the cervical mucus to become drier, which can diminish the chances of fertilization.

ZINC

Zinc helps support the functioning of the pituitary gland, exerting a downstream effect on FSH and LH, the hormones that trigger ovulation and progesterone production. Inadequate zinc levels can contribute to symptoms of PMS and/or PMDD.[14]

Earlier in this section, we discussed several foods that contain zinc, including shellfish, red meat, and some seeds and nuts. A supplement can also serve the Unbalanced Heroine well. I recommend 15 to 25 mg per day.

VITAMIN B6

Earlier in this chapter, we discussed that research has shown that vitamin B6 can help to both decrease estrogen dominance and increase progesterone levels. Taken together, these can potentially ameliorate symptoms of PMS and/or PMDD in addition to reducing the risk of miscarriage risk.[15] Vitamin B6 can also help offset the symptoms of nausea and vomiting during pregnancy.

For the Unbalanced Heroine, I recommend a supplement of 10 mg/day.

L-ARGININE

L-arginine is an amino acid your body converts to nitrous oxide, a chemical that relaxes your blood vessels, increasing blood flow. Athletes tend to supplement their diets with L-arginine to help increase their endurance. Improving ovarian blood flow can help support the production and secretion of progesterone by the corpus luteum.

For the Unbalanced Heroine, I recommend 3 to 6 g of L-arginine per day.

VITEX (CHASTEBERRY)

Vitex agnus-castus, commonly known as chasteberry or vitex, is an herbal supplement that has been used for thousands of years by cultures around the globe to calm sexual desire and to help restore the body's normal levels of progesterone. Studies have shown that vitex can increase the secretion of luteinizing hormone (LH), which in turn boosts progesterone production. Research has indicated that vitex exerts its effects via a series of neurotransmitters, including dopamine, acetylcholine, and/or opioid receptors.

For the Unbalanced Heroine, I recommend a dose of 400 mg two or three times per day.

I do share a few **warnings** about vitex with patients. First, although vitex may begin working in as few as ten days, studies show that women taking the supplement may need to wait for up to six months to experience it benefits. Second, although there are few significant side effects associated with vitex, some of my patients have reported nausea, gastrointestinal upset, skin reactions, and headaches. Women who suffer from menstrual depression or PMDD have also reported an exacerbation of these symptoms. **Vitex is not recommended for women who are pregnant or breastfeeding.**

LICORICE

Research published in the *Journal of Natural Medicine* has indicated that licorice can help counteract symptoms of PMS and PMDD, particularly those caused by fluid retention, including bloating and breast tenderness. Studies have indicated that this is due to the fact that licorice contains isoflavones (phytoestrogens), which can mimic the effects of estrogen.[16] Licorice also blocks aldosterone, an adrenal hormone that increases fluid retention.

For the Unbalanced Heroine, I recommend 400 to 500 mg of powdered licorice per day. **This is one of those supplements that needs to be treated with care, because you can indeed take too much and many hospitalizations have resulted from people eating even just too much black licorice** (I find the taste disgusting). If you are going to take this supplement, make sure you do it under the care of a physician.

VALERIAN ROOT

Although valerian root extract has no direct impact on progesterone production, it can help with sleep-related issues. Valerian has been used around the globe for centuries as a treatment for insomnia, nervousness, headaches, and heart palpitations, and modern research suggests that its effects are rooted in its ability to increase the amount of bioavailable gamma-aminobutyric acid (GABA) in the brain.[17] A neurotransmitter, GABA inhibits communication between nerve cells in the brain, exerting a calming effect.

For the Unbalanced Heroine, I recommend a dose of 100 to 200 mg per day, taken thirty minutes to two hours before bedtime.

Valerian root is not recommended for women who are pregnant or nursing, as its effects on fetuses and infants are unknown. Valerian root may also interact with prescription sedatives, including benzodiazepines and barbiturates, as well as other supplements, including St. John's wort and melatonin.[18]

BOOK RECOMMENDATIONS FOR
UNBALANCED HEROINES

Joseph Campbell, *The Hero with a Thousand Faces* (New York: Pantheon, 1949)

Shawn A. Tassone, MD, PhD, and Kathryn M. Landherr, MD, *Spiritual Pregnancy: Develop, Nurture & Embrace the Journey to Motherhood* (Woodbury, MN: Llewellyn Worldwide, 2014)

UNBALANCED HEROINES

Hermione Granger, *fictional character in J. K. Rowling's Harry Potter series.* Befriended by Harry when he and his friend Ron save her from a mountain troll, Hermione remains at Harry's side through all manner of adventures and travails, using her intelligence, deftness, and vast knowledge to navigate them.

Throughout the series, Hermione struggles with the fact that her parents are not magical—that she is not "pure"—and the criticism that comes her way because of this fact.

In interviews, Rowling has said that she based the character on herself, citing the young Hermione's intelligence and sassiness as well as her underlying insecurities.

Eleanor Roosevelt (October 11, 1884–November 7, 1962), *American politician, activist, and diplomat; longest-serving First Lady of the United States (March 1933–April 1945); later, US delegate to the United Nations (1945–1952).* Although born into immense wealth and privilege, this niece of Theodore Roosevelt endured a tremendously difficult childhood. Her mother died of diphtheria when Eleanor was just eight years old, and a younger brother, Elliot Jr., died of the same disease just months later. Eleanor's father died in 1894 after jumping from a window at a sanitarium where he was being treated for alcoholism. Eleanor's beloved youngest brother, Hall, born in 1891, also suffered from alcoholism for most of his life, dying at the age of fifty.

Eleanor's life with her husband, Franklin Delano Roosevelt, was also fraught with personal difficulty. Despite her feeling that she was ill-suited to motherhood, Eleanor bore six children, one of whom died while he was still an infant. Her marriage also nearly collapsed when, in 1918, Eleanor discovered that Franklin had been having a long-term affair with her social secretary, Lucy Mercer. The Roosevelts remained married, though their union was more a political partnership than a romantic one.

Eleanor was critical of Franklin's decision to carry on his political career after polio paralyzed him in 1921. But she used the stature afforded her by his position and their marriage to advance her own political goals, which included improving working conditions for poor laborers, expanding women's role in the workplace, and advocating for the civil rights of African Americans, Asian Americans, and World War II refugees.

Joan of Arc (c. January 6, 1412–May 30, 1431). Born into a peasant family in northeast France, Joan of Arc claimed to have been called by the Archangel Michael, Saint Margaret, and Saint Catherine of Alexandria to support the as-yet-uncrowned Charles VII in his quest to put an end to English domination during the Hundred Years' War (1337–1453).

Charles sent Joan to the front at the Siege of Orléans, and she rose to prominence after the siege was lifted just days later. Other victories followed, paving the way for Charles VII's coronation and France's triumph. In 1430, however, long before the war ended, Joan was captured by a faction of French soldiers who had aligned themselves with the English. She was tried by a pro-English bishop and convicted of various charges. On May 30, 1431, Joan of Arc was burned at the stake. She was nineteen years old.[19]

The SHINES Protocol: How Do You Care for a Mother?

For the Mother, the focus of the SHINES protocol is self-care. It's about redirecting some of your efforts of protecting and caring for others toward yourself. Whether it's a spiritual practice or an energetic one that requires focusing on your emotional and psychological needs and experiences, a hormonal treatment that can help address your combined imbalances, or planning out a structured and supportive diet and exercise routine, each aspect of the Mother's SHINES protocol prioritizes putting yourself first.

SPIRITUAL PRACTICE

Your spiritual practice may involve as much boundary-setting and *not* doing (in the form of letting others do for you) as active engagement in practices that can help you relax and restore yourself.

MASSAGE

Massage yields a series of physical benefits for the Mother. Just as important, however, it provides an opportunity for complete relaxation in a private and quiet environment. Adding to this, massage requires that you relinquish control to someone else—that you let someone else take charge and take care of you.

DRY BRUSHING

This practice consists of exactly what its name implies: running a soft, dry-bristle brush across your skin. The purpose of dry brushing is to detoxify your body's largest organ—the skin—by exfoliating dead skin and unclogging your pores so that the toxins residing underneath are released.

Taking only minutes a day, dry brushing can relax and invigorate all at once. For the Mother, I suggest purchasing a natural, nonsynthetic bristle brush with a long handle. Make sure the bristles are soft, particularly if you are just beginning the practice. Each day before you shower or bathe, stand in the tub and begin brushing upward from your feet toward your heart in long strokes. (Your skin may be sensitive at first, but with time, its sensitivity to the brush will diminish.) Once you are finished with your legs, brush upward from your fingertips toward your heart, gliding the brush over your shoulder and toward the center of your chest. Then, as you are able, extend the brush down your back, gently pulling it upward toward your neck and shoulders.

Once you have brushed as much of your limbs and torso as feels comfortable to you, take a shower or soak in the tub in either hot or cold water. Each can stimulate your circulation, increasing the flow of energy as it does, in addition to facilitating the removal of toxins through your pores.

TIME WITH (GIRL)FRIENDS

Another spiritual practice I recommend for Mothers is spending time with friends who can relate to your experiences and who may even be suffering from the same symptoms you are. Whether you go out for coffee or stay in for a dinner among (only) friends, this can provide a space in which you can both release some potentially negative energy and feel supported by women who understand what it feels like to be where you are, physically, emotionally, and energetically.

HORMONE MODULATION

For the Mother, hormonal treatment is twofold, involving the reduction of your estrogen levels (and of estrogen dominance) and increasing your progesterone levels.

If you are taking any form of estrogen replacement treatment, evaluating and adjusting your dosage may be the first step. It is important to look beyond the dose itself and directly at its impact on your estrogen levels. Your absorption rate of oral or transdermal medications will vary depending on your tissue's permeability and your overall sensitivity to the medication's active ingredients.

As we discussed earlier, if you are taking birth control pills that contain synthetic estrogen and progesterone, these may have given rise to your archetype. If this is the case, you may want to consider a birth control that contains only progestin (synthetic progesterone). Because it contains no estrogen, this type of medication may help bring your estrogen and progesterone levels closer to balance. At the same time, however, synthetic progesterone may not have the same effects as the progesterone produced by your own body or a bioidentical replacement.

If you are not taking an estrogen replacement or birth control medication, a progesterone supplement may be an effective and generally short-term method for improving your estrogen-progesterone ratio. I recommend bioidentical progesterone replacement medications, which are available in several forms, including tablets, gels, suppositories, and injectables.

If you and your physician decide that a progesterone medication is right for you, make sure he or she closely monitors your progesterone and estrogen levels while you are taking it. Changes normally require between one and three weeks to take hold, so it's best to test your levels at this point and then every several weeks after that.

INFOCEUTICALS

For the Mother, the three most important Energetic Integrators (EI) are EI2, EI8, and EI10.

Operating along the chest meridian, EI2 interacts with your lungs and heart, exerting effects on the circulatory system and subtly influencing the flow of energy through it.

The chest meridian strongly correlates to our most emotional experiences, any of which has the potential to disrupt your estrogen balance. EI2 bioenergetically influences estradiol and estrone, the strongest and the weakest of the three forms of estrogen, respectively. It also helps to balance out the effects of pregnenolone, a naturally occurring steroid and precursor of other hormones, including progesterone.

EI8 helps regulate energetic fields within the liver meridian. It bioenergetically influences those parts of the body that deal with endogenous body waste and exogenous environmental toxins. Exposure to exogenous estrogens can contribute to or exacerbate estrogen dominance, in addition to stressing the liver and diminishing its ability to break down estrogen. Clearing energetic disruptions along this meridian can help regulate this process.

As we have discussed at other points in this book, EI10 appears in the SHINES protocol for each archetype in which menstrual irregularities play a major role. Operating along the circulation/pericardium meridian, it is a critical integrator for the neuroendocrine and circulatory systems and contributes to overall hormone balance.

EI10 bioenergetically influences the hypothalamus, which helps control hormone production by the ovaries. Nerve cells in the hypothalamus release gonadotrophin-releasing hormone, sending messages to the pituitary gland to produce luteinizing hormone (LH) and follicle-stimulating hormone (FSH). EI10 can also bioenergetically influence premenstrual or menopause-related emotional swings or mood disorders, many of which can plague the Mother.

The energetic technique I prefer for Mothers is called the Emotional Freedom Technique, or what is commonly referred to as tapping. As opposed to acupuncture, which uses needles, EFT utilizes gentle repetitive tapping on certain areas of the body. Proponents of the method say that this tapping reduces the stress response on the body. The protocol or method of tapping is very distinctive but easy enough to learn, and I have many friends, colleagues, and patients that utilize this method with great success.

ESSENTIAL OILS

A Mother has the power of the Queen and estranged feeling of the Unbalanced Heroine. While she is trying to rule the land around her, she needs to be organized in her quest for balance. Try these essential oils:

Chamomile	Lemon
Clove bud	Orange
Eucalyptus	

NUTRITION

For the Mother, the role of nutrition is to help diminish the impact of estrogen dominance and support the body's natural progesterone production. This involves embracing certain foods and avoiding others.

FOODS TO EMBRACE TO DIMINISH ESTROGEN DOMINANCE AND SUPPORT PROGESTERONE PRODUCTION

Fiber

As we've discussed in other parts of this book, excess hormones have a tendency to build up in the digestive tract. This is true of estrogen, which is excreted via the bowel. When excess estrogen remains in the bowel for extended periods, it can be reabsorbed and contribute to estrogen dominance. When it is healthy and functioning optimally, a healthy gut can also increase your antioxidant levels and rid the body of some of the free radicals that estrogen produces.

Adding to this, as your progesterone levels increase, you are more susceptible to constipation. This is because the intestines are encased in layers of smooth muscle, and progesterone is a smooth muscle relaxant. Pregnant women are particularly prone to progesterone-based constipation, given their increased levels of the hormone.

I recommend a Mother try to consume at least 25 mg of fiber each day. Within limits, more can be beneficial. Cruciferous vegetables such as broccoli, cabbage, celery, and kale are a great source, as are whole grains and oats, and seeds such as flax and sunflower. Beans, berries, and fruits such as apples and pears contain helpful amounts of fiber, as do nuts such as almonds, pecans, and walnuts.

If you find high-fiber foods unappealing, you may try a supplement. I always recommend trying to get the recommended daily amount from food first. But if you cannot get to 25 mg any other way, I certainly recommend incorporating a supplement into your diet.

When it comes to fiber, I do offer up two notes of caution. The first is that you need to slowly increase the amount of fiber in your diet. Adding too much too quickly can cause your body to produce excess gas, which can lead to mild to severe stomach pain. The second is that cruciferous vegetables can contain phytoestrogens. Some of these, such as lignan, are relatively weak. But they have estrogenic effects nonetheless, so I recommend keeping your consumption of cruciferous vegetables to one serving every other day.

Cruciferous Vegetables

In addition to providing fiber, cruciferous vegetables such as broccoli, Brussels sprouts, cabbage, kale, mustard greens, and turnips contain a compound called indole-3-carbinol (I3C). In recent years, researchers have become interested in I3C as a possible preventive of breast, cervical, endometrial, and colorectal cancers. Studies have also indicated that the compound impedes estrogen receptor cell proliferation in breast tissue.

When you consume cruciferous vegetables, your body naturally produces another compound called diindolylmethane (DIM), which research has shown can help break down estrogen and convert it to its healthy metabolites. DIM has also been shown to have a weak estrogenic effect. This means that it can bind to estrogen receptors, blocking stronger forms of estrogen and thwarting their potentially carcinogenic impact. DIM may also help ease symptoms associated with a Mother's estrogen dominance, including those that mimic PMDD, and breast swelling and tenderness, and is also associated with weight loss. It will also help with the detoxification pathway of estrone and move it more toward a product called 2-methoxyestrone, which is thought to have cancer-protective effects.

Colorful Vegetables

Red and orange vegetables, including peppers and carrots, contain high levels of beta-carotene, a carotenoid compound that has been linked to a reduction in the growth of estrogen-positive breast cancer. High levels of beta-carotene in the body have been associated with reductions as high as 50 percent.

Lean Protein

In addition to helping improve your body composition (by reducing your body fat percentage), a high-protein diet has the added benefit of increasing the amount of the amino acids lysine and threonine in the body. These both help the body metabolize estrogen and support liver function. It is typically recommended to try to consume 1 gram of protein per pound of lean body mass. Most women are safe consuming 100 to 120 g of protein per day and definitely decreasing the amount of processed carbohydrates.

Sulfur

Foods that contain sulfur can help detoxify the liver, improving its ability to get rid of toxins from medications, pesticides, and other external sources. This can make its workload lighter and strengthen its ability to break down estrogen. Foods containing sulfur compounds include onions, garlic, and egg yolks. Lemons and limes also contain sulfur. For a Mother, I recommend drinking a glass of water that contains the juice from half a lemon or lime each morning.

FOODS TO EMBRACE FOR PROGESTERONE SUPPORT

Foods Containing Magnesium

Sufficient amounts of magnesium in your system will help prevent stress-induced inflammation, which in turn supports the healthy functioning of the pituitary gland. This produces LH and FSH, which are carried via the bloodstream to the ovaries, where they drive ovulation and the production of progesterone.

For the Mother, I recommend an intake of between 400 and 800 mg of magnesium per day. Particularly good food sources include:

Dark leafy greens (spinach and chard)
Nuts (almonds and cashews)

Seeds (pumpkin)
Dark chocolate
Yogurt and kefir
Avocados
Bananas
Figs
Fatty fish, including halibut, mackerel, and salmon

Foods Containing Vitamin C

Research has shown that vitamin C can increase both endometrial thickness and progesterone serum levels during the luteal phase. A 2003 study found that women who ingested 750 mg of vitamin C per day experienced both increased progesterone levels and higher rates of pregnancy.

Although vitamin C can have these supportive effects, it is important not to ingest excessive amounts. Taking more than 1,000 mg/day can cause the cervical mucus to become drier, making it more difficult for sperm to travel from the upper vaginal tract to the uterus.

Good food sources of vitamin C include:

Citrus fruits, particularly oranges and grapefruit
Kale
Red peppers (green peppers contain less vitamin C, but are also a good source)
Brussels sprouts
Broccoli
Tropical fruits, including kiwi and guava
Strawberries

Foods Containing Vitamin B6

Research has shown that vitamin B6 can help decrease estrogen dominance and increase progesterone levels, helping to both ameliorate symptoms of PMS and/or PMDD and decrease the likelihood of miscarriage. Vitamin B6 can also help offset the symptoms of nausea and vomiting during pregnancy.

For the Mother, I recommend a vitamin B6 intake of 10 mg/day. Good food sources of vitamin B6 include:

Chickpeas and pinto beans
Tuna and salmon
Turkey and chicken breast
Sunflower and sesame seeds
Pistachios
Prunes

Foods That Contain Zinc

For the Mother, maintaining healthy levels of zinc is particularly important. Similarly to magnesium, zinc helps support the functioning of the pituitary gland, which, as we've seen, secretes FSH and LH, the hormones that trigger ovulation and have the downstream effect of reduced progesterone production. Adding to this, studies have shown that inadequate zinc levels can contribute to symptoms of PMS and/or PMDD.[20]

For the Mother, I recommend 15 to 25 mg of zinc per day. Good food sources of zinc include:

Oysters and shrimp
Red meats, including lamb and beef
Pumpkin, flax, and watermelon seeds
Cashews and peanuts
Wheat germ

Vitamin E

Research into the effects of vitamin E on women diagnosed with luteal phase defect has shown that it can increase progesterone production by the corpus luteum by improving blood flow to the ovaries.

According to a 2009 study, 600 mg of vitamin E administered three times daily significantly increased serum concentrations of progesterone by virtue of its impact on the healthy functioning of the corpus luteum.

For the Mother, I recommend 400 IU of vitamin E per day. Good food sources of vitamin E include:

Sunflower seeds
Almonds
Safflower and palm oils
Asparagus
Red peppers
Avocado
Spinach
Sweet potato

FOODS TO AVOID TO DIMINISH ESTROGEN DOMINANCE AND SUPPORT PROGESTERONE PRODUCTION

Carbohydrates

A Mother would be wise to minimize her intake of carbohydrates or avoid them altogether. If you're eating a diet rich in carbohydrates, your glucose (blood sugar) levels are going to be higher. When this happens, your body responds by telling the pancreas to increase insulin production. Insulin helps your body store calories as fat, which raises both your weight and your body mass index (BMI). Obesity can drive or exacerbate estrogen dominance, given that fat cells will aromatize excess testosterone into estrogen. Fat cells also hold on to excess estrogen in your system.

If your diet is higher in proteins and healthy fats (such as olive oil, flaxseed oil, and coconut oil) and lower in carbohydrates, your insulin levels will decrease, improving your estrogen metabolism.

For a Mother, the best sources of carbohydrates are vegetables and fruits with a low glycemic index. Avoiding processed foods can also make a significant difference. As I tell my patients, I'm a firm believer that if you can grow it, pick it, or kill it, that food is probably a healthy choice for you to eat. Foods that come in a box or a bag should never be your first choice, and if the ingredient list on the packaging contains words you can't pronounce, you're better off avoiding it. It's that simple.

Alcohol

The impact of alcohol on the liver means alcohol interferes with the body's ability to break down estrogen, which can increase a woman's (or man's) overall estrogen levels. For a Mother, I recommend either eliminating alcohol from your diet altogether, or limiting your intake to one glass of red wine per day. If you're in the market for a red wine, Sardinian and Spanish wines happen to be richer in antioxidants than most and, when consumed in moderation, can actually help remove excess estrogen.

Exogenous Estrogens and Phytoestrogens

I recommend that Mothers avoid exogenous estrogens, such as those found in beef, poultry, and dairy products, as well as in plastics and certain cosmetics. Make sure to seek out hormone-free foods and to limit your exposure to plastics containing BPA and/or other known endocrine disruptors.

Mothers should also avoid consuming phytoestrogens, such as those contained in soy. Although there are positive health benefits associated with soy, you will want to make sure you limit your intake of soy products (whether fermented or not) to relatively small amounts. For a Mother, I recommend no more than 15 to 20 grams of fermented soy-derived foods per day. If you enjoy soy milk, I recommend switching to almond or rice milk.

EXERCISE

For the Mother, the purpose of physical exercise is to improve cardiovascular fitness, joint health, flexibility, and energy levels in addition to helping her lose excess fat, which can exacerbate her estrogen dominance. A yearlong study found that women who engaged in three hours of moderate exercise per week had significantly lower levels of circulating estrogens than women who limited their activity to stretching alone. Specifically, women who averaged 171 minutes of moderate exercise spread across five workout sessions per week saw their estrogen levels drop within five months. The researchers discovered that these women experienced increases in their levels of sex hormone binding globulin (SHBG), the blood-borne protein that binds circulating estrogen and makes it inactive.

For the Mother, the first step is to discern the type of exercise that best suits your physical, emotional, *and* logistical needs. Having too little time often proves a constraint for this archetype, as can a lack of energy caused by interrupted sleep as a result of progesterone. This is why for the Mother, in particular, I recommend group exercise. Whether this is a team-based activity such as rowing or softball, a small-group activity such as tennis or golf, or a group fitness class, working out together with friends or colleagues can help keep you accountable and provide you with valuable emotional support.

WALKING

Whether you walk indoors or out, this is a form of exercise you can begin any time and increase in intensity at your pace. In addition to strengthening your bones and improving your balance, coordination, and blood pressure, walking can also help you lose excess fat. While it can be a solitary activity, walking is also an exercise you can undertake with a friend or larger group. There are some great apps for smartphones now that can take you from the couch to running a 5K in about three months. I have personally used them with success (and I hate running).

YOGA AND PILATES

Accessible to Mothers of different athletic abilities whose energy levels may also vary and wane, yoga is a low-impact exercise that promotes muscle strength, balance, and harmonious alignment among all the body's systems.

While practicing yoga together with others can help keep you accountable and provide some important emotional and practical support, you can also undertake this on your own and at your own pace. For Mothers looking to start a practice at home, I recommend Glo.com, which offers thousands of classes based in different styles, with an array of challenges and benefits.

For the Unbalanced Heroine and Mother alike, I recommend practices that can help strengthen the muscles of the abdominal area, hips, and lower back, and one that has proven a favorite is Pilates. Named for its German inventor, Joseph Pilates (whose father was a prize-winning gymnast and mother was a naturopath), Pilates involves performing a series of resistance exercises that emphasize body alignment, muscle stretching and strengthening, balance, and coordination.

Pilates is low-impact and may or may not involve the use of specialized apparatus. It may also be modified for individual practitioners according to their goals, abilities, and physical improvement over time. If you are interested in giving Pilates a try, you may consider trying a mat-based workout first. You may find a series of these workouts, varying in length and practitioner experience level, online at www.pilatesanytime.com.

SUPPLEMENTS

Among the supplements that can help ameliorate a Mother's symptoms are some that can help diminish her estrogen dominance and others that help support her progesterone levels. As with any aspect of the SHINES protocol that has a physiological impact, I strongly encourage you to consult your physician before taking any of these. Although they are unlikely to have as dramatic an impact as a prescription medication, they *can* have significant effects. But once you and your physician have determined they pose no health risk, feel free to try any from this list.

INDOLE-3-CARBONYL (I3C) AND DIINDOLYLMETHANE (DIM)

Studies have indicated that I3C impedes estrogen receptor cell proliferation, at least in breast tissue. In recent years, researchers have become interested in I3C as a possible preventive of breast, cervical, endometrial, and colorectal cancers.

From I3C, your body naturally produces another compound called diindolylmethane (DIM), which research has shown helps break down estrogen and convert it to its safer metabolites. DIM has also been shown to have a weak estrogenic effect. This means that it can bind to estrogen receptors, blocking stronger forms of estrogen and diminishing their potentially carcinogenic impact. DIM may also help ease symptoms associated with a Mother's estrogen dominance, including those that mimic PMDD. It is also associated with weight loss.

While cruciferous vegetables are a wise and nutritionally valuable source of I3C, a variety of I3C and DIM supplements are also available. If you choose to begin taking one of these, I recommend consulting with your physician and considering 100 mg of DIM per day to start. Depending on what ongoing testing reveals, you may increase your dosage over time.

There are some side effects associated with I3C and DIM supplements, including skin rashes, abdominal pain, nausea, and an increase in liver enzymes. DIM may be slightly easier on your digestive system than I3C, because I3C is the unstable precursor to DIM and needs to be activated in the stomach before your body can convert it into DIM.

VITEX (CHASTEBERRY)

Vitex agnus-castus, commonly known as chasteberry or vitex, is an herbal supplement native to tropical and subtropical regions of the globe that has been used for thousands of years by various cultures around the world to help calm sexual desire, as well as restore and maintain a healthy balance of estrogen and progesterone. Studies have shown that vitex can inhibit the secretion of FSH by the pituitary gland, which leads to a decrease in estrogen production by the ovaries. Vitex has also been shown to stimulate the secretion of LH, which triggers increased progesterone production and diminishes various aspects of estrogen dominance.

For the Mother, I recommend a dose of 900 to 1,000 mg each morning.

I do share a few **warnings** about vitex with patients. First, although vitex may begin working in as few as ten days, studies show that women taking the supplement may need to wait for up to six months to experience it benefits. Second, although there are few significant side effects associated with vitex, some of my patients have reported nausea, gastrointestinal upset, skin reactions, and headaches. Women who suffer from menstrual depression or PMDD have also reported an exacerbation of these symptoms. **Vitex is not recommended for women who are pregnant or breastfeeding.**

MACA

An herb grown in Peru, maca has long been used to promote hormone balance (in men and women) as well as reproductive and menstrual health. Each of the thirteen differently colored varieties of maca exerts distinct effects, and many maca-based supplements combine different varieties of the herb. Some of these can raise estrogen levels, which means that for the Mother, it is critical to identify a mix that contains the right varieties of maca in the right ratios to help address your estrogen dominance.

The particular maca supplement I recommend for a Mother is Femmenessence MacaHarmony, a 100 percent organic and vegan mixture of sustainably farmed maca that has been shown to have a balancing effect on women's levels of estrogen, progesterone, and other hormones. I recommend taking the supplement as directed on the label: two 500 mg tablets daily, taken away from meals. Take the first dose in the morning, before breakfast, and the second dose in the early evening, ideally 30 minutes before you normally experience an energy low. Consider taking half the recommended amount for two weeks, then gradually increasing to the standard amount.

Two notes of **caution** with regard to MacaHarmony: First, I recommend that a Mother take this supplement for two to three months and then take a week off. This can help upregulate your estrogen receptors and enhance the supplement's benefits. Second, MacaHarmony can amplify the effects of caffeine. Because caffeine can aggravate symptoms of estrogen dominance, I recommend that Mothers who take this supplement carefully monitor (and limit) their caffeine intake.

BOOK RECOMMENDATIONS FOR MOTHERS

P. D. Eastman, *Are You My Mother?* (New York: Random House, 1960)

Meg Meeker, MD, *Strong Mothers, Strong Sons: Lessons Mothers Need to Raise Extraordinary Men* (New York: Ballantine, 2014)

Heng Ou, *The First Forty Days: The Essential Art of Nourishing the New Mother* (New York: Stewart, Tabori & Chang, 2016)

Christiane Northrup, MD, *Mother-Daughter Wisdom: Understanding the Crucial Link Between Mothers, Daughters, and Health* (New York: Bantam, 2006)

MOTHERS

Maria von Trapp (née Kutschera, January 26, 1905–March 28, 1897). Born in Austria, Maria von Trapp became known in America during the mid-twentieth century as the stepmother and matriarch of the Vermont-based Trapp Family Singers. In 1949, Maria published *The Story of the Trapp Family Singers*, a book that inspired the musical *The Sound of Music*. In the film version of the musical, Julie Andrews famously plays the role of Maria.

Born on a train while her mother was en route to a hospital in Vienna, Maria spent her early years in the Austrian village of Tyrol. An orphan by the age of ten, Maria was educated at the State Teachers College for Progressive Education in Vienna before entering Nonnberg Abbey, a Benedictine monastery in Salzburg, with the intention of becoming a nun.

In 1926, while she was teaching at the monastery, she began to tutor one of the seven children of the widowed naval commander Georg von Trapp. Soon, Maria began to tutor other of Georg's children, and before long, the widower asked her to marry him. Georg was twenty-five years Maria's senior, and by her admission, she was not enthralled by him. "I really and truly was not in love," Maria wrote. "I liked [Georg], but I did not love him. However, I loved the children, so in a way I really married the children. I learned to love him more than I have ever loved before or after."[21]

It was in 1935, when the family faced financial ruin, that a door of opportunity opened for them. Under the direction of a Roman Catholic priest named Franz Wasner, the children began to sing together at concerts in and around Vienna. Before long, they were touring Europe, the United States, and Canada. Although Georg was inducted into the German Navy during the lead up to World War II, the family decided to flee Nazi-occupied Austria, ultimately settling in Stowe, Vermont, in the early 1940s.

Georg died in 1947. But Maria carried on. During the next decade, together with her stepchildren and her three children with Georg, Maria managed the Trapp Family Singers' performances across America and ran a music camp in Vermont. The von Trapp home in Vermont ultimately became a lodge that continues to welcome guests today.

Sojourner Truth (née Isabella "Belle" Baumfree, c. 1797–November 26, 1883). Born into slavery in Esopus, New York, roughly 100 miles north of New York City, Sojourner Truth ultimately escaped to freedom and went on to become one of the most influential abolitionists and women's rights activists of the late nineteenth century. In 2014, *Smithsonian* magazine named her one of the "100 Most Significant Americans of All Time."

Sold away from her parents at auction at the age of nine, Sojourner Truth went on to be enslaved by three different men in New York State before escaping the last of these in 1826. By this time, she had borne five children, one of whom died in childhood. She was able to take only her infant daughter Sophia with her when she escaped. Shortly thereafter, Sojourner learned that her five-year-old son, Peter, had been illegally sold to an enslaver in Alabama. With the help of a couple named Van Wagener who had taken her in, Sojourner successfully sued Peter's new enslaver and was reunited with her son in 1828. Years later, Sojourner was also reunited with her daughters Diana and Elizabeth.

During the 1830s and '40s, Sojourner became both religious and politically active. In 1843, she officially changed her name to Sojourner Truth, telling her friends she'd been called by the "Spirit" to travel and preach in support of the abolition of slavery.[22] In 1844, she became a member of the Northampton Association of Education and Industry in Northampton, Massachusetts. Founded by abolitionists, the organization also supported the causes of women's rights, religious tolerance, and pacifism, and attracted important social activist figures of the day, including William Lloyd Garrison and Frederick Douglass. Drawn to writing and lecturing, Sojourner dictated her memoirs to a neighbor (which were published by Garrison in 1850 as *Narrative of Sojourner Truth, A Northern Slave*) and traveled the lecture circuit. The most widely recognized of her speeches is the extemporaneous "Ain't I a Woman?," which she delivered in 1851 at the Women's Rights Convention in Akron, Ohio.

During the Civil War, Sojourner Truth helped recruit Black troops into the Union Army. Her grandson joined the forces, enlisting in 54th Massachusetts Volunteer Infantry Regiment. (Led by Colonel Robert Gould Shaw, the 54th was the first African American regiment organized in the Northern states.) Sojourner also worked for the National Freedman's Relief Association (with which Douglass was also affiliated) in Washington, DC. In 1864, she met President Lincoln.

After the war, Sojourner continued to speak and agitate for the causes that mattered to her, including women's rights, prison reform, and the end of capital punishment.

Diana, Princess of Wales (née Diana Frances Spencer, July 1, 1961–August 31, 1997). Born in Norfolk, England, to Edward John Spencer, 8th Earl Spencer, and Frances (Roche) Shand Kydd, Diana was the first wife of Charles, Prince of Wales, and heir apparent to the British throne, and the mother of Prince William, Duke of Cambridge, and Prince Harry. During her short life, she became one of the most famous and beloved celebrity figures in the world and devoted much of her time and energy to supporting charitable causes around the globe. In the years after her death, *Time* magazine named her one of the "100 Most Important People of the 20th Century," and the BBC ranked her third among the "100 Greatest Britons," ahead of Queen Elizabeth II and other living monarchs.

Despite never excelling academically, Diana shined in school as a talented pianist, dancer, and student with "outstanding community spirit." After a year of finishing school in her late teens, Diana shared an apartment in London with friends and held a series of jobs, including working as a nanny and a nursery school assistant, the position she held at the time of her engagement to Prince Charles in 1981.

After giving birth to William in 1982 and Harry in 1984, Princess Diana was by all accounts a devoted mother. Sometimes flouting royal protocol, Diana chose her children's first names in addition to insisting on selecting their nannies and schools. She was known for taking her children to school herself whenever she was able and arranging her appearances around the young princes' schedules.

When the discord in Diana's marriage to Charles became evident during the early years of their union, the Princess of Wales did not shy away from the public spotlight or the scrutiny that came with this. Rather, she consistently built upon her engagement in global social and charitable causes that were dear to her. Among the most notable of these were HIV/AIDS prevention and treatment, the removal of landmines and debris from war-torn areas of Africa and Europe, and cancer research and care advancement, as well as fighting homelessness, animal cruelty, and elder neglect.

Having claimed that she'd like to be the "queen of people's hearts," Diana certainly achieved success in this regard.[23] Known around the world for her beauty, gentleness, charm, *and* her strength and grace under fire, her life and sudden death continue to have a significant impact on the public consciousness. In 2017, Princes William and Harry commissioned two documentaries commemorating their mother. *Diana, Our Mother: Her Life and Legacy*, aired on ITV in the UK and HBO in the US in July of that year. *Diana, 7 Days*, which focused on her death and the worldwide outpouring of grief that followed, was aired by the BBC in August.

The SHINES Protocol: How Do You Help a Wisewoman Become an Oracle?

For the Wisewoman, the purpose of the SHINES method is to bring some ease to the heroine's journey. The protocol is designed to help support and sustain you through your transition into menopause and along your extended path, reducing your discomfort at every point.

When I discuss the SHINES protocol with the Wisewomen I treat, I liken it to taking an epidural during labor: Of course you can endure the pain without it. But you don't *have* to. The same holds true for Wisewomanhood and the various aspects of the SHINES protocol, any or all of which can help make the physical aspects of your journey more manageable, and the personal and spiritual elements fulfilling and even transformational.

As you consider seeking out counsel and medical guidance, it is critical to remember that you have no dues to pay. There are no merit badges for enduring unnecessary physiological, emotional, or spiritual suffering. This can be part of a Wisewoman's personal development: honoring your needs first. As you read through the SHINES protocol, remember that the potential effectiveness of each component requires only that you devote your time, energy, and focus to it and to yourself.

SPIRITUAL PRACTICE

For the Wisewoman, I recommend a series of centering spiritual practices that can help you take stock of where you have come from, where you are now, and what lies ahead.

LIFE INVENTORY

Entry into Wisewomanhood signals a sort of checkpoint—a way station at which performing a life inventory can underscore spiritual healing and growth. Whether you're thirty-five or sixty-five, patiently taking stock of the life you've lived from its very beginning can be an exercise not only in reflection, but in self-care and self-respect. Committing your memories, experiences, and life lessons to paper is a way to honor what you've learned and what you've done, and it can help you envision the future you want to live. It can also be a highly effective way to impart your wisdom to your children or grandchildren, your partner, or your friends.

I have always had a huge love for personal narrative or life story. I wrote on the topic for my dissertation, and as I did, I learned just how much we as a culture have lost by failing to maintain the tradition of storytelling that existed when we were a far more verbal society. This has seen us fail to appreciate history as we should, learning from the triumphs and challenges of those who went before us. The stories of famous historical figures have some lessons to teach us about the lives we're living now. But the stories of people we know—our sisters, mothers, aunts, and grandmothers—can serve as an even better guide. Imagine sitting down with your great-grandmother at your fiftieth birthday party. Wouldn't you be interested in hearing what she had to say about living the rest of her life? What if she left pages of her life story behind, beginning with her childhood, adolescence, and the birth of her own child, your grandparent? Wouldn't you be curious to hear the stories of the people who helped shape your physiology and your experience of the world? Wouldn't you be interested in how they dealt with life's trials, including love, work, family, and aging?

When it comes to Wisewomen sharing their stories, I have witnessed the power of narrative being particularly strong. Women I've counseled have told me that hearing other women's stories, even stories that are radically distinct from their own, has helped them feel less alone and less overwhelmed. They often describe this as a void of history having been filled, one they hadn't been aware existed until they entered unfamiliar territory and found themselves without a map.

Many of my patients have written about their immediate experiences of the changes taking hold and the road they traveled to arrive there. Some have chosen to share them, contributing to a certain collective history, while others have chosen to keep their stories for themselves. Journaling is certainly a worthy method of taking inventory of one's life. I know from experience that returning years later to stories we've written can teach us lessons about ourselves in a powerful way.

The most important aspect of performing a life inventory is the writing itself. Commit your story to paper. What's happening now, what happened before. Start at the beginning or wherever feels right, giving voice and space to the life you've lived and the one you're embarking on.

HOT YOGA

Hot flashes are among the most common symptoms Wisewomen experience at various points during their journey. These cause physical discomfort, of course, but their unpredictability and potential severity can also wear on a Wisewoman, emotionally and psychologically. Hot yoga (or Bikram yoga), a practice that consists of 90-minute classes of twenty-six postures in a humid room heated to 95° to 108°F, is a way to help counteract these aspects of hot flashes' impact.

It might seem counterintuitive that a practice that takes place entirely in a heated room would provide this relief. But this idea comes from the ancient healing idea of treating like with like. Hot flashes occur from within the body, the result of surges in vasodilation. The practice of Bikram yoga encourages you to accept the heat rather than resist it, providing you with a space in which you can practice breathing calmly through the discomfort of waves of heat swelling and retreating that result from hot flashes or the physical exertion of the yoga itself. Doing this over and over can help you see hot flashes for what they are: temporary, fleeting instances you can endure without emotional strife or panic. The power of taking ownership of your physical experience in this way can be quite significant, inside the room and out.

The other physical and spiritual benefits of undertaking the practice of yoga should not be underestimated. Designed to increase strength, flexibility, and the functioning of all the body's systems, yoga is also known for its accessibility to practitioners of all ages and skill levels.

MEDITATION

Many of the Wisewomen I've worked with have found guided meditation to be a source of spiritual healing and inner peace. During my years of studying and practicing mind-body medicine, I have developed a series of guided meditations, one of which I wrote specifically for Wisewomen.

Designed to help conjure the images of women who can guide you along your path, the meditation focuses on visualizing women who have come before you and drawing on their wisdom. You may know or have known these women, or not—it's not important. What *is* important is that you remain open to the learning and experience these figures may have to impart and that you ask the question: "What message does this wiser woman have for me?" Ultimately, you are conferring with your wiser self. The visualization and the words of the guided meditation are the tools that help you get there.

To begin, I recommend choosing a specific space in which to

meditate and carefully curating it by bringing in objects that are meaningful to you, items like photographs, pieces of jewelry or clothing, or other small mementoes that remind you of your life's journey and help inspire you to look forward. Arrange these on a low-lying table or on the floor, and at the center of these objects, I recommend placing a candle. Before you begin your meditation, light the candle, which represents the heat that arises and dissipates within you, as well as the life you've lived and are living in the moment. The candle should burn until the meditation is complete. Then blow it out, signaling an end to the ritual as well as your ownership and control of the heat that is part of your ongoing experience. Taking this step is also emblematic of leaving the life you've lived behind and embarking on a new journey that has a light all its own.

HORMONE MODULATION

This aspect of the SHINES method centers on addressing estrogen deficiency. While there is no single solution that suits all Wisewomen, for most Wisewomen, this element of the SHINES protocol begins with estrogen replacement. For patients who still have a uterus, supplemental progesterone is also necessary. Wisewomen may also present with low testosterone (and symptoms that mirror the Nun's; see page 136) and benefit from its replacement as well.

When I counsel a Wisewoman, we begin with her symptoms. If she presents primarily with symptoms related to estrogen deprivation, including hot flashes, vaginal dryness, and mood swings, and has previously had a hysterectomy, estrogen replacement alone may be enough. If she presents with the additional symptom of persistent insomnia, I will consider adding progesterone to her hormone regimen, and if she complains of decreased libido and/or a generalized decrease in physical strength or energy, I will investigate her testosterone levels to see whether a supplement is warranted.

Testing, either blood serum– or urine-based, of hormone levels drives decisions regarding which hormones to supplement. My goal is always to prescribe the fewest hormones in the lowest possible doses. It may be that a patient will experience significant benefits from the three-pronged approach of estrogen, progesterone, and testosterone replacement, but I will monitor her levels and symptoms on an ongoing basis, minimizing or eliminating one of these elements as the assessments dictate. As you and your physician consider hormone replacement, I recommend that you ask them to consider *all* your symptoms and the various options for ameliorating them.

As previously noted, I tend to prescribe bioidentical hormones in my practice. As for estrogen replacement, this comes in custom-compounded and branded formats and may be administered orally or transdermally. (Studies have shown that transdermal estrogen is less likely to break down into the 16α-hydroxyestrone form that may be more carcinogenic, which has made transdermal forms of estrogen more popular among some prescribers.) Branded medications are generally covered by insurance, while custom-compounded medications are not. Depending on your insurance company's formulary restrictions and copay structure, however, custom-compounded medications may be the less expensive option.

For the Wisewoman and any other archetype for whom estrogen replacement therapy may come into play, I recommend taking a progesterone replacement medication as well. While this is necessary for any woman who still has her uterus, I strongly advise women who have had full hysterectomies to add progesterone to their hormone replacement regime. In addition to decreasing the risk of estrogen dominance, progesterone can also help combat insomnia and anxiety more generally. (Again, custom-compounded and branded versions of bioidentical progesterone are available.)

As of the writing of this book, a female-specific FDA-approved testosterone replacement medication has yet to hit the market. Your physician can prescribe a custom-compounded bioidentical option, however, and a pharmacy can create the individualized dose you and your physician determine is appropriate for you.

In the end, hormonal modulation for the Wisewoman is a flexible process that can vary over a period of months or years. While a physician can guide you and assess your hormone levels and symptoms along the way, it is ultimately up to you to take note of your changing body and symptoms and collaborate with your healthcare provider to determine what course is best at any given point.

Progesterone and Wild Yams

Wild yams are commonly used to create so-called natural progesterone oral and transdermal supplements. The yams contain a compound called diosgenin, which can be converted into progesterone via a lab-based chemical restructuring.

Many patients have asked me whether eating wild yams can yield similar progesterone-related effects to these supplements', and the answer, quite simply, is no. For one thing, only twelve of the reported six hundred species of wild yam are considered edible. More important, the body cannot convert diosgenin into progesterone on its own.

If you are interested in natural progesterone supplements, consult with your physician regarding the potential effectiveness of these supplements and ask which brands they recommend.

INFOCEUTICALS

Energetic Integrator 10 (EI10) is best suited to help correct distortions in a Wisewoman's disrupted energy fields. Associated with the heart and circulatory system, this integrator also affects visual and auditory functioning as well as neuroendocrine regulation, including of the ovaries. You may think of it this way: If a mile-long stretch of road were suddenly removed from the highway connecting Austin to San Antonio, EI10 could help bridge the gap, keeping traffic moving smoothly to its destination.

Similar to other energetic integrators, EI10 operates by "echoing" the impact of your hormones as your body has known them throughout your life. Present in different amounts during different stages of development, your hormones—estrogen in particular—have driven major phases of your physiological and psychological development. Your body remembers this, and the influence of those hormones on its integrated functions. This means that when your body ceases to produce estrogen, the communication pathways among the body's systems along which the hormone traveled become compromised.

When estrogen's energetic influence is suddenly diminished and the flow of energy within and among the body's twelve meridians is interrupted, EI10 can help restore it, supporting this element of the body's overall balance.

There is a lot of evidence out there showing the effectiveness of acupuncture and Chinese herbal medicine in treating hot flashes and other menopausal symptoms. As I say to all my patients, there are many potential therapies out there because it is not a one-size-fits-all process.

Essential Oils

To restore the balance of the Wisewoman, seek out essential oils that have an estrogenic effect, such as:

Clary sage	Lavender
Fennel	Neroli
Jasmine	Rose

NUTRITION

According to the US Department of Health and Human Services, the average life span for women in America is 81.2 years. With the onset of menopause now hovering near fifty-one, hundreds of thousands of women will enter into this phase during the next few years alone. Pharmaceutical companies have been and continue to be eager to profit from the "quick fix" promised by hormone replacement therapy, and for some Wisewomen, medication may be a critical aspect of the SHINES protocol. Diet, in combination with other elements of the SHINES protocol and on its own, can also have a significant impact.

Before we take a closer look at diet and the Wisewoman archetype, it is important to recall that it may be natural for your body to hold on to excess body fat (particularly abdominal fat) during this phase. There are two major reasons for this. The first is that fat aromatizes estrogen, making it available to the various organs and systems debilitated by estrogen deficiency. The second is that extra weight can help strengthen your bones. During and after menopause, estrogen deprivation puts you at a higher risk for osteoporosis, a danger your body may be trying to stave off by carrying more weight than it's accustomed to.

All this is to say that while you may feel exasperated at your body retaining a little extra fat even when you change your diet and exercise habits, it may help to remember that it is working to protect you. As I tell my patients: You know what you're eating and how your workouts are going. If you've optimized these as best you can, try not to worry about extra weight. Just keep going with an eye to feeling healthier and more balanced on every level—physically, spiritually, and emotionally.

FOODS TO EMBRACE

Soy

When it comes to balancing out estrogen deficiency, one of the foods physicians and other healthcare practitioners focus on most is soy. Rich in isoflavones, including genistein and daidzein, which the body can convert into weak forms of estrogen, soy can help elevate your estrogen levels and diminish the symptoms of deficiency. These may include everything from hot flashes to vaginal atrophy. In order for soy to exert these effects, you need to consume roughly 60 grams of soy protein per day—the equivalent of five to six glasses of soy milk.

Before we dive deeper into the various forms of soy protein and which of those I recommend, it is important to note that consuming large amounts of soy can pose a danger to women who have battled breast cancer or are at increased risk for the disease. As previously noted, even weak estrogens can bind to estrogen receptors, including those in breast tissue, and have stimulatory effects. Be aware, too, that soy is a crop that has been genetically modified, so choose your sources wisely and consume soy in moderation. If you or other women in your family have a history of breast cancer, it is best to discuss the incorporation of soy into your diet with your physician.

In addition to an increased risk of cancer, some studies have shown that soy products containing genetically modified plant material can damage the thyroid. Some of my patients have also tested positive for soy allergies. If you are concerned that you may have a soy allergy yourself, I encourage you to ask your physician to test you for it.

For all that these risks merit consideration, the most important thing to note about soy may be this: Fermented soy products are believed to pose far fewer concerns than unfermented soy, affording consumers more of the benefits and fewer of the risks. Examples of fermented soy, many of which are widely used in Asian cultures, include:

Fermented soy milk

Miso

Natto

Soy sauce

Tempeh

Examples of unfermented soy products include tofu, soy protein isolates (such as those found in bars and shake powders), edamame, soy flour, and processed foods that contain soy derivatives or soybean oil. Many of these products have become increasingly popular during the past decade.

For Wisewomen, I recommend consuming fermented soy, including fermented soy milk (which you can mix with berries and other fruits), and making sure any soy product you choose is organic in order to avoid potential hazards associated with genetically modified soybeans.

Foods Rich in Vitamin B12

Vitamin B12 (also known as cobalamin) can have a positive impact on sleep. For Wisewomen suffering from insomnia, whether due to nighttime hot flashes, a progesterone deficiency, or generalized stress or anxiety, foods rich in B12 can be a useful complement to other aspects of the SHINES protocol. Among these foods are:

Red meat, including beef, beef liver, and lamb

Fish, including salmon, mackerel, and sardines

Poultry

Eggs

Dairy products, including cheese

One important note is that acid inhibitors such as Zantac, Pepcid, and Prilosec (and their generics) can also inhibit absorption of vitamin B12. If you are taking one of these medications, you may want to eat additional portions of foods rich in B12.

Foods Containing L-Tryptophan

A precursor to melatonin, the amino acid L-tryptophan (commonly referred to simply as tryptophan) can help with sleep and with mood more generally. Related to the production of serotonin, tryptophan can help alleviate depression symptoms that can accompany the onset of menopause. Foods high in L-tryptophan that I recommend for Wisewomen include:

Turkey

Eggs

Cheese

Salmon

Soy (including fermented soy)

Spinach

Seaweed

Pineapple

In addition to these foods, the familiar rule that a glass of warm milk can help you fall asleep may actually hold true. Many Wisewomen I've counseled have told me that late-night mugs of warm milk have been helpful both for the tryptophan they contain and the ritual that accompanies their preparation.

For patients who can't drink milk, I recommend a good old-fashioned mug of chamomile tea. Back in the day when I was a youngster, my grandmother used to think three things cured everything: a good bowel movement, Vicks, and chamomile tea. Her tea was made from bulk chamomile flowers that she would steep herself, and I remember that tea used to make me feel like the world was a better place.

Although chamomile tea does not contain tryptophan, it has soothing properties all its own that can also help decrease general restlessness and insomnia. I take this note from my patients and my grandmother, who brewed whole chamomile flowers into tea for me to drink as a cure for everything from my upset stomach to my hyperactivity. If chamomile tea is unappealing, hops-valerian tea is another option.

Foods Containing High Levels of Omega-3 Fatty Acids

During the past several years, I've been pleased to see a medical and cultural shift away from fat-restrictive diets and back toward diets containing "good fats," including omega-3 unsaturated fatty acids. These have been shown to help support cardiovascular health, stabilize blood sugar levels, boost immunity, and improve mood, among other benefits. For the Wisewoman, consuming 2 grams of omega-3 fatty acids daily can help reduce menopause-related symptoms, including hot flashes and vaginal dryness as well as hypertriglyceridemia, joint pain, depression, and osteoporosis.

Known as "essential" fatty acids because the body does not produce them on its own, the omega-3 fatty acids ALA (alpha-linolenic acid), DHA (docosahexaenoic acid), and EPA (eicosapentaenoic acid) are found primarily in seafood, sea vegetables, some nuts and seeds, and grass-fed meat. For the Wisewoman, I recommend consuming 2 grams (2,000 mg) of omega-3 fatty acids per day, with as much as possible coming from food sources. Among the best of these sources are:

FISH
Wild-caught salmon (and salmon oil) and tuna
White fish, including herring and mackerel
Sardines and anchovies
Cod liver oil

NUTS, SEEDS, AND OILS
Walnuts, Brazil nuts, cashews, hazelnuts,
  butternuts (white walnuts)

Flaxseeds (and flaxseed oil—see page 301), hemp
   seeds, chia seeds
Coconut oil
Fish oil (see page 301)

VEGETABLES
Brussels sprouts
Kale, spinach, watercress
Seaweed, algae
Algal oil (vegetarian)

ADDITIONAL SOURCES
Natto
Egg yolks

Regardless of whether you are actively trying to lose weight, lean protein sources are an important element of the Wisewoman's diet. Even for women who are relatively thin, maintaining a healthy body mass index (BMI) of 18.5 to 24.9 is particularly important during and after menopause. (BMI has come under some intense scrutiny, but using it as a general guide is a good place to start.) But substituting healthy lean proteins for those containing saturated fat and avoiding processed carbohydrates and refined sugars can be a healthy counterbalance.

WATER

For the Wisewoman, remaining sufficiently hydrated is important. Dehydration can worsen the decreased vaginal lubrication associated with estrogen deficiency, as well as general skin thinning and wrinkling, so ensure that you drink *2 to 3 liters of water per day*.

The question is, how much is "enough"? When it comes to making these recommendations, I tend to be conservative. I don't encourage my patients to wander around with gallon jugs of spring water, forcing themselves to constantly drink it. I simply advise them to try to drink eight 8-ounce glasses each day, and to increase this amount if they intensify their workout regimens or routinely experience excessive sweating.

Remember, too, that we get water from a variety of sources, including the food we eat. The key is to remain mindful of the potential for dehydration and its negative effects, and to substitute water for juice or soda whenever possible.

DARK CHOCOLATE

Dark chocolate (at least 70 percent pure cacao) can yield a series of benefits for the Wisewoman. Researchers at institutions including the Cleveland Clinic and the American Cancer Society have found that when consumed in moderation, dark chocolate can help boost your mood, improve your cardiovascular health by lowering your blood pressure and improving circulation, and help protect all your body's systems from potentially disease-causing free radicals.[24] These potential benefits arise out of the antioxidant effects of the flavanols found in the chocolate. At roughly 170 calories an ounce, dark chocolate contains 2.2 grams of protein and 3.1 grams of fiber, as well as significant amounts of iron and magnesium.

Antidepressant Medications, Menopause, and Weight

Sometimes, a Wisewoman may choose to take an antidepressant to help combat not only depression, but also the physiological symptoms of menopause, including hot flashes and night sweats. This is particularly common among women for whom estrogen replacement therapy is not a viable option. Examples of popular antidepressant medications include venlafaxine (Effexor), fluoxetine (Prozac), sertraline (Zoloft), paroxetine (Paxil), desvenlafaxine (Pristiq), and citalopram (Celexa).

Any antidepressant may affect your appetite, and weight gain can be a side effect of taking almost any of them. Amitriptyline (Elavil) is an example of a tricyclic antidepressant that has been known to produce larger increases in weight gain than others. There are other antidepressants and antianxiety medications that have reported weight loss rather than weight gain, like Wellbutrin.

If you're interested in antidepressant therapy, certainly discuss this with your physician. Consider your options and be aware of all the potential side effects, including weight gain and decreased libido. Consider also how an antidepressant will integrate into your SHINES protocol and complement its other aspects.

FOODS TO AVOID

Caffeine

Across the board, I recommend that Wisewomen try to avoid caffeine or at least decrease the amount they consume. Data indicates that caffeine can contribute to an increased frequency in hot flashes and night sweats. Caffeine can make a poor night's sleep that much worse, especially when it's consumed after three o'clock in the afternoon.

Some studies indicate that caffeine consumption can also worsen symptoms of menopause, including anxiety, mood swings, and even bone loss.[25]

Alcohol

I also encourage Wisewomen to reduce their alcohol intake. Alcohol is a natural vasodilator and therefore a potential contributor to hot flashes and night sweats, and has also been shown to impair rapid eye movement (REM) sleep cycles. As with caffeine, consuming alcohol later in the day can worsen its impact. Studies have shown that having a high glycemic index four hours before bedtime can prolong the onset of sleep.

Taking Control

The guidelines contained in this section can go some distance to helping you plan out your daily meals and routines. I hope they also encourage you to try foods that perhaps you haven't before. Taking the time to investigate and explore new options can be a type of spiritual practice in its own right—a way to honor your changing body's needs to serve your larger life.

You may want to consult with a nutritionist who can help tailor your new diet to suit your lifestyle. Your physician may also be helpful. Recently, I counseled Sylvia, a fifty-five-year-old patient who was seeking help to alleviate a series of menopause-related symptoms, including insomnia, severe fluctuations in mood, hot flashes, night sweats, and decreased libido. Given Sylvia's family history of breast cancer, I was reluctant to prescribe hormone therapy, so she and I focused on the other elements of the SHINES protocol, including nutrition. Sylvia was relatively thin, but had a BMI over 40, so I knew she would benefit from incorporating nutrient-rich lean protein sources into her daily routine.

We landed on a diet of 2,000 to 2,500 calories per day that incorporated cold-water fish, fermented soy products (including tempeh and soy milk powder, which I recommended she mix with berries to make it more palatable), and five daily servings of different-colored fresh fruits and vegetables. I also recommended that she consume at least 30 mg of fiber per day to help decrease her estrone levels, protecting her against the hormone's potentially carcinogenic effects.

EXERCISE

For the Wisewoman, exercise is critical to help maintain or improve her cardiovascular health and overall body composition, but also to help strengthen her bones and protect her major joints. For this reason, weight-bearing exercise that helps increase muscle mass and preserve joint health should be at the center of a Wisewoman's workout regimen.

This is not to say that cardio will not play any role. But consider two images: one of a marathon runner and one of a short-distance sprinter. The marathon runner is likely to be very thin, her body burning fat and catabolizing muscle as it struggles to keep up with its daily functioning and the extreme demands of her training (see page 120 for a refresher on catabolism). The sprinter, on the other hand, is likely to be far more muscular. Even if her training regimen causes her body to burn fat, keeping her BMI low, the short, intense bursts of speed also help her body build muscle. This occurs particularly in her legs, but also in her arms and abdomen and elsewhere throughout her body. The sprinter is very likely to have stronger bones than the marathon runner, given the stress her muscular frame continuously places on them. For the Wisewoman, weight-bearing exercise that supports and sustains muscle mass will go the longest distance toward helping her maintain her overall physical health in the long term.

This is why I advise Wisewomen to avoid extreme workouts and instead follow a simple, intuitive rule: Keep it primal. Just as I recommend eating primarily what you could grow, pick, or kill, I borrow from longtime extreme fitness trainer Mark Sisson's work, covered in his book *Primal Endurance*, which describes the major pillars of ideal exercise goals and routines: Move around a lot at a slow pace, lift heavy things (but not too heavy), and run really fast every once in a while.

The first, as Sisson describes, is to "move around a lot at a slow pace." This is what our ancestors did as they hunted and gathered and scouted out new terrain. They did this without ever worrying about keeping their heart rate at 80 percent of its maximum for a period of time. They may have walked 8 miles each day, but we can safely assume they didn't run 26.2. And neither, I submit, should you.

The second is to "lift heavy things." Again, our ancestors were forced to do this for survival. Whether they were carrying children, weapons, firewood, or animal carcasses, using their bodies as means of transporting essentials was unavoidable. Using their muscles in this way helped promote muscle regeneration and growth. We may compare this to modern-day weight-bearing exercise, including those forms that rely on body weight alone, such as lunges and squats.

The last is to "run really fast every once in a while" in the manner of hunters and gatherers who occasionally had to sprint to catch their prey or avoid being someone else's. As we discussed, sprinters are far more likely to have the kind of healthy muscles that are ideal for the Wisewoman, whose bones need strength and density. Like weight-bearing exercise, exerting your muscles to an "extreme" degree not for hours but merely seconds at a time can help promote regeneration and growth.

The bottom line is this: If your goal is to live a longer, healthier life, don't damage your body with exercise. Don't stress your body any more than you must. Support your body's natural tendency to regenerate, rebuild, and repair. Avoid driving it to cannibalize itself.

YOGA

Yoga is the ultimate body-weight workout, helping to promote muscle strength, balance, and overall alignment among all the body's systems. For the Wisewoman, the elements of improved muscle tone, joint health, and balance are particularly important during and after menopause. When guided by a properly qualified instructor, yoga is a relatively safe form of exercise. It also enables you to go at your own pace, physically challenging yourself more or less according to your body's needs and your inclinations.

Hot yoga (also known as Bikram yoga) in particular can be a valuable and significant spiritual practice. But any type of yoga, whether practiced in a heated room or not, can provide the critical physiological benefits described here. At Glo.com, you will find thousands of classes based in different styles, some of which are more physically demanding than others. You may find that a few or more of these classes are suited to your goals and abilities.

ISOMETRICS AND RESISTANCE EXERCISES

Isometrics are a low-impact *and* highly effective way of toning your muscles. They moderately elevate your heart rate, increase your blood flow, and burn calories. Even football great Herschel Walker has claimed that he always eschewed weight lifting in favor of doing thousands of sit-ups and push-ups each day. Add lunges and squats to a few rounds of these, and over time, you will begin to see the difference they can make.

You may also want to consider light resistance exercises, such as those that use resistance bands or light weights.

CARDIO AND SHORT-BURST EXERCISE

For the Wisewoman, I recommend *some* cardiovascular activity to help burn fat and improve cardiovascular health. But as we've discussed, I do not recommend excessive or extreme workouts that have you running the risk of burning muscle along with fat.

Some options you may consider are biking, either on your own or at the gym on a stationary bike, walking at a brisk pace, and swimming. Depending on the intensity of the exercise, an effective session may last between 10 and 30 minutes or slightly longer.

As for short-burst exercises, doing the equivalent of short sprints as part of a circuit or walking or swimming session can give your routine—and your mood—a little boost.

ADDITIONAL RECOMMENDATIONS

The first of these comes from my own experience. As I write this, I'm thinking about the Peloton indoor exercise bike that recently arrived at my house and the nervousness that takes over when I imagine trying to keep pace with the New York City spin class that is live streamed onto its video screen. Although I'm not in menopause and will never experience its equivalent, I am still a man of a certain age, and I need to accept that doing what I can to keep up with the hard-bodies for 15 to 20 minutes may be all I can do—and may also be what's best for my body. I know it will be a mental struggle, with my brain insisting I should be able to keep up with the class for the duration. This is where my hard-earned wisdom comes in and saves me from myself.

Your wisdom can do the same for you, reminding you that depending on your age, your body may not be able to do what it could when you were twenty-five. With each decade, injuries become more likely and recovering from them takes longer, so let one of the things you've learned in your life be that it's okay to start slow. Remember also that you always need to keep your long-term goals of muscle, bone, and joint health in mind.

My second recommendation is that you find a guide. Whether a knowledgeable physician or a personal trainer, find someone to help get you started by recommending appropriate cardio, isometric, and/or weight-bearing exercises and teaching you how to use any relevant tools or equipment. They can also help you track your overall progress and suggest modifications to your workouts as improvements in your physical and emotional health take hold.

SUPPLEMENTS

I recommend that Wisewomen try a few specific supplements. Before you do, however, I strongly encourage you to consult a physician, nutritionist, or healthcare provider who has sufficient experience with supplements to help you decide which—if any—are right for you, and how much of any given supplement you should plan on taking for how long. This healthcare professional can also help you steer clear of potentially problematic interactions between supplements and/or any other medications you may be taking.

MACA

Maca, an herb indigenous to Peru, has long been used to promote and protect hormone balance (in men and women), and in certain permutations, it can help reduce the intensity of menopausal symptoms. Each of the thirteen differently colored varieties of maca exerts distinct effects, and many maca-based supplements combine different varieties of the herb.

For the Wisewoman, I recommend a particular formulation of maca called Femmenessence MacaPause. Created specifically for women in menopause, MacaPause contains significant concentrations of highly bioavailable maca and helps decrease a series of menopausal symptoms that includes hot flashes, night sweats, decreased libido, vaginal dryness, and occasional insomnia. MacaPause has also been shown to support bone and heart health, two factors that Wisewomen must always consider. I recommend the standard dose: two capsules twice daily, taken away from meals. Take the first dose in the morning, before breakfast, and the second dose in the early evening, ideally 30 minutes before you normally experience an energy low. (For women who are more sensitive to higher clinical dosages, consider **taking just one** capsule in the morning and one in the early evening.)

All maca products can cause some level of gastrointestinal distress because they contain fiber. If you decide to give maca a try, I recommend starting off slow in order to give your system time to acclimate to it. Consider taking half the recommended dose for two weeks, then gradually raising this amount. You may find that your symptoms abate when you take less than the full dose. Assuming your system tolerates the maca well, I suggest continuing to take the supplement at the near full or full dose for four to six weeks in order to give yourself enough time to determine whether it is having the intended positive effect.

Two notes of **caution** with regard to MacaPause: First, I recommend that a Wisewoman take this supplement for two to three months and then take a week off. This can help upregulate your estrogen receptors and enhance the supplement's benefits. Second, MacaPause can amplify the effects of caffeine. So while a Wisewoman is always wise to limit or avoid caffeine, taking extra caution around caffeine when taking this supplement is a good idea.

Other maca-based products include a series of blended powders, capsules, and extracts. When considering alternatives, it is important to ascertain the level of "pregelatinized" (bioavailable) maca it contains, and if other ingredients have been blended in. Some of these added ingredients may negatively interact with other supplements or medications you are taking, so again, plan on seeking advice from your physician, nutritionist, or other healthcare provider before you incorporate maca into your SHINES protocol.

BLACK COHOSH

The second supplement I recommend for the Wisewoman is black cohosh, a flowering plant also known as black bugbane and fairy candle, among other names. The roots and rhizomes of the plant are used for medicinal purposes, and black cohosh is widely considered a safe and effective alternative to estrogen replacement therapy for the treatment of menopausal symptoms, including hot flashes, night sweats, and insomnia. There has, however, been some concern among scientists and healthcare providers that black cohosh may contain phytoestrogens; research into this has been inconclusive. Although no definitive link between black cohosh and an increased risk of breast cancer has been discovered, if you or your family members have a history of breast cancer, I certainly advise you to discuss this with your healthcare provider before starting this supplement.

There are several black cohosh supplements on the market. These come in capsule, tablet, liquid tincture, and extract forms. A product I often recommend to patients is called Oona. Containing both black cohosh and vitex (chasteberry), Oona helps reduce the frequency and intensity of hot flashes, night sweats, interrupted sleep, and moderate mood swings.

One note of caution: Black cohosh can have a negative impact on liver function. If you suffer from hepatitis or cirrhosis of the liver, avoid any herbal supplement containing black cohosh.

FLAXSEED, FLAXSEED OIL, AND FISH OILS

As we discussed in the Nutrition section (page 286), flaxseed, flaxseed oil, and fish oil are all good sources of omega-3 essential fatty acids, and each has its own benefits, including improved heart health and cognitive functioning.

You may take flaxseed in one of two ways. The first is to eat the seeds themselves. But eating them whole won't help. Your body cannot digest the shell, which means that unless you grind up the seeds to release their oil, you won't get what you need. Once the seeds are ground, your body can digest the fiber. I recommend that patients add ground flaxseed to their smoothies or salad dressings.

There are several flaxseed oil options available on the market;

these come in both lignan (fiber)-free and lignan-rich varieties, and in capsule and pourable-oil forms. I recommend oil over capsules for simplicity. In order to ingest the recommended tablespoon per day, you would need to take between ten and fifteen capsules. Adding the oil to a shake, smoothie, or dressing is easier—and more appealing. You may also take the oil directly, though it does have a bit of a grassy taste.

Taking pure flaxseed oil can give you the recommended amount of omega-3 fatty acids each day. But for Wisewomen, I recommend Udo's Oil Omega 3-6-9 Blend, which contains the recommended amounts of both omega-3s and omega-6s. Created by Dr. Udo Erasmus, author of the widely popular 1993 book *Fats that Heal, Fats that Kill*, this supplement combines fresh flax, sesame, and sunflower seeds with oils from evening primrose, rice germ, oat germ, and coconut to create an ideally balanced mix of omega-3 and omega-6 fatty acids.

Fish oil is another option for Wisewomen who are looking to increase their intake of omega-3. Although this is a good option for women who don't want to incorporate fish into their diets, the most common complaint I hear is that once the capsules are in the stomach, they can release a fishy odor you can taste. To mitigate this, I recommend freezing the capsules. This way, the oil will not be thawed until it has passed through your upper digestive system. I also recommend patients choose a brand called Nordic Naturals. Flavored with lemon, the oil inside these capsules emits a more pleasant aroma.

An alternative to fish oil is krill oil. Made from the tiny crustaceans that comprise most of a whale's diet, krill oil has less of an aftertaste than traditional fish oil and is also more environmentally sustainable. (Only 1 percent of the world's total supply of krill are utilized for oil extraction each year.) Adding to this, krill oil contains an antioxidant called astaxanthin, which prevents the oil from spoiling when stored in your cupboard.

Two important recommendations regarding flaxseed oil, fish oil, and others:

1. With the exception of krill oil, I recommend purchasing only *refrigerated* products. Oils can become rancid, and because they are contained in capsules (or shells, in the case of flaxseed), you will not know. Look for products with expiration dates that are one to two months from the date of purchase.

2. Be mindful that your liver is responsible for processing these oils and that they may cause GI upset, including dyspepsia and diarrhea. Start slow, taking less than the recommended dose in order to give your body a chance to gradually adjust.

CALCIUM AND VITAMIN D

Calcium and vitamin D are important supplements for maintaining bone health and density. But Wisewomen need to be wary of taking too high a dose of either.

In the past, physicians recommended daily doses of calcium as high as 1,200 mg. For the Wisewoman who is at an elevated risk for kidney stones, however, this can be too much. I recommend 600 to 800 mg per day of calcium, with a maximum dose of 1,000 mg.

As for vitamin D, taking too much can result in vitamin D toxicity, symptoms of which include hypercalcemia (a buildup of calcium in the blood), nausea, vomiting, frequent urination, and diminished kidney function. Reaching toxic levels requires taking roughly ten times the dose I recommend, which is 5,000 IU per day. But when my patients are taking vitamin D, I closely monitor their levels. Should you and your physician or healthcare provider decide that a vitamin D supplement is right for you, make sure they closely monitor your levels at this dosage. (A more standard dosage is 1,000 IU per day.)

ST. JOHN'S WORT

Used around the world to treat a variety of medical conditions, in the United States St. John's wort is most commonly used to treat mild to moderate depression, including menopause-related depression. Although research into its efficacy has yielded mixed findings, some studies have shown that a St. John's wort supplement may be as effective as certain tricyclic antidepressants and selective serotonin reuptake inhibitors (SSRIs).[26]

As with any supplement, it is critical that you consult with a physician, naturopath, nutritionist, or other knowledgeable healthcare practitioner before you begin taking St. John's wort. It may interact or interfere with medications or other supplements, which can have a deleterious impact on your physiological or psychological health. The supplement can have negative side effects of its own as well, including anxiety, interrupted sleep, and GI distress. Again, close monitoring is key.

DHEA (AND VAGINAL DHEA)

Known as the "hormone of youth" because its levels of production drop off after we turn thirty, DHEA (dehydroepiandrosterone) is a hormone produced by the adrenal glands that can convert into estrogen and testosterone. Men and women may benefit from a DHEA supplement in different ways. For the Wisewoman, DHEA capsules may alleviate menopausal symptoms, including hot flashes, vaginal dryness, and weight gain. Exerting both androgenic and estrogenic effects, it may also increase your libido. DHEA's estrogenic effects mean, however, that women with a personal or family history of breast cancer must discuss the relevant risks with their healthcare provider.

For the Wisewoman who decides that DHEA is right for her, I recommend a dose of 10 to 25 mg per day. In addition to its capsule formulation, DHEA comes in the form of a vaginal cream. Applied directly, it can help with lubrication in the short term, as well as vaginal dryness and other symptoms of vaginal atrophy in the longer term. The dosage in this form typically is around 6.75 mg. As with the capsule formation, I strongly encourage you to consult your healthcare provider before using a DHEA cream.

BOOK RECOMMENDATIONS FOR WISEWOMEN

Christiane Northrup, MD, *Women's Bodies, Women's Wisdom* (New York: Bantam, 2010)

Mache Seibel, MD, *The Estrogen Window: The Breakthrough Guide to Being Healthy, Energized, and Hormonally Balanced—Through Perimenopause, Menopause, and Beyond* (New York: Rodale, 2016)

WISEWOMEN

Dr. Maya Angelou (April 4, 1928–May 28, 2014). Raised in Missouri, Arkansas, and California, Maya Angelou was an author, poet, and civil rights activist. Best known for her works of autobiographical fiction, including *I Know Why the Caged Bird Sings* (1969), which received international acclaim, Angelou was also awarded a Pulitzer Prize, three Grammy Awards, and, in 2011, the Presidential Medal of Freedom.

Jane Goodall (b. April 3, 1934). Jane Goodall set out to Tanzania in 1960 to study wild chimpanzees. She immersed herself in their lives, bypassing more rigid procedures to make discoveries about primate behavior that have continued to shape scientific discourse. A highly respected member of the world scientific community, she advocates for ecological preservation through the Jane Goodall Institute.

Margaret Thatcher (October 13, 1935–April 8, 2013). British politician who served as prime minister of the United Kingdom from

1979 to 1990. Commonly known as the "Iron Lady," Thatcher was the first woman to lead a major political party (the Conservative Party) in the United Kingdom, and is widely regarded as one of the most influential statespeople in British history. Although she came under fire for her economic policies, which supported deregulation and privatization, during the early 1990s, Thatcher also called for NATO to crush the Serbian assaults on Bosnia and Herzegovina, comparing these to the "worst excesses of the Nazis." As a child, Thatcher had saved her allowance to help fund the journey of a Jewish teenage girl whom Thatcher's family was helping escape from Nazi Germany. In her memoirs, Thatcher described this event as among the most significant of her formative years.

The SHINES Protocol: How Do You Slow Down a Workaholic?

For the Workaholic, the purpose of the SHINES method is to help bring cortisol levels back into balance by reducing levels of psychological and physical stress and improving the ratios of cortisol to other hormones. The Workaholic's SHINES protocol also focuses on ensuring that your body receives the nutrients and other physical support it needs so that during the process of bringing your cortisol levels back into balance, you are less and less susceptible to the negative effects of cortisol-driven catabolic processes (see page 120 for more on catabolism).

SPIRITUAL PRACTICE

At the center of the Workaholic's spiritual practice is learning to slow down. Experience with this archetype has taught me that this can be difficult for Workaholics to do. For you, who is hardworking, successful, and driven in various aspects of your life, the idea of slowing down can inspire fear. It can be daunting for you to forgo certain tasks and slow the pace at which you do others, and to take time out to focus exclusively on your physical and emotional well-being. But this is the critical spiritual aspect of your journey toward balance. An essential part of this is controlling your surroundings and learning how to create space for your health.

PRACTICING DETACHMENT

To detach is to remove yourself, even for minutes at a time, from all that comprises your daily routines. This includes people and technological devices alike. Detaching means finding a quiet space in which you can be alone, without your phone, and practicing simply *being* with yourself in that space. Here, in the absence of any background noise or external demands, you can observe what is happening in your body and mind without rushing to adjust, fix, or avoid it. Spending even a few moments in detachment helps you achieve a clearer understanding of the impact of the various sources of stress you're under and can inspire you to take steps toward meaningful self-care.

It can also help you on a physical level. When you are in this space, be conscious of your breath. Breathing deeply and deliberately expands your chest, stimulating the vagus nerve and the parasympathetic nervous system, calming you down. This lowers your blood pressure and slows your heart rate, interrupting the relentless physical and emotional stress Workaholics tend to endure every day.

Emerging from this space can be equally instructive: You will find that the world is still there, awaiting your return.

This is not to say that detachment comes easily. Workaholics can tend to equate detachment with nothingness. And nothingness can seem frightening. But as James S. Gordon, psychiatrist, author, and founder of the Center for Mind-Body Medicine, has explained, while we're all worrying about making sure our cups—our lives—are as full as possible, we would do well to learn to empty them. If we did this, Gordon contends, we would be better at appreciating their contents.

Over time, you may build up to detaching for longer and longer periods, from two minutes to ten to sixty. But to begin, choose a place where you know you will be comfortable and undisturbed, leave all potential distractions behind, and simply *try*. If you find the silence itself too distracting, you may consider using a guided meditation (provided you remain out of reach of phone calls and texts). Deepak Chopra and Tara Brach both offer series of free guided meditations on their websites.[27]

PRACTICING FORGIVENESS

In my own experience and in my clinical practice, I have found that underlying the drive to work harder and harder can be a resistance to face certain issues in our lives, including internal and interpersonal emotional conflicts. For the Workaholic, practicing forgiveness can be both spiritually healing and fortifying in itself, and a way of diminishing the drive to maintain a grueling schedule and lifestyle more generally.

The act of forgiveness is one you need to show yourself as well as others—and it is possible that neither will come easily. Whether this involves letting go of expectations, regrets, or past insults or injuries, deliberately freeing yourself of anger, resentment, and fear can alleviate the psychological stress that can contribute to sustained high levels of cortisol.

EMBRACING UNCERTAINTY

In my experience treating Workaholics, I have found that a prevailing characteristic of this archetype is the desire to *control*. Whether it applies to circumstances, outcomes, or other people, the desire to control can be pervasive and can add to the stress of a Workaholic's daily life.

Letting go of this desire or need for control and embracing uncertainty can have healing effects for the Workaholic. An exercise I recommend comes from my friend and author Dr. Gabrielle Pelicci. It's simple: Whenever you are clinging to a need to control a given situation or outcome, ask yourself, "What's the worst that will happen if it doesn't go my way?" If you don't make a deadline at work, or if you don't get that promotion, or if you don't lose 10 pounds by Christmas? Consider these possibilities and then ask yourself—really ask yourself—what's the *worst* that will happen? Maybe your boss or client will be annoyed. Maybe you won't get that raise. Maybe your clothes will still fit the way they do now. The point is, unless you're dealing with a clear and present life-threatening danger, chances are you're going to be okay, no matter whether the situation goes exactly your way.

Consistently acknowledging that you are not, in general, in life-threatening situations can be a healing and supportive exercise in itself. Over time, confidently embracing uncertainty can decrease the likelihood that you will experience fight-or-flight responses and can help reduce your body's cortisol production.

AROMATHERAPY

Studies have shown that aromatherapy can help reduce cortisol levels.[28] One way of administering this is via certain essential oils, the scents of which are believed to have various health benefits, including improved cardiac health, mood, and skin health. Among the essential oils I recommend for the Workaholic are balsam fir, ylang-ylang, lavender, neroli, and marjoram. You can add any of these oils to bathwater, apply them directly to your skin, or warm them, releasing the scent into your surroundings.

An alternative to essential oils is scents that elicit good memories. Although I recommend this in particular for the Workaholic, this form of aromatherapy can provide a pleasant, calming experience for any of us. I use it myself. One of my favorite smells is that of Sedona, Arizona. Each year, I travel there with my family. We disconnect as soon as we arrive, removing ourselves from school and work and the internet, and we spend our time relaxing and enjoying each other's company. Sedona has a distinct smell to it—a mix of pine trees, manzanita, and the desert's red dirt—that balsam fir oil approximates. When I warm the oil, the smell takes me to Sedona. Even if only for a moment, I am transported, and I experience the calm I know so well there.

Perhaps there is a smell that can do this for you. It could be food, or a certain flower, or a particular perfume. Whatever it may be, the critical aspect is that taking a deep breath of it leads you to reexperience a pleasant moment in your life, taking you there for an instant and inspiring the calm and happiness you knew then.

HORMONE MODULATION

There are no medicinal hormone treatments that lower your cortisol, per se. However, there are certain hormone-based treatments that can help balance out your levels of cortisol relative to other hormones—in particular, DHEA and estrogen. Improving the ratios of cortisol to each of these hormones can, together with the other aspects of the SHINES protocol, help alleviate the symptoms of cortisol excess.

DHEA

DHEA (dehydroepiandrosterone) is an androgenic hormone—a precursor to both testosterone and estrogen—that has the ability to offset the effects of cortisol. Where cortisol has catabolic effects, often breaking down the body's tissues, DHEA has anabolic, or building, effects. Studies have shown that DHEA can increase the body's ability to transform food into energy, burn off excess fat, and reduce inflammation throughout the body, which can help stave off chronic diseases, including heart disease and certain types of cancer. DHEA's anabolic effects also help improve bone density, muscle mass, and skin quality, offsetting cortisol's destruction of these tissues. Often referred to as "the fountain of youth," DHEA peaks in your twenties and declines with age.

When I test patients' cortisol levels, I also look at their DHEA. If this is low, or on the low side of "normal," I often recommend incorporating a DHEA supplement into their treatment protocol. DHEA supplements are available over the counter and are made from either soy or wild yam. I start with a dosage of 10 to 25 mg.

In some cases, however, a Workaholic's DHEA levels may already be elevated, her body having increased production of the hormone in response to her high cortisol. In these instances, supplementing with DHEA is not advisable.

ESTROGEN AND PROGESTERONE

I also test patients' estrogen levels when assessing them for cortisol excess. If you're a Workaholic who is also estrogen dominant (a Queen archetype), you may benefit from a supplement of diindolylmethane (DIM) or indole-3-carbinol (I3C). These supplements, like the cruciferous vegetables from which they're derived, can help break estrogen down into its healthy metabolites and minimize the effects of estrogen dominance, including severe PMS or PMDD. (For more on these supplements and the impact of cruciferous vegetables on estrogen dominance, see the section on the Queen archetype, page 226.)

Workaholics can also benefit from increased progesterone. As noted, progesterone exerts an overarching calming effect on the body. In particular, progesterone helps with sleep, which can aid in lowering cortisol all on its own. Increasing progesterone levels can also help diminish symptoms of estrogen dominance.

In the final analysis, the hormonal modulation element of the Workaholic's SHINES protocol focuses not only on cortisol, but also on the hormones that influence and are influenced by it. Hormones are highly integrated and interactive. This is why an assessment of cortisol excess requires a comprehensive look at your various hormone levels and cross-archetype symptomology. This can help guide both the hormonal modulation and remaining aspects of your SHINES protocol.

INFOCEUTICALS

For the Workaholic, Energetic Integrator 9 (EI9) is what I recommend to help restore equilibrium to the archetype's disrupted energy fields. EI9 operates along the "triple warmer meridian," which begins at the tip of the ring finger and runs up through the wrist, forearm, and shoulder before entering the pericardium (the sac that surrounds the heart), rising up to the collarbone, and looping around to the back of the ear. EI9 affects all the body's major cavities, including the cranium, thorax, abdomen, and pelvis. It also helps to maintain the body's thermal equilibrium, which in the Workaholic can be thrown off by cortisol's power to keep the body in fight-or-flight mode, constantly generating heat.

EI9 also addresses energetic disturbances associated with other adrenal-overload-related conditions, including thyroid disorders, postpartum depression, and autoimmune diseases such as fibromyalgia.

Energetically, the Workaholic needs to learn one simple word: NO. The Workaholic is the way they are because they always say yes, both internally and externally. They are a product of their own dreams and desires and the desires of those around them. Learning to say NO now may save you from more problems in the future.

ESSENTIAL OILS

Those who push the envelope and don't sleep may find that their cortisol levels have crept up, and coupled with the inherit high cortisol levels from times of high stress, we want to introduce some essential oils that will possibly lower levels and induce relaxation. I suggest trying the following:

Frankincense	Myrrh
Lavender	Patchouli
Lemongrass	Vetiver

NUTRITION

For the Workaholic, the nutrition element of the SHINES protocol centers on foods that can help the body rebuild from the catabolic effects of cortisol excess. Workaholics who have been keeping up with relentless schedules and sleeplessness *and* whose bodies have long been catabolizing muscle and collagen need to avoid sugar and carbohydrates (for a refresher on catabolism, see page 120). Workaholics need to turn to nutritionally valuable foods to help restore their physical health and bring their cortisol and other hormones back into balance.

In addition to committing to a diet of certain foods, it can also benefit the Workaholic to practice mindfulness around eating. In any given moment, whether you're preparing or consuming meat, vegetables, or fruit, think about the substance itself. Think about the animal, pausing for a moment to consider its life and sacrifice. Consider the seed that grew into the fruit or vegetable you're holding: Think about where it came from, who planted it, who tended to it and harvested it.

This simple act of slowing down and considering what's in front of you can be a meditation in itself and help you be more thoughtful about the fuel your body is running on.

FOODS TO EMBRACE

Lean Proteins

Workaholics whose bodies have burned through their sugar-based energy reserves and begun breaking down tissues to sustain their constant activity need to consume higher amounts of protein than many of the other archetypes. In general, I recommend between 0.5 and 1 g of protein per pound of body weight per day, depending on your level of physical activity. If your daily life is hectic and your sleep is poor, but you do not exercise regularly, this number should be closer to 0.5 g; if you work out, it should be closer to 1 g. Good sources of lean protein for the Workaholic include:

Fish, including salmon and tuna
Lean meats, including ground beef and pork loin
Eggs
Low-fat or nonfat dairy products, including milk, yogurt, and cottage cheese
Beans and lentils
Nuts and nut butters
Seeds
Protein powders, such as vegan pea, rice, or powdered peanut options

Healthy Fats

Healthy fats—omega-3 and omega-6 monounsaturated and poly-unsaturated fats—can be a great source of energy for the Workaholic. In a catabolic state, the body can break these down rather than muscle or collagen. Healthy fats have also been shown to decrease inflammation, which excess cortisol tends to cause, as well as being good fuel for the brain. Broken down into ketone bodies, the brain's preferred fuel source, healthy fats can help with memory and mental clarity.

Good sources of healthy fats include:

OILS

Coconut oil

Olive oil

Oil blends, including Udo's Oil Omega 3-6-9 Blend,
  a mixture of omega-3, -6, and -9 fatty acids

NUTS AND SEEDS

Walnuts, almonds, and pistachios

Nut and seed butters, including almond, cashew,
  and sunflower seed

Flaxseed

Sunflower seeds

Chia seeds

OTHER FOOD SOURCES

Avocados

Olives

Fish, including salmon and tuna

Tofu

Eggs

Healthier skin is a good indication that you are ingesting sufficient amounts of these healthy fats. The largest organ in your body, your skin, is also among the last to receive nutrients. If your diet does not contain sufficient amounts of healthy fats, your skin will likely be dry and flaky. The more of these fats you consume and that do their part to help protect your tissues from destructive catabolic processes, the healthier your heart, liver, and muscles will be, the more functional your body will begin to be overall, and the more pliable and faster-healing it can become.

Fruits and Vegetables

Various fruits and vegetables contain nutrients that can benefit the Workaholic. The best are those that contain relatively low amounts of sugar. Although any fruit or vegetable is preferable to packaged food filled with processed sugar, I encourage the Workaholics I consult with to seek out cruciferous vegetables that are low in sugar and high in fiber and antioxidants, such as broccoli and Brussels sprouts, as well as fruits that are lower in sugar and higher in fiber, such as grapefruit.

FOODS TO AVOID

A common problem among Workaholics is a dependency on caffeine. This increases cortisol production, raises your heart rate, and drives up your blood pressure. Caffeine also escalates diuresis, which leaves you chronically dehydrated. In addition to causing headaches, long-term dehydration can also weaken the skin and other tissues.

While I do not insist that Workaholics give up their coffee or tea altogether, I do recommend decreasing your caffeine intake over time or mixing up your coffee routine with some lower-caffeine options like green tea or matcha. Be careful not to replace caffeine with sugar. As your cortisol-excess-related symptoms gradually abate in response to the various elements of the SHINES protocol you've put into practice, you are likely to feel less and less dependent on caffeine. This will make substituting lower-caffeine or caffeine-free options that much easier.

EXERCISE

At first, it may seem counterintuitive to discuss the benefits of exercise for the Workaholic. After all, exercise increases cortisol levels. Exercise is also a form of stress in itself, and *lowering* a Workaholic's stress levels is central to this archetype's SHINES protocol. Even with all this, however, exercise can yield physiological and psychological benefits for women seeking to bring their cortisol levels into balance.

When it comes to physical exercise, the key for the Workaholic is moderation. As I tell my patients, as frustrated as you might feel by the few extra pounds you're carrying, do *not* overdo it. Do not try to force yourself to do high-intensity workouts that burn a thousand calories or more. Do not run five miles a day or force yourself to work out for hours at a stretch. For the Workaholic, I recommend exercising for 30 to 40 minutes, and to think of these workouts as a means to relieve and repair your body—a way to strengthen the muscles, bones, and other tissues that have been under attack.

Another note about exercise for the Workaholic: Try to do it during the morning hours. For most of us, our cortisol peaks in the afternoon or early evening, and exercising will raise it even more. Elevated levels of cortisol late in the afternoon or evening can contribute to difficulties falling asleep and staying asleep, and as we've discussed, getting enough sleep can dramatically impact a Workaholic's physiological and psychological symptoms.

Adding to this, exercising first thing in the morning can help the body metabolize fat. When you wake up, your body is in a fasting state. When your cortisol levels rise and signal the liver to release glucose to feed your muscles and your liver does not have glycogen available, your body enters a state of ketosis. In this state, your body burns fat rather than sugar. For anyone seeking to diminish excess abdominal fat, this shift to ketosis can be advantageous.

WALKING

One of the most beneficial forms of exercise for the Workaholic is walking. I recommend going outside whenever possible. I also recommend seeking out a route along which you enjoy the scenery and that instills in you a sense of calm.

You may also combine walking with meditation. For the Workaholic, I recommend a series of guided walks by author and spiritual teacher James Endredy in his book *Earthwalks for Body and Spirit*.

KAYAKING

Being out on the water can have calming, healing effects all its own. Kayaking does not require a lot of experience or even owning your own equipment. If you live near a body of water, you can likely rent a kayak for a few hours at a time.

Solitary and meditative, kayaking is also a gentle aerobic exercise you can do at your pace. It can help you strengthen not only your upper body but your core—the literal and figurative seat of your formidable inner power.

WEIGHT LIFTING

Anabolic (tissue-building) exercises can also yield significant benefits. If you're consuming lean proteins and steadily improving your sleep, weight lifting can help rebuild your muscles. Importantly, for every pound of muscle your body gains, your body—at rest—burns an additional 50 calories per day. Adding 10 pounds of muscle means burning 500 calories per day, or 3,500 calories (1 pound) per week.

As you incorporate the various aspects of the SHINES protocol into your daily life, changing your diet, sleep, and exercise habits and employing hormone modulation techniques as appropriate, you will shift your body's metabolic pathways away from destroying muscle and collagen and toward breaking down fat and other substances for energy. This will create the opportunity for your body to rebuild and repair.

Weight lifting can also be aerobic. Doing this for 30 to 45 minutes in sets with 1 to 2 minutes' rest in between can raise your heart rate as it also helps build muscle mass. If you're new to weight lifting and are interested in giving it a try, I recommend reading fitness expert, entrepreneur, and author Bill Phillips's *Body for Life: 12 Weeks to Mental and Physical Strength*. In it, Phillips encourages shorter workouts of 30 to 45 minutes and emphasizes the importance of strength training. He also incorporates research on healthy eating and how this can have a transformative physiological and psychological impact.

SUPPLEMENTS

The supplements that can yield the most benefits for the Workaholic are known as adaptogens. These are plants and plant-based substances known for their ability to help support the adrenal system and the body's ability to manage stress, fend off fatigue, and counter the normal effects of aging. Adaptogens take their name from their ability to help the body "adapt" to the ever-changing elements of its environment.

An important note about adaptogens is that they're unlikely to give you a big boost. Rather, they are silent helpers, building up in your system over time and working in the background to protect your tissues and organs from the destructive impact of excess cortisol.

Used for centuries in traditional Chinese and Ayurvedic medicine, adaptogens have significantly increased in popularity in Western cultures during the past several decades.[29]

GINSENG

Among the most popular adaptogens is Asian ginseng. Containing chemical components called ginsenosides, Asian ginseng is touted for its power to support physical stamina and the body's immune system in addition to slowing various aspects of the aging process and alleviating symptoms of certain respiratory and cardiovascular disorders.[30] Ginseng is also believed to help diminish anxiety and relieve symptoms of depression. Some studies indicate that the herb also helps minimize hot flashes.[31]

A word of warning regarding ginseng: Make sure you are taking the right type. The terms "red ginseng" and "white ginseng" both refer to preparation of Asian ginseng. "Panax ginseng" refers to American ginseng, and "Siberian ginseng" refers to another adaptogenic herb called eleuthero, which is not actually related to ginseng at all.

As with any supplement, I recommend researching your options and ensuring that the brand you choose produces quality products. While the most expensive option is not always the best, make sure that any supplement you take contains the ingredients you're looking for—and few, if any, others. For ginseng and other adaptogen supplements, I recommend Nature's Way and Designs for Health brands.

ASHWAGANDHA

Sometimes called Indian ginseng (though it is not ginseng at all), ashwagandha has been used for centuries in Ayurvedic medicine for its immune-system-boosting effects.[32] An all-around adaptogen that can help users cope with daily stress and offset the physiological effects associated with stress and cortisol excess, ashwagandha has also been shown to help improve sleep and cognitive functioning, in addition to reducing inflammation.

ASTRAGALUS

Long used in Chinese medicine as an immune booster, this adaptogen is known for its ability to help protect against the physically and psychologically destructive effects of stress. The herb may also minimize the impact of excess cortisol by limiting the hormone's ability to bind to cell receptors.

Astragalus is known for its antiviral, anti-inflammatory, antibacterial, and antioxidant properties. It can also help lower blood pressure and strengthen the immune system.[33]

RHODIOLA (GOLDEN ROOT)

After ginseng, rhodiola is perhaps the most widely studied adaptogen. Like some of the other adaptogens we've discussed, rhodiola can help minimize the effects of long-term stress. It has been shown to help restore normal patterns of eating and sleeping in addition to reducing fatigue and oxidative stress (the body's inability to counteract or detoxify the harmful effects of free radicals). Native to the arctic areas of Asia and Eastern Europe, rhodiola has also been found to directly decrease the cortisol response to awakening stress.[34]

Rhodiola can also help burn belly fat. The herb contains a compound called rosavin, which has been shown to stimulate an enzyme called hormone-sensitive lipase. This enzyme can break down fat stores in adipose tissue, such as the fat that builds up in the abdominal area. In one 1999 study, subjects on a restricted-calorie diet who added a daily dose of rhodiola experienced more than twice the weight loss of subjects who did not include the adaptogen, and also showed a significant decrease in body fat.[35]

MUSHROOMS

For me, mushrooms are among the most underappreciated sources of potential adaptogenic support for the Workaholic. Not the psychedelic, "Lucy in the Sky with Diamonds" type, nor the white button variety you can find in blue plastic crates in the produce section of your supermarket, but medicinal mushrooms, including reishi, shiitake, maitake, turkey tail, and agarikon.

If you are interested in a mushroom-based supplement, I recommend mycologist Paul Stamets's Host Defense Series. Available in liquid, capsule, and spray formats, the Host Defense products combine the supportive enzymes, antioxidants, polysaccharides, and prebiotics found in mushrooms into specialized supplements. For the Workaholic, I recommend the CordyChi capsules, a blend of cordyceps and reishi mushrooms designed to help promote a healthy response to stress factors as well as support the body's overall immune system. For more on mushrooms' potential benefits, visit www.fungi.com.

BOOK RECOMMENDATIONS FOR WORKAHOLICS

Alan Christianson, NMD, *The Adrenal Reset Diet: Strategically Cycle Carbs and Proteins to Lose Weight, Balance Hormones, and Move from Stressed to Thriving* (New York: Harmony Books, 2014)

Jonathan Fields, *Uncertainty: Turning Fear and Doubt into Fuel for Brilliance* (New York: Portfolio, 2011)

Amy Myers, MD, *The Autoimmune Solution: Prevent and Reverse the Full Spectrum of Inflammatory Symptoms and Diseases* (New York: HarperOne, 2015)

WORKAHOLICS

Madonna (née Madonna Louise Ciccone, b. August 16, 1958). Born in Bay City, Michigan, Madonna is an American singer, songwriter, actress, and entrepreneur. One of the most successful musical artists of all time, Madonna has released a series of number one hits, won seven Grammy Awards, earned a Golden Globe for her performance in the 1996 film *Evita*, and runs her own entertainment company, Maverick. She is also a philanthropist, donating to a series of charities and founding the Raising Malawi organization in 2006.

Oprah Winfrey (b. January 29, 1954). This American media mogul, talk-show, host, actress, producer, and philanthropist is commonly regarded as the most influential living woman in the world. In 2013, Oprah was awarded the Presidential Medal of Freedom, and ranks among the nation's richest women with a net worth of roughly $3 billion.

Born into poverty in rural Kosciusko, Mississippi, to an unmarried teenage mother, Oprah was shuffled among family members during her early years and suffered sexual abuse at the hands of family members and friends. Her oratory talent and beauty were irrepressible, however, and despite the difficulties that characterized her childhood and adolescence, she won the Miss Black Tennessee beauty pageant at age seventeen. Oprah was awarded a full scholarship to Tennessee State University, and after she graduated, she began working in radio. Soon, she made the move to television, where she became known for her ad-lib reporting on the local news. By the age of thirty-two, Oprah had her own groundbreaking daily talk show, *The Oprah Winfrey Show*. The show quickly outpaced *Donahue* in the ratings. Oprah's ascendancy had begun.

The SHINES Protocol: How Do You Preserve a Saboteur?

I named this archetype for the psychological and physiological "sabotage" that helps drive and sustain its symptomology. In some cases, a Saboteur is not even aware that either is happening. Certainly, she cannot know when her body is robbing itself of critical energy and altering her hormone production in ways that may have negative downstream effects.

The SHINES protocol focuses on eliminating these sabotaging behaviors on every level. Each aspect is designed to help you acknowledge and address your physical, emotional, and spiritual needs. Over time, the protocol can help reverse the negative impact of your body's and mind's previous self-destructive patterns and help you emerge from the labyrinth armed with a new perspective on self-care and the tools to help you embrace positive change.

SPIRITUAL PRACTICE

For the Saboteur, the aim of a spiritual practice is to *restore*—to help you heal from the trials you've endured and instill in you the importance of separating yourself from the external and tending to yourself, body and mind. Given that physical, emotional, and even spiritual fatigue is already plaguing you, the practices I suggest require little energy. You can begin them from right where you are. I often advise women that the best spiritual practice for the Saboteur is the practice of saying NO. Too often women are made to be not only the head of the household but also the breadwinner, planner, executor, and savior. When you are burning the candle at both ends, and doing so with a blowtorch, it can be helpful to set up some boundaries. For those who are used to constantly doing, saying NO will take practice for you to find that one thing that is important for you to focus on. And that one thing to focus on is you.

MINDFUL BREATHING

Deep, abdominal breathing is a practice you may engage in anytime to stimulate your vagus nerve and diminish your body's fight-or-flight responses. Doing this also slows your heart rate, helps aerate your lungs, and relaxes your body overall. Given these effects, deep breathing can also reduce your cortisol levels. Doctors often prescribe deep-breathing exercises for patients who have undergone surgery to help stave off pulmonary infection and offset the effects of the physiological and emotional stress inevitably associated with the trauma.

Dr. Andrew Weil, author and director of the University of Arizona's Center for Integrative Medicine, has published widely on the health benefits of breathing exercises. "Practicing regular, mindful breathing exercise can be calming and energizing," Weil notes, "and can even help with stress-related problems ranging from panic attacks to digestive disorders."[36] For the Saboteur, I recommend two of Dr. Weil's exercises in particular.

THE 4-7-8 (RELAXING BREATH) EXERCISE

You can do this exercise anywhere, anytime. The steps are simple and easy to follow. Dr. Weil recommends you do this exercise sitting up with your back straight, particularly as you learn it.

> Place the tip of your tongue on the roof of your mouth, just behind your front teeth. You will be opening and closing your mouth throughout the exercise, but your tongue will remain still in this position.
> Exhale through your mouth. Try to completely empty your lungs.
> Close your mouth and inhale through your nose, mentally counting to 4.
> Hold your breath for a count of 7.
> Audibly exhale through your open mouth to a mental count of 8.
> Begin again. Do 4 complete breaths.

The ratio of your inhalation, breath-holding, and exhalation is critical. Be especially mindful of this, and be patient with yourself if getting it right requires practice.

BREATH COUNTING EXERCISE

This exercise combines the benefits of deep breathing and meditation. It encourages you to breathe deeply, aerating your lungs and stimulating your vagus nerve, and also to focus exclusively on the task at hand—to breathe mindfully, exhaling each breath for a particular length of time.

As with the 4–7–8 exercise, you may engage breath counting

anytime, anywhere. Dr. Weil recommends doing this exercise in a seated position, with your back straight and head angled slightly forward.

> Close your eyes and take a few deep breaths. These may vary in depth and rhythm.
> Begin counting to yourself as you exhale. To begin, internally count to 1 as you exhale.
> On the next exhale, count to 2. And on the breath after that, count to 3.
> Continue until you reach a count of 5 on the exhale. Never go higher than 5. Instead, return to 1 and repeat the cycle.

Plan to do this exercise for ten minutes at a stretch. At one or more points, you may find yourself counting all the way up to eight, ten, or even higher. This is a sign that your mind has wandered. Bring it back to the task at hand and start over, continuing the exercise for the minutes you have left.

BE IN THE NOW

Another practice that can calm the Saboteur is very intentionally being in the *now*. This means focusing exclusively on your internal experience in *this very moment*, regardless of what is happening in the world around you. Doing this forces you to recognize that in this very moment, there is no threat at hand. Although any stressful circumstances of your life that have contributed to the rise of your archetype may continue, in any given present moment, you maintain the ability to simply and safely *be*.

Acknowledging this and spending time in a space where any stress or threats are at bay can be a restorative practice in its own right. Author and speaker Eckhart Tolle, one of the most widely known authorities on the positive spiritual impact of being in the now, has explained it this way: "Your outer journey may contain a million steps; your inner journey only has one: the step you are taking right now."[37]

In any given moment, practice being exactly—and only—where you are. Combined with deep breathing exercises, this seemingly simple act of freeing yourself from the onslaught of the various stressors that have been driving your body's fight-or-flight responses can have restorative and spiritually healing effects.

RECOGNIZE THE SELF

Different from intentionally being in the present but potentially also healing and restorative for the Saboteur is a practice I call "recognizing the self." This involves looking back from where you are now and performing an inventory—patiently, carefully, and with respect and care for yourself considering the people and events of your life that have led you to where you are now.

For the Saboteur in particular, acknowledging all you have endured and giving yourself time and space to feel whatever comes up as you survey your personal history can have a calming and restorative impact on you, spiritually and physically. Looking at pictures can help you recall the various experiences that have led you to where you are. When you do, give yourself the space to feel what you did in those moments, whether this was happiness or anger or misery, and acknowledge the joy, pain, or loss you have felt since. Honoring your experiences in this way and giving yourself credit for enduring them can calm you in body and mind and help generate emotional and spiritual energy that will serve you well on your journey toward balance.

HORMONE MODULATION

The Saboteur is typically suffering from a series of hormone deficiencies, including cortisol, progesterone, estrogen, and testosterone.

But the hormonal aspect of the SHINES protocol does not involve introducing a series of hormone replacement medications. In fact, it does not involve hormones at all.

For the Saboteur, I recommend taking an adrenal complex supplement for a relatively short period of time; this may range from a few weeks to a few months. Typically made from the desiccated adrenal glands of cows, pigs, and sheep, adrenal support supplements can improve the overall functioning of the adrenal glands and help boost the production of cortisol and other hormones.

A note of caution: For all that your body may respond positively to the actual adrenal compound contained in these supplements, it is imperative that your physician monitor your condition and progress while you are taking one. If an adrenal complex is going to help you, it will do this relatively quickly—again, within a few months—and you should stop taking it at that point. This will help avoid undesirable side effects. Among these are the risk of infection, particularly in patients with severely low immune function.

If you are interested in trying an adrenal complex, discuss this with your physician. Map out a plan for monitoring your progress at the outset and be alert for any sign of infection. As with any supplement, I also strongly encourage you to research the brand you are buying and review the ingredients very carefully, including the geographical region from where they're sourced. For adrenal extract in particular, it is best to avoid supplements containing ingredients from countries where bovine spongiform encephalitis (BSE, or "mad cow disease") has been reported. Among these are several European countries, including Great Britain, France, and Holland, as well as some countries in Asia.

INFOCEUTICALS

For the Saboteur, the most helpful Energetic Integrators are EI9 and EI10.

EI9 addresses energetic disturbances associated with adrenal overload. It can help bolster your immune system, improve temperature regulation, and relieve symptoms of extreme fatigue. Operating along the "triple warmer meridian," which begins at the tip of the ring finger and runs up through the wrist, forearm, and shoulder before entering the pericardium (the sac that surrounds the heart) and rising up to the collarbone and looping around to the back of the ear, EI9 bioenergetically affects all the body's major cavities. These include the cranium, thorax, abdomen, and pelvis.

EI9 also helps to maintain the body's thermal equilibrium, addressing energetic disturbances associated with other adrenal-overload-related conditions, including thyroid disorders, postpartum depression, and autoimmune diseases such as fibromyalgia.

EI10 energetically influences the neuroendocrine system. Associated with the hypothalamus, adrenal cortex, and ovaries, EI10 "echoes" the impact of the hormones without introducing any actual hormones into your system. When hormone deficiencies compromise or block the flow of energy within and among your twelve energy meridians, EI10 can help restore this.

I'm not one to throw around the words *detoxification* and *toxins* because I think they are widely overused. However, in the case of the Saboteur, I want you to consider that your body is full of toxic energy from stress and the stories you have been telling yourself: "I'm tired, I suck, and I'm overweight. I wish this wasn't my life." In this case it is bringing you back into the light—literally. Getting you into an infrared sauna or into some sort of home red-light therapy that possibly involves sweat and pulling things out of you. One aspect of this is giving you 15 to 30 minutes with yourself and your own thoughts in the heat and allowing your body to relax and open to the possibilities while getting rid of waste it doesn't need. Infrared saunas are not cheap, so there are also red-light panels you can buy that go on the back of bedroom/bathroom doors.

ESSENTIAL OILS

Low cortisol for the Saboteur is often the end result of extended periods of burning your candle not only at both ends, but with a blowtorch. These essential oils will not only support the adrenal glands, but can possibly help with the symptoms of low cortisol:

Lavender	Spruce
Nutmeg	Sweet orange
Pine	Valerian
Rosemary	

NUTRITION

For the Saboteur, supportive nutrition involves the body *and the mind*. More than the food that will help support your body's overall functioning and return you to balance, eating well requires mindfulness. It requires focusing on yourself, including recognizing the depleting physiological and psychological patterns of behavior that have driven the rise of your archetype. Again, you may or may not have been aware of these patterns. But once aware, it is critical that you do what you are able to avoid engaging in them going forward. As with your spiritual practice and other elements of the SHINES protocol, the goal is to refuel and restore. To heal.

Similar to Workaholics, Saboteurs tend to cannibalize their own tissues, including muscle. For this reason, protein is an especially important component of the Saboteur's diet. I recommend roughly 1 gram of protein per pound of body weight. For a 150-pound woman, I suggest aiming for 120 to 150 grams of protein per day.

Carbohydrates also play an important role in the Saboteur's daily diet, comprising 30 to 40 percent of your daily caloric intake. Switch to natural carbohydrates such as fruits and vegetables rather than refined carbohydrates such as pasta, bread, and crackers (particularly white varieties of any of these) that are likely to exacerbate abdominal weight gain.

For Saboteurs in particular, I advise consulting with a nutritionist. This can alleviate some of the work associated with planning your meals each day and can help you maintain your forward, healing momentum. It will also give you some accountability and positive reinforcement of efforts made if you have a qualified guide.

Food Sensitivity Testing

For the Saboteur, I suggest consulting with a physician or nutritionist who can perform food sensitivity or allergy testing. A significant percentage of my patients who have presented with this archetype have developed food sensitivities of which they're unaware. And these are exerting serious negative physiological and psychological effects. The major food "offenders" are gluten and dairy.

Different providers use various types of food sensitivity assessment methods, including stool and blood testing. Depending on your symptoms and diet, the physician or nutritionist you consult should help you determine which test will yield the information you need.

FOODS TO EMBRACE

Lean Proteins

Lean proteins are an essential component of the Saboteur's restorative diet. Seek out simple, nutrient-rich options that are unlikely to contain antibiotics, hormones, or other toxins (including pesticides), the elimination of which will stress your already overtaxed system. I recommend fish and lean meats, as well as nut and seed proteins. I do not recommend dairy proteins for the Saboteur because lactose sensitivity or intolerance tends to be characteristic of the archetype. Good sources of protein for the Saboteur include:

Salmon

Lean meats, including chicken, turkey, and organic grass-fed beef

Seeds, including pumpkin, chia, and flax (see page 301 for preparation methods)

Healthy Fats

Healthy fats, such as the omega-3 and omega-6 monounsaturated and polyunsaturated fats found in a Mediterranean diet, are a healthy addition to the Saboteur's restorative regime. Remember: Cholesterol is both a fat and critical to hormone production. Making healthy, easily digestible fats part of your daily nutritional intake can help support your adrenal function. It can also help your tissues and organs, including your heart, liver, and skin, repair from the long-term, catabolic effects of cortisol excess.

Good sources of healthy fats include:

OILS

Coconut oil

Extra-virgin olive oil, cold-pressed

Oil blends, such Udo's Oil Omega 3-6-9 Blend, a mixture of omega-3, -6, and -9 fatty acids

OTHER FOOD SOURCES

Avocados

Olives

Nuts, including almonds and walnuts

Seeds, including flax and pumpkin

Colorful Vegetables

Vegetables rich in antioxidants such as vitamins A, C, and E and beta-carotene as well as copper, zinc, and selenium are a valuable addition to the Saboteur's diet. These unrefined carbohydrates are also a healthy source of calories and fiber.

I recommend seeking out colorful—and different-colored—vegetables. Shoot for five colors each day. Among good choices for the Saboteur are:

Bell peppers in yellow, orange, and red
Broccoli
Brussels sprouts
Carrots
Eggplant (including the skin)
Sweet potatoes
Butternut squash

One note of caution: It is important for the Saboteur to avoid ingesting toxic pesticides. Whenever possible, seek out organic produce options.

Fruits with Low Glycemic Indexes

Various fruits can be helpful for the Saboteur. Rich in many vitamins and minerals, including a series of antioxidants, they are a nutritionally valuable source of unrefined carbohydrates and fiber.

Although most any fruit has nutritional value, the best choices for the Saboteur are fruits with lower glycemic indexes. Sweeter fruits, such as bananas and pineapple, that have higher glycemic indexes can raise your blood sugar, triggering your body to produce more cortisol. When your adrenals are already severely fatigued, adding this pressure can exacerbate the "pregnenolone steal" (see page 127) and have other downstream effects.

This is not to say you should avoid *all* fruits with relatively high glycemic indexes. Have half a banana, if you crave one. But on a regular basis, try to steer yourself toward fruits that are less sweet.

Good fruits for the Saboteur include:

Apples
Dried apricots
Cherries
Grapefruit
Oranges
Pears

Foods That Promote Gut Health

A healthy gut is an important element in any archetype's overall well-being. But for the Saboteur who can be prone to gastrointestinal distress, incorporating specific foods that help support and improve the gut's functioning and condition is particularly important.

The most effective additions to your diet will be probiotics. In addition to various yogurt- and animal-milk-based products, there are also nondairy options available. I recommend:

Almond milk- or coconut milk–based yogurt
Kombucha, a fermented beverage made from black tea
Kvass, a fermented beverage popular in Slavic countries made from rye (black) bread

If you are not lactose sensitive or intolerant, I recommend:

Kefir, a fermented milk drink made from cow, goat, or sheep milk

Bone Broth

One of the most nutritious elements of an animal is its bone marrow. Consumed in broth form, it can help boost the immune system, support healthy cholesterol levels, and reduce inflammation, particularly in the gut. Bone broth may also help strengthen your bones and teeth in addition to promoting muscle protein synthesis and weight loss. For Saboteurs looking for an energizing alternative to coffee, bone broth can be a good choice.

The health benefits of bone broth derive largely from the amino acids it contains, including arginine, L-glutamine, and cysteine. It also contains collagen, fat, and key minerals, such as calcium, magnesium, potassium, and phosphorus. Bone broth made from fish bones also contains iodine.

When made with vegetables, bone broth also contains carbohydrates and electrolytes, both of which can help with dehydration.

You can drink bone broth like a tea or cook with it in any recipe that calls for stock or broth.

Seaweed

Seaweed is another food from which the Saboteur may derive significant benefits. In addition to the antioxidant vitamins A and C and calcium, seaweed also contains iodine. Critically important to maintaining healthy thyroid function, iodine can help stave off several of the Saboteur's symptoms, including muscle weakness, fatigue, and weight gain.

Seaweed is now available in a variety of formats, including chips and crackers. Seaweed is a key component of sushi, and can also be made into salad on its own.

Raw Honey

When I consult with patients, I generally advise them to avoid sugar. It yields few, if any, health benefits, and when consumed in excess, it can have significant negative effects. For the Saboteur looking for a relatively healthy sweetener option, I recommend raw honey.

Unlike refined sugar, raw honey has some health benefits. Studies have shown that people who substitute raw honey for refined sugar lose weight more easily. Research has also indicated that raw honey boosts immunity, helps alleviate allergy symptoms, and aids in wound healing by boosting the body's production of hydrogen peroxide, a natural antibacterial agent. Also important, raw honey is full of polyphenols—plant-based antioxidants that have been shown to support cardiovascular health.

Raw honey can also promote sound sleep. Consuming a tablespoon before bedtime restores the liver's glycogen supply, preventing the brain from triggering hunger signals. Raw honey can also cause the release of melatonin. It does this by causing a small spike in insulin, triggering the release of tryptophan. This converts to serotonin, which then converts to melatonin.

One note of caution about raw honey is that you must source it carefully. It can contain botulism toxin.

FOODS TO AVOID

Processed Flour

I always recommend that Saboteurs go through the kitchen cupboards and removing everything in a bag or a box that's made with flour. Whether it's bread or Bisquick, replace it with whole foods. Gluten-free foods made with almond flour, rice flour, or tapioca starch are all good alternatives.

Sugar

In addition to flour, sugar is another "poison" it's worth your effort to avoid. This can be easier said than done. Foods that few of us consider "sugary" can contain high amounts.

Take spaghetti sauce, for example. For years, I've had a favorite store-bought brand. It's thick and rich. It's also sweet, but it was only recently that I checked the ingredients and saw that sugar ranked among the first. Peanut butter is another example of a food you may not think of as containing large amounts of sugar. Many of the most commercially popular brands do, however.

Another note of caution: Foods that are sweetened with agave nectar or monk fruit extract or another natural sweetener still contain sugar and can still exert some or all of the negative effects of refined sugar. If you're trying to limit your intake of sugar, I recommend using stevia-based sweeteners. Derived from the stevia plant, these are healthier options than artificial sweeteners such as aspartame and saccharin, and contain no calories. Some research has indicated that these sweeteners may mimic the effects of sugar on your body, however, including raising cortisol levels. For the Saboteur, then, it is important to use even these sweeteners only in moderation.

Caffeine

As challenging as it may be to avoid caffeine, doing this is critically important for the Saboteur. Caffeine can exacerbate the destructive effects of physiological and psychological stress, including increasing cortisol levels, and can diminish the restorative impact of other aspects of the SHINES protocol.

If you're reliant on caffeine, using it to help you get going in the morning and carry on through the afternoon, try to gradually reduce your dependency on it. Quitting caffeine cold turkey can cause severe headaches and leave you feeling severely fatigued. Instead of doing this, try transitioning away from it over time by mixing caffeinated coffee with decaf, or, if you drink tea, exchanging half of your traditional black teas for decaffeinated black or herbal varieties.

EXERCISE

For the fatigued Saboteur, exercise can prove physically and psychologically challenging. For this reason, I do not recommend forcing yourself into a high-intensity training program. Rather, I suggest focusing on the element of movement—flexing your muscles and joints, increasing your blood flow, facilitating deep breathing. Isometric exercises may figure into your exercise regime, while weight lifting may not. Similarly, a brisk walk outside may serve you well, where running several miles could do more harm than good.

Before you embark on a new exercise program, I recommend spending some time in reflection, considering the various events and circumstances in your life that have contributed to the Saboteur archetype taking hold. Similar to the "life inventory" that is an element of the spiritual aspect of the SHINES protocol, this reflection involves looking back to the time when certain events or circumstances began to drive the stress underlying your archetype and perhaps altered or interrupted your exercise routine. Doing this can inspire you to reclaim some time and energy for yourself. It can also help you determine what kind of exercise is appropriate for you and your lifestyle *now*. This may be very different from what worked for you many months or years before.

The most important note about exercise may be that you *not overdo it*. Remember: Your SHINES protocol is designed to help you heal and restore yourself both physiologically and psychologically. (Also important, if you are suffering from a medical condition or recovering from surgery, you will want to confirm with your physician that any exercise routine is appropriate for you.)

TAI CHI

One exercise I recommend for the Saboteur is tai chi. Mixing movement with meditation, tai chi involves moving deliberately and intentionally. It also requires that you focus on what is happening in your mind and body, including your breath.

SWIMMING

Swimming can yield physical and psychological benefits for the Saboteur. An aerobic exercise, swimming does not involve the breakdown (catabolism) of your muscles. Adding to this, it's an exercise you can start slowly, building up the intensity of your regimen over time.

In addition to its physical benefits, swimming can also have a calming and restorative psychological impact. It frees you of the weight the world places on your shoulders. When you are under water, the noise of the world is also shut out. All you can hear then are the sounds of your own breath and of the water as you move through it.

SUPPLEMENTS

Among the supplements I recommend for the Saboteur are certain vitamins, minerals, and herbs that have adaptogenic and other supportive properties. Before introducing a supplement into your daily routine, I recommend consulting with a physician, nutritionist, or other knowledgeable healthcare provider to help you decide which supplements may be right for you. It is also important to confirm that your body is healthy enough to benefit from supplements, and that you take them in the amounts and for the duration of time that serves you best.

ADAPTOGENS

Just as they can help support the Workaholic, adaptogenic supplements can also yield restorative benefits for the Saboteur. Adaptogens are plants and plant-derived substances that can help support the adrenal system and the body's ability to manage stress and fend off fatigue. Some research suggests that adaptogens can also diminish the effects of aging.

LICORICE ROOT

Licorice root (*Glycyrrhiza glabra*) can help address the Saboteur's hormonal imbalances by bringing cortisol levels back within normal range. It does this not by increasing cortisol production, but by slowing the rate at which the body breaks down the hormone.

Again, for the Saboteur who is likely suffering from a series of hormone deficiencies, including low levels of cortisol, raising its levels can reduce the pressure on your adrenal glands to increase production of the hormone. **This is one of those supplements that needs to be treated with care, because you can indeed take too much and many hospitalizations have resulted from people eating even just too much black licorice.** (I find the taste disgusting.) If you are going to take this supplement, make sure you do it under the care of a physician.

ASHWAGANDHA

Also called Indian ginseng (though it is not ginseng at all), ashwagandha has been used in Ayurvedic medicine for its immune-system-boosting effects and to help diminish the effects of stress, including increased cortisol production. Studies have shown that ashwagandha can also help improve sleep and reduce inflammation,[38] a condition that tends to plague the Saboteur.

RHODIOLA (GOLDEN ROOT)

Rhodiola is another adaptogen used to help minimize the effects of long-term stress. Studies have shown that it can help users combat fatigue and diminish the effects of oxidative stress (the body's inability to counteract or detoxify the harmful effects of free radicals). This herb has also been found to directly diminish the body's cortisol-production response to awakening stress.

Rhodiola can also help burn belly fat. The herb contains a compound called rosavin, which stimulates production of an enzyme called hormone-sensitive lipase. This enzyme has been shown to break down fat stores in adipose tissue, including those that tend to build up in the abdominal area. In one 1999 study, dieters who incorporated a daily dose of rhodiola into their supplement routine lost more weight and body fat than dieters who did not.

MACA

For the Saboteur suffering the effects of chronic stress and fatigue, any of your hormones may be out of balance or operating at diminished levels. Maca can help restore overall equilibrium among these as the elements of the SHINES protocol begin to exert various healing effects. An herb grown in Peru, maca has long been used to promote hormone balance (in men and women). Each of the thirteen differently colored varieties of maca exerts distinct effects, and many maca-based supplements combine different varieties of the herb.

The particular maca supplement I recommend for a Saboteur is Femmenessence MacaHarmony. I recommend the standard dose: two capsules twice daily, taken separate from meals. Take the first dose in the morning, before breakfast, and the second dose in the early evening, ideally 30 minutes before you normally experience an energy low.

BETAINE

Also known as trimethylglycine (TMG), betaine is a plant-based amino acid derivative that has been shown to support muscle gain[39] and fat loss. Betaine can also help protect cardiovascular health by breaking down the naturally occurring amino acid homocysteine. In high levels, homocysteine can damage blood vessels and contribute to conditions including vascular disease and stroke.

For the Saboteur, I recommend a daily betaine supplement of between 600 mg and 1,000 mg before meals, ideally in combination with pepsin for maximum efficacy. It should also be noted that some betaine supplements also include the enzyme pepsin.

Betaine, a by-product of sugar beet processing, is available over the counter in powder, tablet, and capsule form. I also recommend taking betaine with a methylated B-complex vitamin, one that contains folic acid (1,000 to 2,000 mcg), riboflavin (25 mg), vitamin B6 (10 to 25 mg), and vitamin B12 (also called methylcobalamin or, in its synthetic form, cyanocobalamin, 1,000 mcg).

ZINC

Zinc aids in the synthesis of a series of hormones, including progesterone and cortisol.[40] A deficiency in this mineral can therefore exacerbate the hormonal deficiencies and imbalances (including estrogen dominance) associated with the Saboteur archetype.

BOOK RECOMMENDATIONS FOR SABOTEURS

James L. Wilson, ND, DC, PhD, *Adrenal Fatigue: The 21st Century Stress Syndrome* (Walnut, CA: Smart Press, 2001)

Alan Christianson, NMD, *The Adrenal Reset Diet: Strategically Cycle Carbs and Proteins to Lose Weight, Balance Hormones, and Move from Stressed to Thriving* (New York: Harmony Books, 2015)

SABOTEURS

Carol Peletier, *fictional character from* The Walking Dead *comic book series and American television series of the same name.* Though initially portrayed in both the *Walking Dead* comic and television series as an abused housewife, in the television version, Carol is depicted as a practical and stern but ultimately compassionate character whose postapocalyptic "hero's journey" involves fleeing from zombies (called "walkers") with her husband and daughter, losing them both, and ultimately becoming a leader among the country's survivors.

Claire Underwood, *fictional character from the Netflix series* House of Cards. As the wife and right-hand woman of Frank Underwood, a Washington politician who becomes vice president and then president of the United States, Claire is overworked and overworking, but ultimately claims her own strength and achieves political stature. From her position as a lobbyist leading an environmental non-profit, Claire rises to become Second Lady of the United States, then US ambassador to the United Nations, vice president of the United States, and, finally, the nation's forty-seventh president.

The SHINES Protocol: How Do You Get a Nun Back in the Game?

For the Nun, the journey begins with the insight that your archetype is, in itself, a calling. You have been called to a journey of introspection and self-discovery—to a period of time during which you can arrive at a better understanding of how the circumstances of your life have affected your spiritual, emotional, and physical well-being. Your journey may involve a significant shift in your perspective on what it is that you want to devote your physical, emotional, and spiritual energy to, or even significant changes in your life. Whatever it entails, what is most important about your inner Nun's "pilgrimage" is that it is about *you*.

The Nun is a natural counselor. She represents love and safety and peace. With every step you take, pause to consider how such a force—one that now resides within you—can offer up emotional and energetic support, offering you both solace and guidance. Imagine sharing your worries, questions, and fears in the sacred space she creates. What would you say? Perhaps you are unhappy in your relationship. Perhaps you feel unloved, or fear feeling this way. Perhaps you are angry at yourself or someone else. Whatever it is you yearn to share, you can share it safely, without fear of judgment. Doing this consistently and with care and self-respect is a critical aspect of the self-discovery at the heart of the Nun's journey.

Many women who present with the Nun archetype report diminished sexual desire. For some women, this is not a pressing concern. For others, it is. Either way, any physiological or psychological condition that can significantly diminish your sexuality merits your consideration. Perhaps you feel unattractive or uneasy in your body. Perhaps you've been betrayed by a partner and are carrying around the pain of that wound, or perhaps career, financial, or other stress has diminished your inclination or ability to experience sexual desire or arousal.

If you're experiencing this and it is a concern for you, I encourage you to not only look inward, but also speak outwardly about it. Talk to your physician, who can offer perspective on the physiological underpinnings of the condition. Talk to a trusted friend or counselor with whom you may share some of the emotional difficulties that may be claiming your energy and focus and diminishing your interest in physical intimacy in the process. If you are in a relationship, also speak to your partner. Of course, this can be difficult. It requires vulnerability and can inspire insecurity and defensiveness. Still, it is important. The longer a lack of intimacy goes unacknowledged, the harder it can be to breach and the more distance it can create.

Above all, remember that your journey is about carefully evaluating the various physiological and emotional circumstances that have shaped and continue to shape your experience of the world around you. Again, you may rely on your own counsel as you navigate your way back to balance, calling up your inner Nun's ability to soothe and to guide without judgment or criticism. Ultimately, the aim of each element of the SHINES protocol is to support your passionate and joyful engagement in your life.

SPIRITUAL PRACTICE

EMOTION EXPLORATION

The first practice I recommend for the Nun comes from the bestselling author, speaker, and awakening coach Arjuna Ardagh. In his

2008 book, *Leap Before You Look*, Ardagh describes a solitary exercise involving music that is designed to help you access past and present emotional experiences by evoking feelings including joy and grief, resentment and anger.

This is how it works: First, find a series of songs that evoke emotion in you. Together, these should take between 35 and 40 minutes to play and inspire a range of feelings, from ecstasy to sadness to rage. Put these songs into a list so that they play in order, without your intervention, and listen to them in private, where you can feel free to enter into your emotions as they come up and act in any way that feels right to you. Cry, scream, dance, lie still. Do whatever you're inclined to, using your entire body to express what's going on inside you.

Ardagh claims this practice is quintessentially feminine (though he recommends it for men and women alike). For the Nun in particular, this is important.

HORMONE MODULATION

In adult women, "normal" testosterone levels range from 15 to 70 ng/dl. (The normal range for an adult male is 270 to 1,070 ng/dl.)[41] The range for adult women represents nearly a fourfold difference, which means your testosterone levels could *quadruple* and you would still be within the "normal" range.

Once again, when any one of your hormones falls within "normal" range, it does not mean that level is normal for *you*. This is certainly true of testosterone. If your levels are on the low side of the normal range and we double them, they will still be "normal," but you will feel better.

Testosterone replacement in women poses a challenge for healthcare providers because there is no commercially available medication we can prescribe for it. (There are more than ten testosterone replacement medications for men.) This means that doctors need to prescribe female patients custom-designed medications and closely monitor their androgen levels for the duration of time they're using them.

This type of hormone modulation therapy can have side effects. Some are reversible. These include acne, irregular menstrual cycles, and a reduction in breast size. Any of these will resolve within a relatively short period of time following termination of treatment.

Other side effects are irreversible. These include clitoromegaly (enlargement of the clitoris), which only surgery can reverse. Deepening of the voice is an additional permanent side effect, as is hirsutism (increased body and facial hair growth). Electrolysis (laser hair removal) is required to permanently prevent this.

All this said, I encourage you—as I encourage my patients—to not fear testosterone replacement therapy. The key is to find a knowledgeable and *experienced* practitioner who will prescribe the proper medication at the dose that's right for you and appropriately monitor your progress. I recommend starting off slowly, at a low dose and with a form of the medication you can easily stop.

HORMONE MODULATION OPTIONS FOR THE NUN

While there are a number of forms of reliable testosterone replacement options for men, including capsules, lozenges, pills, gels, injections, and subdermal pellets, for women, there are just four: transdermal creams, sublingual pills, vaginal suppositories, and subdermal pellets (which I do not recommend). Each form has benefits and drawbacks.

Transdermal Creams

My preferred androgen-replacement option is specially compounded transdermal cream. The dosing is relatively easy to control and adjust as necessary. Also, daily application is required to maintain higher levels of circulating testosterone. This means that in the event a patient experiences unwanted side effects, I advise that they simply discontinue application, and we reassess. In general, any issues swiftly resolve. Adding to this, it is extremely unlikely that any properly compounded cream will raise your testosterone to dangerous levels. Other options can carry this risk.

Sublingual Pills

Sublingual pills are an option I also recommend. Similar to transdermal creams, these require daily application, and their effects are relatively easy to manage.

One downside to sublingual pills is that they're flavored. Some of my patients complain that the taste is unappealing, and that taking the pills each day becomes too unpleasant a chore. In some cases, the pills can also cause irritation on the underside of the tongue. This generally occurs after a few weeks of use. The majority of my patients who experience this irritation switch to another form of medication.

Vaginal Suppositories

For women who do not want to use a transdermal cream or sublingual pill, suppositories are another option. Dosing via suppositories is reliable and relatively easy to manage. Similar to transdermal creams and pills, terminating suppository usage swiftly diminishes adverse effects.

The most common complaint I've received from patients who use these suppositories is that application can be awkward or messy.

Subdermal Pellets

Although some women choose this form of androgen replacement, in my practice, I do not recommend it. Not only are subdermal pellets more expensive than creams, pills, and suppositories, they can also be dangerous for female patients. Inserting them under the skin requires an in-office procedure that exposes the patient to the risk of pain, bleeding, bruising, and infection. Potentially worse than this, once the pellets are inserted, they cannot be removed.

The fact that the pellets cannot be removed can create a number of difficulties. The first is that there is no way to reverse any adverse effects. Some of these will diminish or resolve altogether once the pellets' period of effectiveness is over, but others will not. Again, some of the adverse effects of testosterone, including deepening of the voice and clitoromegaly, are permanent.

Dosing also poses a challenge. Pellets release large amounts of testosterone during the first few weeks of implantation, causing testosterone levels to spike. This can make you feel significantly more energetic and physically strong. After this, however, your levels begin to taper off, becoming generally unsteady during the three to four months of the pellets' effectiveness. Once this wears off, your testosterone levels are likely to sink to their original low point, prompting you to begin the cycle again.

Pellets are also problematic for the Nun because they're designed for men and therefore simply deliver too much testosterone. In my practice, I have treated women who have had pellets inserted by another practitioner and whose testosterone was dangerously far outside the "normal" range.

Here are the top ten reasons why I advise against using hormone pellets:

1. **They're expensive:** Pellets cost somewhere between $300 and $400 every three months (somewhere around $100 to $125 per month). Bioidentical creams and troches at reasonable compounding pharmacies are around $45/month, and if you buy three months at a time, they are usually closer to $39/month. Pellets, delivering the same medicine, cost about three times more than compounded creams.

2. **They contain hormone levels that are dangerously high:** Pellets will be advertised as maintaining a level hormonal balance. But if you really think about it, there is absolutely no way this can be true. There is no guarantee that the same amount of hormone will be released daily for three months. Absolutely none.

Most commonly, what I see is that in the first month of pellets, levels will go dangerously high; for many women, three to four times the high end of normal. This is followed by two months of a steep fall in levels. So, patients initially feel good because their levels are surging and super high, then start having withdrawal symptoms and thinking, "Shit, I need my pellets again." The problem is that many women feel these withdrawal symptoms not because their levels are low, but because their levels were so high initially that even a small drop can trigger symptoms. I have seen hundreds of women whose hormone levels are still super high but who are having symptoms of low hormone levels.

3. **Using them involves a surgical procedure:** Pellets have to be put under your skin every three months. The provider has to dig a pocket in the fat of your butt cheek to get that pellet in. This results in bruising and pain, and can lead to infection—I can't tell you how many infected butt cheeks I've seen over the years . . . it's a lot. How many infections, bruises, and painful side effects happen with creams? None.

4. **Once they're in, they don't come out:** Well, that's not totally true—sometimes they actually do pop out on their own—but the reality is, they aren't made to come out. So if the levels of hormone are too high and end up causing side effects, such as pain, bleeding, headache, weight gain, water retention, lethargy, clitoromegaly (enlarged clitoris, which is permanent), deepening of the voice (also permanent), mood swings, irritability, anxiety, and high blood pressure, you're likely stuck with them for three to six months and sometimes longer.

5. **They must be replaced every three months:** You are told you have to go to the office every three months to have new pellets put in. Simply put, why would you do anything that required you to have a small in-office surgical procedure four times a year? It makes absolutely no sense whatsoever. The costs alone should have been a deterrent, but the idea of your doctor digging a pocket in your butt cheek every

three months should be even more reason for you to say no.

6. **Their absorption rates are irregular:** Pellets are promoted as being the ultimate in stability and stable absorption rates, but as I've explained, that simply isn't true. They aren't made with some genius device that releases stable hormone levels every day, and in fact, I have seen quite the opposite. The medication is released as a high dose initially, then slows over time. I haven't seen one study that shows stable hormone levels with pellets that is either legitimate or reproducible. The reason? There aren't any.

7. **Show me the money:** I'm gonna be honest here: If I used pellets in my practice, I'd be rich. The number of women I see in my practice who are receiving hormones is in the thousands, and if I was doing pellets on them, I'd make a ton of money. This is a cash cow for doctors' offices. Every three months, hundreds of women have to come in to have pellets placed, and they are all paying up. In my opinion, the offices offering pellets aren't doing so because they think it's an amazing treatment—they've just seen the bottom line.

8. **Who is putting them in?** If I haven't made friends to this point, then this is where I might make enemies: Simply put, overall, the people putting pellets in their patients have absolutely no idea what they are doing. Why do I say this? Because the majority of providers offering pellets are armchair quarterbacks, physicians who dabble in hormones, or physician extenders who, like many practitioners, took a weekend course in hormone therapy. You see, the companies that sell the pellets offer courses that a physician can attend for a weekend and then magically come out a hormone expert. I just think this is a horrible recipe for failure. Expertise comes with years of study coupled with years of patient encounters, not a weekend course where you learned about hormones from another nonexpert. Yeah, it's harsh, but I'm not one to sugarcoat things, and the reality is, pellets are being inserted by people who simply don't have the expertise. If

they were hormone experts, they wouldn't be using pellets in the first place.

9. **It's a club:** The offices offering pellets have to pay to play. They have to pay a monthly fee to use the pellet company's name and they have to buy their pellets. Because they are invested, they are obviously biased toward this form of treatment and, in my opinion, are going to push pellets.

10. **You're a number:** If and when these practitioners draw your blood, they take the results and feed the numbers into a program from the company that produces the pellets, which then spits out a protocol of what to do with the dosage. Experts don't use protocols, and we don't treat you like you fit into a tidy formula. Hormones never work this way, and they never will, and the reason for this is that we are all different. To try to simplify our vast hormonal network into a series of protocols is a serious detriment to you as an individual. Hopefully you can see this.

Addyi: The "Female Viagra"

In 2015, the FDA approved a medication called Addyi to treat hypoactive sexual desire disorder (HSDD) in premenopausal women. The pink tablets contain no hormones, and their mechanism of action exerts no effect on hormones in the body. Nor does the medication affect blood flow to the genitals, as Viagra does for men. Rather, Addyi has action within the central nervous system, affecting certain postsynaptic receptors in a way that helps balance your levels of dopamine and norepinephrine, which influence sexual excitement, and decreases levels of serotonin, which influences sexual satiety and inhibition.[42]

According to the FDA, in clinical trials, Addyi increased the number of "satisfying sexual events" by

(continues)

between 0.5 and 1 each month over a placebo. The drug was also reported to have increased subjects' "sexual desire" score by between 0.3 and 0.4 over a placebo (on a scale of 1.2 to 6), and decreased their sexual-desire-related "distress score" by between 0.3 and 0.4 (on a scale of 0 to 4).[43]

In other words, the impact was relatively insignificant.

Adding to this, research showed that Addyi's potential side effects were quite serious. The most notable among these was a negative interaction between the medication and alcohol. Patients must completely abstain from drinking when taking Addyi, or risk a significant hypotensive event (a severe drop in blood pressure that could cause a loss of consciousness). Addyi also interacts with other medications and herbal supplements, and on its own can cause dizziness, nausea, tiredness, dry mouth, and difficulty falling asleep or staying asleep.

Lastly, this medication is basically in the category of antidepressants and anxiolytics. So, while male sexual enhancement medications are geared toward performance, this medication is geared toward mood, and in my opinion, this medication is saying, "It's all in your head."

INFOCEUTICALS

Energetic Integrator 11 (EI11) is best suited to help correct distortions in the Nun's disrupted energy fields. Although it contains no testosterone, this integrator "echoes" the impact of the hormone, helping to restore the flow of energy your androgen deficiency has disrupted.

Associated with the stomach meridian, this integrator influences digestion and the liver's processing of heavy metals and environmental toxins, in addition to exerting effects across the pelvic region or sacral chakra, including on the reproductive organs. The sacral chakra corresponds to the domain of emotions, encompassing those related to relationships (with people as well as the material elements of our lives, such as money), sex, and sexuality. Given the Nun's tendency toward solitude, reestablishing the energetic flow of her sacral chakra can be an important aspect of restoring not only her physiological balance, but also her broader emotional and psychological balance and her relationships with her partner, family, friends, and larger life.

ESSENTIAL OILS

The power of testosterone and personal power inspires the Nun. The following essential oils can be used to aid in assisting the power behind the drive you might want to get your day going:

Chamomile
Clary sage
Fennel
Frankincense

Geranium
Sandalwood

NUTRITION

For the Nun, nutrition can play three important roles. The first is to directly help raise testosterone. Certain vitamins and minerals can raise your levels, and these nutrients are best obtained via foods that contain them.

The second is to help decrease your estrogen levels. Provided that you are not suffering from estrogen deficiency, decreasing your estrogen levels is a helpful strategy for lowering your levels of the sex hormone binding globulin (SHBG), which binds free testosterone and diminishes the hormone's impact. Here we borrow from the nutritional guidelines for the Queen archetype (see page 224), which is primarily characterized by estrogen dominance.

The third role of nutrition in the Nun's archetypal journey is to help improve fat-to-muscle ratio. In particular, diet can help reduce abdominal fat, which is commonly referred to as a "testosterone killer." Although there is some debate around whether visceral abdominal fat (which surrounds your organs) causes low testosterone or the other way around, studies have demonstrated a correlation between waist-to-hip ratio (WHR) and testosterone levels in men, and emerging research suggests a similar correlation in women. In men and women alike, higher levels of visceral fat correspond to higher levels of estrogen, which can exacerbate testosterone deficiency.

We also know that in both sexes, testosterone has a lipolytic potential, meaning it can break down fat cells. We know, too, that visceral abdominal fat releases cholesterol and free fatty acids into the bloodstream, prompting the body to produce a protein called cytokine, which triggers low-level inflammation. High levels of visceral fat can also lead to increased production of a hormone called angiotensin, which causes blood vessels to constrict and blood pressure to rise and contributes to insulin resistance. In addition to being a factor in weight gain, insulin resistance is directly related to low testosterone in men and women.

While the nutritional aspect of the Nun's SHINES protocol is geared toward helping minimize excess fat and improving your fat-to-muscle ratio, it may or may not involve caloric restriction. But it certainly prioritizes lean proteins and "good fats" in addition to eliminating processed carbohydrates and sugar whenever possible.

FOODS TO EMBRACE

Foods High in Vitamin D

Research into low testosterone has linked it with a vitamin D deficiency. Foods rich in vitamin D that I recommend for the Nun include:

Egg yolks (also rich in omega-3 fatty acids)

Tuna (also rich in omega-3 fatty acids)

Enriched nondairy milks, such as almond milk and
cashew milk

Foods High in Zinc

Studies have shown that if you have low testosterone, zinc can help boost your body's natural production of the hormone. For Nuns whose zinc levels are low, good food sources include:

Oysters and other shellfish, including lobster and
Alaskan king crab

Grass-fed beef (chuck roast or ground beef patty)

Chickpeas

Cashews

Mushrooms

Spinach

Almonds

Whole almonds contain a set of nutrients vital to testosterone production, including vitamin E, calcium, magnesium, and potassium. They are also rich in arginine, an amino acid that is involved in increasing blood flow to the genitals in men and women. Increasing your arginine levels can enhance stimulation and sensation during the sexual arousal phase.[44]

Although almonds are a source of quality protein and contain high levels of unsaturated fatty acids, they are also a significant source of calories. For the Nun, I recommend consuming no more than twenty-five each day.

Cruciferous Vegetables

In addition to providing fiber, cruciferous vegetables such as broccoli, Brussels sprouts, cabbage, kale, mustard greens, and turnips contain a compound called indole-3-carbinol (I3C). I3C has been shown to increase the efficiency of estrogen metabolism by the liver (by virtue of its impact on the enzyme that drives this process), bringing down the body's overall estrogen levels. This decrease in turn reduces the body's SHBG levels, which can result in an increase in free testosterone. In recent years, researchers have also become interested in the way the compound impedes estrogen receptor cell proliferation and have looked into I3C as a possible preventive of breast, cervical, endometrial, and colorectal cancers.

Consuming cruciferous vegetables also triggers the body's natural production of a compound called diindolylmethane (DIM). Research has shown that this compound also helps break down estrogen, contributing to a lowering of SHBG levels and a corresponding rise in testosterone.

One word of warning regarding cruciferous vegetables: They can contain phytoestrogens, which can exert estrogenic effects. For the Nun, who may already be estrogen dominant, I recommend limiting your consumption of cruciferous vegetables to one serving every other day.

Foods Containing "Good" (Unsaturated) Fats

It is important for the Nun to rely on unsaturated fats rather than carbohydrates—particularly processed carbohydrates—for fuel. While I do not recommend cutting out carbohydrates altogether, relying more heavily on healthy fats (including omega-3s) than carbohydrates can help decrease your levels of visceral abdominal fat and increase your muscle-to-fat ratio. Omega-3 fats in particular have an overarching balancing effect on your hormones and contribute to the health of your skin, including your vaginal mucosa.

For the Nun, good sources of unsaturated fats include various nuts, seeds, and oils, as well as foods high in omega-3 fats.

Oils I recommend:

Nut oils, including coconut oil[*]
Rapeseed oil

Although avocados do not contain omega-3 fatty acids, they are a great source of unsaturated fat, fiber, and a number of supportive vitamins and minerals. Containing no cholesterol and few carbohydrates, avocados are high in vitamin B, magnesium, manganese, potassium, and vitamin K.

If you use butter, I recommend switching to a grass-fed butter, clarified butter, or ghee. Although all of these contain saturated fats, they have benefits over traditional, grain-fed butter that are relevant for the Nun. Grass-fed butter contains five times the amount of a fatty acid called conjugated linoleic acid (CLA), which research has shown can help with weight loss. Grass-fed butter is also significantly higher in omega-3 fatty acids and vitamin K2. Both clarified butter and ghee are believed to lower LDL (so-called bad cholesterol) levels and protect the arteries from hardening.

EXERCISE

For the Nun whose energy levels are low and who is experiencing generalized muscle weakness, exercise can pose a significant challenge. The good news is that even moderate exercise can help increase your testosterone levels, improve your overall health, and bring your hormones into balance.[45]

The first step in the Nun's exercise regime is to simply start moving. Any aerobic activity, whether it's walking, jogging, bicycling, or swimming, will help boost your adrenal glands' testosterone produc-

---

[*] If you are experiencing vaginal dryness, you may consider applying coconut oil directly to the vulva. This can help with lubrication in the short and longer term.

tion. To start, do what you can. And no more. Trust that over time, your energy levels can improve, and your fatigue dissipate.

Gradually increase the intensity and duration of your workouts as you are able. Do this without judgment and with a forgiving spirit. But dedicate yourself fully to the form of exercise you choose. Create a regular schedule for your workouts and commit to it. Regard the time and space you set aside for them as sacred and inviolable. If it helps you stick to your routine, consider enlisting the help of a trainer or coach, or joining a group that will hold you accountable for showing up for each session.

When combined with other elements of the SHINES protocol, a primarily aerobic workout regime will help you burn fat and improve your muscle-to-fat ratio. Incorporating an interval-training element (brief anaerobic "spurts") into your workout routine when you're able can improve this even further.

WALKING AND RUNNING

Beginning where you are can mean starting slow. We've talked about the immediate availability of walking. Whether you walk outdoors or on a treadmill at home or at the gym, start off with walking until you feel fatigue. Over time, you can increase your distance and pace.

When you feel ready, you may also introduce higher-intensity and even muscle-building anaerobic interval training into your workouts. You may consider running or sprinting short distances. You may also seek out hills along your outdoor route or set your treadmill at an incline. Either of these will require that you push yourself a little harder, helping you to burn fat and build muscle at a faster pace. Of course, you can keep these intervals to durations that are manageable for you, increasing these at the rate that feels right for you.

RESISTANCE TRAINING

Increasing your muscle mass can help boost testosterone production. And for the Nun, resistance training can be a great place to begin.

Resistance training requires no equipment. Isometric exercises such as push-ups, squats, and lunges are all examples of exercises you can do with no equipment (although you can incorporate exercise bands), at your own pace, and when it's convenient for you. Gradually increasing these in number and intensity can have a significant impact over time.

Last, you can transform some of your aerobic exercises into resistance exercises. Momentarily increasing the intensity with which you walk or cycle—inserting anaerobic "bursts" into your usual routine—can engage your muscles enough to kick off the muscle-building cycle of damage and repair.

CYCLING

Cycling is a low-impact exercise, rendering it easier on your knees and hips, and it's a relatively easy activity to begin. If you are suffering from low energy levels, cycling is a workout you can build at your own pace.

Whether you cycle indoors or outdoors, you can gradually increase the intensity of your workout. Like walking, cycling provides opportunities for incorporating muscle-building anaerobic intervals. By seeking out hillier terrain, a spin class, or a video you can watch while you ride a stationary bike at home, you can increase the rate and power of your pedal strokes. For anywhere from a few seconds to a few minutes, you can take your workout to a higher level. Again, you can control whether and to what extent you push yourself, remaining attentive to what your body is telling you.

SUPPLEMENTS

Three overarching objectives drive this element of the Nun's SHINES protocol: boosting testosterone levels, enhancing sexual desire and arousal, and helping to restore overall hormonal balance.

MACA

An herb grown in Peru, maca has long been used to promote hormone balance (in men and women) as well as reproductive and menstrual health. Each of the thirteen differently colored varieties of maca exerts distinct effects, and many maca-based supplements combine different varieties of the herb. Some of these can raise estrogen levels, which is why it's critical to use a supplement that contains the right types of maca in the right ratios to address your estrogen dominance.

The particular maca supplement I recommend for a Nun is Femmenessence MacaHarmony, a 100 percent organic and vegan mixture of sustainably farmed maca that has been shown to have a balancing effect on women's levels of estrogen, progesterone, and other hormones. I recommend taking the supplement as directed on the label (one 500 mg tablet in the morning and one in the evening).

Two notes of **caution** with regard to MacaHarmony: First, I recommend that a Nun take this supplement for two to three months and then take a week off. This can help upregulate your estrogen receptors and enhance the supplement's benefits. Second, Maca-Harmony can amplify the effects of caffeine. So while a Nun is always wise to limit or avoid caffeine, taking extra caution around caffeine when taking this supplement is a good idea.

Maca is an herb I rely on in many of the archetypes. Although it has not been shown to boost testosterone production per se, maca is associated with increased energy levels and stamina as well as enhanced sex drive in women and men. (Maca has also been shown to help alleviate premenstrual and postmenopausal symptoms.)

Different maca-based powders, capsules, and extracts contain different strains of the herb and exert particular effects. For the Nun, I recommend two different maca blends. If you are premenopausal, I recommend Femmenessence's Maca Harmony Menstrual Health. In addition to supporting overall hormonal balance, this particular maca blend also helps improve energy levels, mood, and bone health. If you are postmenopausal, I recommend Femmenessence's MacaPause. This blend helps alleviate common menopause-related symptoms such as hot flashes and interrupted sleep in addition to improving your energy levels and libido and reducing vaginal dryness.

Given their fiber content, all maca products can cause some level of gastrointestinal distress. A maca blend may also interact with other supplements or medications you are taking. Before you incorporate it into your daily routine, seek advice from your physician, nutritionist, or other healthcare provider. I also recommend beginning with a relatively low dose of maca in order to give your system time to acclimate to it.

I recommend the standard dose: two capsules twice daily, away from meals.

First dose in the AM before breakfast
Second dose in the early PM, ideally 30 minutes
    before you normally experience an energy low

Consider taking half the recommended amount for two weeks, then gradually increase to the standard amount. Assuming your system tolerates the maca well, I suggest continuing to take the supplement at the near-full or full dose for four to six weeks. Maca can require this much time to exert its impact.

HORNY GOAT WEED

Also known as barrenwort, bishop's hat, and fairy wings, horny goat weed is an herb belonging to the genus *Epimedium*. Found primarily in China, horny goat weed has been used for centuries in Eastern medicine as an aphrodisiac for women and men.[46] Popular now in the West, horny goat weed supplements are available in a variety of forms, including liquid extract and capsules.

Although their specific mechanisms of action are unknown, the flavonoids contained in horny goat weed have been shown to help increase blood flow, which can enhance sexual arousal in women and men. These have also been shown to help prevent osteopenia and osteoporosis by stimulating the proliferation of cells called osteoblasts, which play a critical role in bone restructuring.[47]

YOHIMBE

Derived from the chemical yohimbine, extracted from the bark of yohimbe trees indigenous to Africa, this supplement may help enhance your libido and levels of sexual arousal. Yohimbe has been shown to increase both blood flow and nerve impulses to the vagina, which can intensify sexual excitement. It has also been shown to counteract the negative sexual side effects of SSRIs.[48] If you're interested in adding a yohimbe supplement to your daily regime, be sure to confirm the ingredients and review them with your physician. Certain ingredients in yohimbe supplements can interact with prescription medications. Also important to consider are the supplement's potential side effects, which include rapid heart rate, anxiety, high blood pressure, cold sweats, vomiting, nausea, stomach pain, and insomnia. If you experience any of these side effects, immediately cease taking the yohimbe and consult your physician.

TRIBULUS

Commonly found in dry climates around the globe, *Tribulus terrestris* is a weedy plant covered in spines. Chemicals contained in its fruit, leaves, and roots are used in the creation of powder- and capsule-based supplements. Tribulus (also known as cat's-head, puncture vine, and devil's eyelashes, among other names) is used in Eastern and Western medicine to treat kidney, bladder, and urinary tract issues, digestive difficulties, and circulatory problems. Studies have shown that tribulus can also have a positive impact on sexual desire and arousal in women with hypoactive sexual desire disorder.[49]

Tribulus's mechanism of action is unclear. Several studies have indicated that the herb does not directly boost testosterone levels in women or men. Research has shown, however, that the herb may enhance androgen receptor density in the brain, which can amplify the effects of testosterone on libido.

One important side effect of tribulus is its impact on blood sugar levels. If you are diabetic and rely on blood-sugar-regulating medications, taking the supplement may necessitate that your physician adjusts your dose. Also, tribulus should be taken only in the short term. For the Nun, I recommend a period of no longer than eight weeks.

RESVERATROL

Found in the skins of red grapes, mulberries, and blueberries, and in nuts such as peanuts and pistachios, resveratrol is a chemical compound produced in plants in response to injury, including bacterial and fungal attacks. Although resveratrol's potential benefits for humans remain a matter of debate, recent research suggests it may have a positive effect on testosterone levels.

Like chrysin, resveratrol may help reduce the aromatization of testosterone into estrogen, increasing the levels of free testosterone in the bloodstream. It may also activate the body's androgen receptors, enhancing testosterone's effects. Resveratrol may also reduce inflammation, which has a negative impact on metabolism and contributes to muscle deterioration.[50]

One limitation of resveratrol is its bioavailability. When you consume it via food, drinks, or supplements, resveratrol is absorbed by the intestines and conjugated by the liver. Check each supplement for bioavailability. Standard doses of resveratrol are between 250 and 600 mg per day. For the Nun, I recommend a dose of about 250 mg/day. (If you're hoping to get your resveratrol from red wine, I have some bad news: The average bottle contains only 2 mg.)

There are few side effects associated with resveratrol itself. Like other supplements, however, it may interfere with prescription medications that are processed by the liver. Resveratrol supplements can affect circulating amounts of blood thinners, birth control pills, and antibiotics.

BOOK RECOMMENDATIONS FOR NUNS

Susan Rako, MD, *The Hormone of Desire: The Truth About Testosterone, Sexuality, and Menopause* (New York: Three Rivers Press, 1996)

Kathy C. Maupin, MD, *The Secret Female Hormone: How Testosterone Replacement Therapy Can Change Your Life* (Carlsbad, CA: Hay House, 2014)

NUNS

Saint Teresa of Ávila (b. Teresa Sánchez de Cepeda y Ahumada, March 28, 1515–October 4, 1582). Born in what is now Spain, Teresa of Ávila was an influential mystic, Carmelite nun, theologian, and author during the Counter-Reformation (also called the Catholic Reformation) of the late sixteenth and early seventeenth centuries.

Teresa of Ávila's religious career began in or around 1535, when she entered the Carmelite Convent of the Incarnation of Ávila. (She did this against her father's wishes; her mother had died in 1529, when Teresa was just fourteen.) Within two years, Teresa became seriously ill. She remained an invalid for three more, during which time she developed a deep love for contemplative prayer. Once her health was restored, however, Teresa abandoned this practice. It was not until 1555, when she experienced a religious awakening, that she embarked on the spiritual, theological, and philosophical work and writing that would prove so influential.[51]

In the world of modern theology, Teresa of Ávila's ascetic doctrine is regarded as the quintessential explication of the contemplative life, and her writings rank among the most widely read. These include *The Way of Perfection* (1583), *The Interior Castle* (1588), *Spiritual Relations, Exclamations of the Soul to God* (1588), *Conceptions on the Love of God* (date unknown), and the autobiographical *Life of the Mother Teresa of Jesus* (1611). Teresa was canonized by Pope Gregory XV in 1622. Pope Paul VI named the saint a Doctor of the Church on September 27, 1970.

Mother Teresa (Saint Teresa of Calcutta) (b. Anjezë Gonxhe Bojaxhiu, August 26, 1910–September 5, 1997). Born in what is now the Republic of Macedonia, Mother Teresa lived briefly in Ireland before moving to India, where she spent most of her life and engaged in her most influential work. In 1950, Mother Teresa founded the Roman Catholic Missionaries of Charity, which operates soup kitchens, orphanages, schools, and clinics for needy patients suffering from such diseases as HIV/AIDS, leprosy, and tuberculosis. As of 2012, the organization was staffed by more than 4,500 Catholic nuns and was active in more than 130 countries.[52]

In addition to her work at the helm the Missionaries of Charity, Mother Teresa also engaged in serious, dangerous work on the ground. During the 1982 Siege of Beirut, for example, she brokered a temporary cease-fire between the Israeli Army and Palestinian guerillas so that she and representatives from the American Red Cross could evacuate young patients trapped in a front-line hospital.[53]

Although frequently the object of criticism and scrutiny, Mother Teresa also received a number of honors and awards. These include the 1962 Ramon Magsaysay Award for Peace and International Understanding and the 1979 Nobel Peace Prize. The Roman Catholic Church canonized her on September 2, 2016.

The SHINES Protocol: How Do You Relax a Warrior?

For the Warrior, the purpose of the SHINES protocol is not only to bring her testosterone and other hormones into balance, but also to help her harness her physical, spiritual, and emotional energies and redirect these in ways that serve her when she's off the battlefield—when she's a mother, a partner, a sister, a friend. Many of the elements of the SHINES protocol focus on solitary, centering practices. Over time, these can draw a Warrior's attention away from her daily battles, refocusing in on her true self and the deeper fears and desires that drive her.

SPIRITUAL PRACTICE

When I open a discussion about spiritual practices with a Warrior, I often refer to the work of Chögyam Trungpa, the founder of Shambhala Buddhism. Trungpa regards the essence of warriorship not as aggression, but rather as the essence of human bravery. As he writes in his 1984 book, *Shambhala: The Sacred Path of the Warrior*, "The key to warriorship and the first principle of Shambhala vision is not being afraid of who you are. Ultimately, that is the definition of bravery: not being afraid of yourself."[54]

For me, Trungpa's words are apt for the Warrior. Prone to getting caught up in her daily outward battles, she can neglect to turn her focus inward. But doing this is critical to the Warrior's journey. Less than victory, this is about how the Warrior shows up to battle— whether she is centered in her convictions, whether she feels rooted in her beliefs, whether she feels courageous, sure of herself, well-rested, balanced.

Beginning here, the first step along the Warrior's spiritual journey involves venturing inward, centering her calm focus on herself and being lionhearted enough to face and grapple with the emotional elements and underpinnings of her archetype and tending to these. As you consider the following suggestions for spiritual practices, consider these questions: Where is there fearfulness inside you? Do you fear missing out on something? Are you afraid of success? Are you afraid of digging too deep? Are you afraid of being alone? Are you afraid of asking questions about yourself? Your larger life? What is it you're afraid of?

WALKING MEDITATIONS

Solitary walks can be a very effective way for you to distance yourself from the battles that take so much of your time, focus, and energy, and instead to turn your focus on yourself. And combining walks with meditative practices can help you work through your inner Warrior's inclinations toward aggression or competition.

JOURNALING

Whether you're an avid diarist or have never kept a journal in your life, taking time each day to record some of the details of your thoughts, feelings, and physical symptomology, as well as your external encounters with the world around you, can help you focus on yourself. Over time, the ritual of journaling can make this shift in attention feel more natural and occur more spontaneously.

SACRED QUESTS

An essential aspect of the Warrior's spiritual practice is redirecting her often high levels of physical energy and strength. While quietly and deliberately focusing inward can yield significant results, so, too, can setting your sights on a distant goal—a holy grail, if you will—and undertaking the quest to achieve it.

Your goal will be unique to you. All that matters is that it's important to you and that you believe you can—and will—attain it. Maybe it's weight loss. Maybe it's a better relationship with your family. Maybe it's improved physical condition, whatever that looks like for you. It may also involve a new hobby or entering a sphere of competition. Taking on your quest directs your energy and purpose.

HORMONE MODULATION

There is no "anti-testosterone" prescription I can write for a Warrior, meaning there are no hormone-based or other medications you can take to lower your testosterone levels. Rather, the hormone modulation element of her SHINES protocol involves addressing and treating the root cause of the excess.

If your imbalance has arisen out of exposure to exogenous testosterone, hormonal modulation involves limiting or eliminating your contact with it. If you come into frequent contact with a man who uses topical testosterone creams or gels, we will discuss how to keep yourself safer. If you have been working with a healthcare practitioner who has prescribed injectable testosterone or subdermal pellets that have caused your levels to rise too high, to the point where you're suffering undesirable, adverse effects, we will consider options for diminishing or eliminating the impact of these medications.

Given the strength of injectable testosterone and subdermal pellets, I don't recommend either of these medications to my patients who are suffering from testosterone deficiency. This said, injectable testosterone *can* be moderated such that it potentially delivers an appropriate dose. If you have been diagnosed with low testosterone and are taking an injectable medication to address it, it may be advisable to continue the medication at a lower dose, adjusting it over time as necessary. Subdermal pellets, on the other hand, cannot be moderated. Not only do these cause huge spikes and decreases in your testosterone levels that leave you with exaggerated symptoms of both excess and (relative) deficiency, they also cannot be removed once inserted. This means the pellets continue to exert their effects for months. If pellets have given rise to your Warrior archetype, the SHINES protocol can help offset their impact.

In any of these scenarios, the end game may not involve eliminating your exposure to exogenous testosterone altogether. The goal of this element of the SHINES protocol (and of the protocol more generally) is to help bring your testosterone and other hormones into *balance*. You may, in fact, need and benefit from a customized testosterone replacement medication. After all, testosterone helps supports physical and mental fitness in addition to a healthy libido. But in women in particular, too-high levels of testosterone are neither healthy nor sustainable. The work, then, is to find a replacement therapy that helps support your energy levels and muscle strength but stops short of exerting the significant androgenic effects we've reviewed in this chapter.

If you're a Warrior who has been diagnosed with PCOS, certain hormone-based medications can help alleviate the symptoms of this condition. The most common are birth control medications. By effectively interrupting the signals between the pituitary gland and the ovaries, birth control pills prevent follicle-stimulating hormone (FSH) and luteinizing hormone (LH) from triggering the ovaries' production of estrogen and testosterone, respectively. Birth control pills also raise your level of production of sex hormone binding globulin (SHBG), a protein that binds to testosterone and estrogen in the bloodstream, rendering them inactive. In addition to birth control medications, you may also benefit from taking progesterone. This can offset the effects of estrogen dominance, which PCOS also causes.

Although hormone-based medications can help alleviate some of the symptoms of PCOS, including excess testosterone production, weight loss is the best means of bringing your inner Warrior back into balance. While weight loss is rarely easy for anyone, it can be particularly difficult if you're suffering from PCOS. This is because in addition to the hormonal imbalances to which the condition gives rise, PCOS can also cause insulin resistance and hyperinsulinemia, a condition in which insulin levels in the blood tend to be high relative to your glucose levels. Hyperinsulinemia is associated with both weight gain and high levels of testosterone, which may be caused in part by your body's natural effort to regulate insulin.

Because Warriors tend to benefit from having a plan of attack—clearly drawn schematics, if you will—I recommend taking a very structured approach to weight loss. This begins with the basics: reduce calorie consumption and increase calorie expenditure. For the Warrior who is battling PCOS, I recommend aiming for a calorie deficit of between 300 and 500 calories per day. Just as important, I recommend a ketogenic diet, which focuses on "good" fats and proteins while limiting carbohydrates. (I advise Warriors who are trying to accelerate weight loss to reduce their intake of carbohydrates to just 50 g/day.) The big idea behind the ketogenic diet is that it helps force the body to burn fat rather than carbohydrates. For the Warrior whose weight gain (and increased testosterone) is tied to insulin resistance, shedding excess fat is particularly important. The Nutrition section on page 372 contains specific suggestions of foods to embrace and avoid.

As for exercise, I always remind Warriors that the most important thing is to *begin*. Start where you are without pressure or judgment. Take walks or short bike rides, participate in a low-impact cardio class at home or at the gym, but begin. Make a commitment to yourself to make the time in your day, and stick to it. The Exercise section on page 376 will help guide you toward a workout that can work for you.

In addition to diet, exercise, and nutritional supplements, insulin-resistant Warriors can often benefit from certain oral anti-diabetes medications, such as glimepiride or metformin. As they increase your insulin sensitivity, these drugs can also facilitate weight loss. There are side effects associated with all antidiabetes medications, however, so weighing these against any benefits is critical.

INFOCEUTICALS

For the Warrior, Energetic Integrator 11 (EI11) can help resolve the energetic disturbances testosterone excess can cause. Exerting effects along the stomach meridian and within the pelvic region (sacral chakra), this integrator impacts digestion and liver function, including the processing of heavy metals and environmental toxins, in addition to influencing the reproductive organs and, in particular, testosterone.

As we also discuss in the Infoceuticals section for the Nun archetype (see page 352), the influence of EI11 on the sacral chakra is particularly important to consider. The sacral chakra corresponds to the realm of feelings and emotions, including those associated with relationships and relating as well as to sex and sexuality, and disruptions within it can indicate troubled relationships with partners, friends, and family, and even certain practical elements of our lives, such as money and career. For the Warrior who is struggling not only on the physiological front but also on the emotional and practical fronts of her life, restoring a steady and balanced flow of energy within this sensitive region can bring some ease and calm.

ESSENTIAL OILS

Warriors want to avoid essential oils that may have a testosterone-boosting effect. If one can safely increase estrogen levels, this will increase the levels of SHBG and lower active testosterone. Consider trying:

Lavender   Spearmint
Peppermint   Tea tree oil

NUTRITION

The goal of the nutrition aspect of the Warrior's SHINES protocol is twofold: lower testosterone levels and help the body shed excess fat. While not every Warrior will be concerned with weight loss, any can benefit from the guidelines regarding which foods to embrace and which to avoid.

FOODS TO EMBRACE

Fiber

One important aspect of fiber consumption is that it can increase your SHBG levels. As we discussed earlier in this chapter, the more SHBG is circulating in your system, the more it will bind to free testosterone, rendering the hormone inactive.

Another advantage of fiber that is of particular importance to Warriors suffering from PCOS is that it can help keep your blood sugar levels in balance. Consuming fiber-rich foods with low glycemic indexes can, over time, reduce your insulin resistance and its downstream effects on your testosterone levels. Significant, too, is that fiber-rich foods help you feel satiated, an aid to Warriors working to shed excess weight.

For all Warriors, I recommend sources of fiber with low glycemic indexes. Among the most beneficial are:

Grapefruit and oranges
Pears and apples (both with the skin on)

Prunes

Dates

Bran

Oatmeal

Barley

Winter squash

Beans

Raw nuts

I also recommend *slowly* increasing the amount of fiber in your diet in order to avoid gastrointestinal distress.

Phytoestrogens

For Warriors who are not also estrogen dominant (Warriors suffering from PCOS are likely to be) or at increased risk for breast cancer, I recommend increasing your consumption of phytoestrogens. This can help reduce your levels of circulating testosterone by raising your SHBG levels.

Several foods contain phytoestrogens. The most potent is soy. Rich in isoflavones such as genistein and daidzein, which the body can convert into weak forms of estrogen, soy can help elevate your levels of circulating estrogen and SHBG.

For any Warrior, I recommend organic fermented soy (and fermented soy products) over conventional (non-organic) unfermented versions. Widely popular in the United States, unfermented soy products are coming under increased scrutiny for their potential to contribute to digestive, metabolic, and circulatory dysfunction. Adding to this, genetically modified soy has been linked to food allergies, thyroid damage, and digestive disorders. Examples of unfermented soy products include tofu, soy milk, edamame, and soy flour, as well as processed shakes and bars that contain soy derivatives or soybean oil.

Fermented soy, by contrast, has been linked to improved digestive health and increased delivery of key minerals, including calcium, iron, magnesium, and zinc. Adding to this, the fermentation process itself increases the product's levels of such nutrients as thiamin and biotin, rendering it a healthier food overall. Examples of fermented soy I recommend for the Warrior include:

Fermented soy milk
Miso
Natto
Soy sauce
Tempeh

Again, before incorporating soy into your diet, I recommend discussing any potential risk factors, including allergies, with your physician.

Other phytoestrogen-containing foods I recommend for the Warrior include:

Barley
Flaxseed
Lentils
Oatmeal
Sesame Seeds
Yams

Reishi Mushrooms

Revered in its native China and other parts of Asia for its healing powers, this "mushroom of immortality," as it has been called, can also help reduce the conversion of testosterone to dihydrotestosterone (DHT), a metabolite of the hormone that is responsible for some of the negative side effects of testosterone excess, such as male-pattern balding. Studies have shown that reishi mushrooms (*Ganoderma lucidum*) reduce levels of the 5α-reductase enzyme, which drives the conversion.[55]

FOODS TO AVOID

Cruciferous Vegetables

One group of foods I counsel Warriors to consume in limited quantities are cruciferous vegetables. Broccoli, kale, cabbage, Brussels sprouts, and others contain a compound called indole-3-carbinol (I3C), which has been shown to increase the efficiency of estrogen metabolism by the liver (by virtue of its impact on the enzyme that drives this process). As it helps reduce the body's overall estrogen levels, I3C also contributes to a drop in the body's SHBG levels. This results in an increase in free testosterone. Consuming cruciferous vegetables also triggers the body's natural production of a compound called diindolylmethane (DIM). Studies have shown that DIM has a similar effect on estrogen and SHBG as I3C.

For the Warrior who is also estrogen dominant, it is important to keep in mind that cruciferous vegetables can also contain phytoestrogens that exert estrogenic effects. For this reason, too, limiting your consumption of these can be a wise choice. Obviously, I am not saying that cruciferous vegetables are bad, but I am trying to increase the levels of SHBG temporarily with the goal of decreasing the negative effects of free testosterone.

Asparagus

Containing the testosterone building blocks of folic acid, potassium, and vitamin E, asparagus stimulates the production of testosterone. While you need not avoid asparagus altogether, I advise consuming it infrequently and in relatively small quantities.

Avocados

Although avocados are a great source of unsaturated fat, fiber, and various vitamins and minerals, they are also high in vitamin B, magnesium, manganese, potassium, and vitamin K—the building blocks of testosterone. Like asparagus, avocados can stimulate the production of testosterone, and Warriors would do well to limit their consumption of them.

Garlic

Research into the effects of garlic on testosterone has indicated that it boosts the effectiveness of the hormone by reducing the body's cortisol levels. Its effect on cortisol seems to be linked to a compound called allicin, which is found in the powder form of garlic as well as in fresh garlic cloves themselves. Again, while the relatively limited and infrequent consumption of garlic is unlikely to significantly contribute to your testosterone excess, I recommend Warriors avoid consistent exposure.

EXERCISE

For any Warrior, exercise is an important element of the SHINES protocol. Regardless of whether weight loss is one of your goals, exercise helps improve or maintain your healthy body composition, bone and muscle health, and overall energy levels, each of which is a critical component of your overall well-being and hormonal balance.

Whether you're a fanatical athlete looking forward to your next Tough Mudder or your low energy levels have kept you from working out for some time, one or more of the Warrior exercises I recommend here can work for you. As we discussed earlier in this section, depending on the conditions that have given rise to your archetype, you may feel more or less ready to commit to a regular workout routine, but the important thing is to begin. Read on with this in mind, remembering that you may choose to start off slow and gradually increase the intensity of your regime as your strength and endurance improve.

SWIMMING

Swimming is one of my favorite exercises for the Warrior because at any stage along your journey, it can deliver significant benefits. Part resistance training, part aerobic exercise, this low-impact workout can be appropriate for Warriors seeking a high-intensity, high-calorie-burning activity and those looking to gradually build up to a more demanding regime.

From the start, your workouts will be more or less exacting depending on the strokes you choose and whether you use equipment such as a kickboard. Explore your options, taking note of how each feels and for how long you are able to sustain it.

One Warrior patient of mine recently told me that when she first started swimming, she felt exhausted after just seven minutes in the pool. Five months later, she could swim forty-five minutes at a stretch. She had also lost 15 pounds. While other elements of the SHINES protocol were contributing to her improved overall health, hormonal rebalancing, and increased energy levels, she attributed her enhanced performance in the pool to her commitment to the workout. "Letting myself start slowly paid off," she noted.

BIKING

Similar to swimming, biking is both (generally) aerobic and low-impact. You can also take it at your pace. Whether you ride outside or on a stationary bike, you can vary your workouts from relatively short and less intense to longer and more intense.

Ultimately, biking can be a very effective method of creating calorie deficits. Again, because it's low-impact, increasing the intensity of your workouts involves making them longer, which you can do at relatively low risk to your major joints.

WEIGHT LIFTING AND RESISTANCE TRAINING

The benefits of weight lifting and resistance training reside in their ability to help build and sustain muscle tone. Whether you're looking to improve your muscle-to-fat ratio or are already quite lean, getting into the habit of routinely performing exercises that will help you sustain a healthy body composition is critical to your long-term health and overall hormonal balance.

For the Warrior, the best way to approach weight lifting and resistance training is to focus on involving as possible many of your major joints. Exercises such as lunges and squats, as well as certain strengthening yoga poses (including Warrior 1 and Warrior 2), can help improve the strength and flexibility of your hips. Weight lifting can also help strengthen your lower body. Consider using lighter weights and higher reps.

SUPPLEMENTS

This aspect of the Warrior's SHINES protocol aims not to lower total testosterone, per se, but to diminish the free amounts of the hormone and limit the conversion of testosterone to DHT, a potent metabolite that contributes to the rise of side effects, including hirsutism, acne, and androgenic alopecia (male-pattern baldness).

RED CLOVER

Similar to reishi mushrooms, a red clover supplement can help reduce the conversion of testosterone to DHT.[56] This means that while the supplement may not influence your body's production of testosterone, per se, it can help diminish some of the less desirable side effects of an excess, including male-pattern balding.

There are two notes of caution regarding red clover. The first is that the supplement can help sustain high levels of luteinizing hormone

(LH), which, in turn, can help maintain higher levels of testosterone. LH stimulates ovary- and ovarian cyst–based theca cells to produce testosterone. This is particularly important for Warriors who have PCOS, whose LH levels are likely already elevated. The second is that red clover contains isoflavones, which the body can convert to phytoestrogens. Warriors who are also estrogen dominant and/or whom excess estrogen puts at increased cancer risk should consult with their physician before incorporating red clover into their daily regimen.

VITEX (CHASTEBERRY)

Vitex agnus-castus, commonly known as chasteberry or vitex, is an herbal supplement that has been used for thousands of years by cultures around the globe to help maintain a healthy balance of estrogen and progesterone. Studies have shown that vitex can inhibit the secretion of follicle-stimulating hormone (FSH) by the pituitary gland, which leads to a decrease in estrogen production by the ovaries. Vitex has also been shown to stimulate the secretion of luteinizing hormone (LH), which triggers the formulation of a corpus luteum and increases progesterone production.

I do share a few **warnings** about vitex with patients. First, although vitex may begin working in as few as ten days, studies show that women taking the supplement may need to wait for up to six months to experience it benefits. Second, although there are few significant side effects associated with vitex, some of my patients have reported nausea, gastrointestinal upset, skin reactions, and headaches. Women who suffer from menstrual depression or PMDD have also reported an exacerbation of these symptoms. **Vitex is not recommended for women who are pregnant or breastfeeding.**

Although it has no direct effect on testosterone, Vitex can help bring levels of the hormone back into balance by boosting the body's production of progesterone. This helps lower the body's production of estrogen, which in turn decreases its production of testosterone.

Another note of warning regarding Vitex is that similar to red clover, it can raise luteinizing LH levels.[57] Research indicates, however, that this is most likely to occur in women *whose levels are not already elevated.* This means that Warriors battling PCOS whose LH levels are high due to the condition are unlikely to experience this effect. For Warriors who do not have PCOS and decide to try vitex, I advise consistent monitoring of LH levels.

Some researchers have asserted that vitex works by reducing levels of prolactin, a hormone produced by the pituitary gland that is present in both men and women. Others have argued that vitex exerts its effects via a series of neurotransmitters, including dopamine, acetylcholine, and/or opioid receptors.

INOSITOL

A vitaminlike substance found in plants such as cantaloupe, beans, brown rice, and sesame seeds, inositol helps the body balance a variety of chemicals, including those associated with psychological and physiological conditions from depression to high cholesterol to cancer.

Inositol has been shown to lower blood serum testosterone in women. Studies indicate it can also increase insulin sensitivity. In Warriors battling PCOS, hyperinsulinemia (insulin insensitivity) is linked to elevated testosterone.[58]

If used as directed, inositol has relatively few side effects. (Excessive dosages can cause diarrhea, headache, fatigue, and dizziness.) Water-soluble, inositol and its metabolites are excreted by the kidneys. Inositol is not recommended for patients already taking an antidepressant, as it can increase serotonin levels.

For the Warrior, I recommend 500 mg of inositol twice per day.

SPEARMINT TEA

Commonly used in Middle Eastern countries to treat excessive male-pattern hair growth (typically on the face, chest, and back) in women, spearmint tea has been shown to have antiandrogenic properties. Research indicates that spearmint tea can reduce a woman's levels of free testosterone, diminishing the various effects of excess.[59]

FLAXSEED AND FLAXSEED OIL

Flaxseed is another potentially supportive supplement for the Warrior. Studies have indicated that flaxseed's high lignan (fiber) content is likely responsible for its antiandrogenic properties. Lignan has been found to increase levels of SHBG, which reduces free testosterone. Researchers have also speculated that lignan may also inhibit the production of 5α-reductase, the enzyme responsible for converting testosterone to DHT.[60] As we discussed earlier in this section, impeding this conversion can diminish the effects of testosterone such as excessive body hair growth and acne.

LICORICE

In addition to helping regulate symptoms of PMS and PMDD, studies have shown that licorice (*Glycyrrhiza glabra*) can also reduce total testosterone levels and diminish effects of excess, including hirsutism.[61] Researchers have attributed this to the steroid glycyrrhizin and glycyrrhetic acid licorice contains. Each has been shown to have antiandrogenic properties.[62]

Like some of the other supplements we've discussed here, licorice contains phytoestrogens, which can exert a mild estrogenic effect. **This is one of those supplements that needs to be treated with care, because you can indeed take too much and many hospitalizations have resulted from people eating even just too much black licorice**

(I find the taste disgusting). If you are going to take this supplement, make sure you do it under the care of a physician.

SAW PALMETTO

Extracted from a small palm tree indigenous to the eastern United States, saw palmetto is commonly used to counteract the symptoms of PCOS-related and non-PCOS-related elevated testosterone in women, including hirsutism, acne, and male-pattern baldness. Similar to reishi mushrooms, red clover, and flaxseed, saw palmetto may block the production of 5α-reductase, the enzyme that helps convert testosterone to DHT. Researchers have noted that this may be related to the phytosterols (cholesterol-like compounds) saw palmetto contains.[63]

BOOK RECOMMENDATIONS FOR WARRIORS

Eckhart Tolle, *The Power of Now* (Novato, CA: New World Library, 2004)

Angela Grassi and Stephanie Mattei, *The PCOS Workbook: Your Guide to Complete Physical and Emotional Health* (San Francisco: Luca Publishing, 2019)

To learn more about the role of testosterone in your overall hormonal makeup and well-being:

Kathy Maupin, MD, *The Secret Female Hormone: How Testosterone Replacement Can Change Your Life* (Carlsbad, CA: Hay House, 2014)

Susan Rako, MD, *The Hormone of Desire: The Truth About Testosterone, Sexuality, and Menopause* (New York: Harmony Books, 1999)

WARRIORS

Wonder Woman, *fictional character of DC Comics fame.* Making her first appearance in 1941, Wonder Woman is a cofounder of DC Comics' Justice League, the other super-hero members of which include Superman, Batman, the Flash, and the Green Lantern. Endowed with superhuman strength, speed, endurance, and intelligence, Wonder Woman wields a series of weapons, including the Lasso of Truth, indestructible bracelets, and a projectile tiara.

Wonder Woman was cocreated by artist Harry G. Peter and writer and psychologist William Moulton Marston (known as Charles Moulton), who credited his wife, Elizabeth Marston, and lover Olive Byrne with inspiring the character's physical appearance. Moulton was also reportedly inspired by the writings of a series of early twentieth-century American feminist writers, most notably the sex educator, writer, nurse, and birth control pioneer Margaret Sanger.

Ann Richards (September 1, 1933–September 13, 2006), *American politician; forty-fifth (and first publicly elected female) governor of Texas (1991–1995).* Staunchly Democratic, Ann Richards was known for being outspoken on the issues that mattered to her, including women's health and reproductive rights. She is also credited with reforming the Texas prison system during her tenure as governor, including by establishing a substance abuse program for inmates, and with attempting to curb the proliferation of high-powered assault weapons by backing proposals to limit the sales of semiautomatic weapons and cop-killer bullets. At the age of sixty-three, Richards was diagnosed with osteoporosis after losing ¾ inch in height and breaking a hand and ankle. In 2004, she cowrote an account of her battle with the disease titled *I'm Not Slowing Down*, in which she also shared tactics for other women suffering from it.

Richards is the recipient of the Texas NAACP Presidential Award for Outstanding Contributions to Civil Rights and the National Wildlife Federation Conservation Achievement Award, among others.

Eva "Evita" Perón (May 7, 1919–July 26, 1952), *First Lady of Argentina, as wife of President Juan Perón, from June 1946 until her death* *in 1952*. Born into poverty, Evita was the youngest of five children. She moved at the age of fifteen to Buenos Aires to pursue an acting career. At a charity event in the city in 1944, she met her future husband, Colonel Juan Perón.

As Argentina's First Lady, Evita assumed a position of power within the pro-Peronist trade unions, which she used to advance a platform of workers' rights. She also ran the nation's Ministries of Labor and Health and her own Eva Perón Foundation, in addition to championing women's suffrage (granted in Argentina in 1947) and founding the Female Peronist Party. In 1951, Evita announced her candidacy for vice president, quickly earning the support of the low-income and working-class Argentines whose causes she espoused. The Argentine military (and bourgeoisie) pressured her to withdraw her candidacy, and this, combined with her deteriorating health, led her to do just that. A short time later, Evita succumbed to cancer. She was just thirty-three years old.

The SHINES Protocol: How Does an Underdog Emerge Victorious?

For the Underdog, the purpose of the SHINES protocol encompasses supporting the health and healthy functioning of your thyroid. But it also extends beyond this, addressing the spiritual, energetic, and nutritional aspects of your life that influence and are influenced by your thyroid's role in the regulation of your body's functions, including metabolism, cardiac, and digestive function.

When I discuss the SHINES protocol with Underdogs, I always emphasize that the journey toward balance can be a slow—if steady—one. I also stress that while prescription thyroid hormone replacement can be critically important to helping ameliorate your symptoms, it is only one aspect of the holistic protocol I've designed to help you reclaim your physiological and psychological energy and help you live the life you're meant to.

SPIRITUAL PRACTICE

The Underdog's spiritual practices center on the throat (fifth) chakra. Also known in Hindu tradition as Vishuddha, the throat chakra is closely associated with the endocrine system, and the thyroid gland in particular.

The throat chakra is also associated with an individual's creativity and personal expression. For this reason, a reluctance or inability to speak out on behalf of oneself or others—to speak your truth—correlates to a "closure" or blockage of the throat chakra. This, in turn, is believed to contribute to a series of health problems rooted in the neck, throat, and mouth, including depressed thyroid function.

For the Underdog, engaging in practices that open the throat chakra can help restore the flow of energy through this vital region and support the health and function of the thyroid. These practices involve using the voice, the breath, and the body more generally.

BREATHING EXERCISES

From yogic tradition comes many breathing exercises that can yield benefits for the Underdog. The following exercise is one of my favorites.

Three-Part Breathing (Dirga Pranayama)

A relaxing but disciplined exercise that involves inhaling and exhaling through your nose, three-part breathing begins with placing one hand on your chest and the other on your belly, roughly at the level of your navel. Breathe in for a count of 5, filling your chest, then your upper abdomen, then your belly, letting this fully expand. Then exhale, beginning with your belly, for another count of 5. Once you are comfortable with the pattern, you may take your hands off your body. You may also try increasing the length of your exhalations. (These should take no longer than twice as long as your inhalations.)

HUMMING AND SINGING

Something as simple as humming along to a tune can help exercise your voice and restore the flow of energy through your throat chakra. Do this intentionally, paying attention to the vibration, and you will feel the ease it can inspire.

Singing can have a similar effect. Whether it's in the car, in the shower, or onstage at karaoke night, try out your voice. Without hesitation or self-consciousness, let your voice out—let it carry forth unimpeded, and allow this to induce a sensation of release.

YOGA POSES

Certain yoga poses are particularly helpful for opening the throat chakra. According to author and Vedic educator Michelle Fondin, some of the poses best suited for restoring energetic flow to this region and stimulating the thyroid and parathyroid are Ustrasana (Camel Pose), Setu Bandha Sarvangasana (Bridge Pose), and Halasana (Plow Pose).[64]

Ustrasana (Camel Pose)

This pose involves kneeling on the mat, resting the palms of your hands on your heels (if necessary, place your toes on the mat to reduce the distance to your heels), and arching your back as you let your neck relax and your head fall backward. Keep breathing throughout, holding the pose for 10 to 15 seconds.

Setu Bandha Sarvangasana (Bridge Pose)

This pose begins with lying on your back on the mat, palms of your hands flat on the mat next to you and your legs outstretched. Next, bend your knees, bringing your feet closer as you keep the soles of your feet on the mat. From here, gently press your heels into the mat as you lift your lower back as high as possible and hold it aloft for 10 seconds. You may also bring your palms together under your back for increased opening of the throat and chest.

Halasana (Plow Pose)

An inversion that opens the throat chakra from the back rather than the front, plow is a relaxing pose often performed at the end of class. It begins with lying flat on the mat, with your legs outstretched and your arms relaxed at your side, palms facing down. Using your core muscles, lift your legs (keeping them straight if possible) and hips such that the toes begin to come up and over the head. Ultimately, the goal is to touch the floor behind your head with your toes while keeping your legs outstretched. Take it slowly, supporting your lower back with your hands as necessary as you go, and try to come out of the pose as you went in. You may hold Plow Pose (breathing calmly through it) for 20 seconds or longer, if it's comfortable.

As you enter into these poses, remain conscious of each inhale and exhale, feeling the breath helping to release any tension in the throat chakra and introduce a feeling of openness and ease.

HORMONE MODULATION

Prescription thyroid hormone replacement medication is generally necessary for women (and men) who have been diagnosed with clinical hypothyroidism. Depending on the root cause of the condition, dependency on medication may be temporary or permanent. If you have had a total thyroidectomy, for example, prescription thyroid medication is a must. If you have had a partial thyroidectomy, you are also likely to rely on a thyroid hormone prescription, though the duration of this dependency may depend on the degree to which your thyroid returns to a healthy level of functioning. If you have experienced damage to your thyroid due to radiation, disease (including Hashimoto's thyroiditis), or injury, or if your pituitary gland has suffered damage that results in an inability to produce thyroid-stimulating hormone (TSH), you are also likely to need prescription medication.

As noted, prescription thyroid hormone replacement medication may also benefit Underdogs who suffer from subclinical symptomatic hypothyroidism. Whether this is associated with early- to mid-stage Hashimoto's thyroiditis or other autoimmune disease, a secondary imbalance, nutritional deficiency, or other condition, temporary or permanent treatment with prescription thyroid hormone replacement can be an important element of an Underdog's journey toward balance and overall well-being.

One note about thyroid function and metabolism: Although thyroid medication can improve your metabolism, taking it does not guarantee you will lose weight. As I explain to my patients, the power of the medication lies in its ability to restore your energy levels to the point where you want to be more active.

There are four types of thyroid hormone replacement medications. Three are synthetic, and one is natural (meaning made in a laboratory from animal-based elements). Of the synthetic varieties, most contain only an artificial version of T4 called levothyroxine. (These are the most commonly prescribed for clinical and subclinical hypothyroidism.) Others contain only T3, and some contain both. Natural, animal-based thyroid replacement medications contain both T3 and T4.

Taking into consideration the nature and severity of your hypothyroidism, your physician can help you determine which is likely to work best for you. Be sure to confirm how best to take the medication, including at what time or times of day. In general, thyroid replacement medications should be taken on an empty stomach to maximize absorption. (Waiting 30 minutes to eat should suffice.)

If you begin taking prescription thyroid replacement, I also recommend consistent monitoring of not only your TSH but also your Free T4 and Free T3 levels. In my practice, I ask that patients check in every 6 to 8 weeks for testing.

SYNTHETIC T4 REPLACEMENT (LEVOTHYROXINE)

The most commonly prescribed thyroid replacement therapy, levothyroxine is marketed under the brand names Synthroid, Tirosint, Unithroid, Levoxyl, and Levothroid. Although levothyroxine is completely "man-made," its biological impact is exactly the same as the hormone produced by your own body. Also, while all brands of levothyroxine are bioequivalent, meaning there is little difference in their composition, I recommend sticking to a single brand whenever possible, as the dosing may vary slightly among them.

SYNTHETIC T3 REPLACEMENT (LIOTHYRONINE)

Marketed under the brand name Cytomel, synthetic T3 has the same biological impact as your own. At first blush, a T3 replacement may seem the most effective way of mimicking or supporting healthy thyroid function. But in reality, a T3-only replacement can be problematic because it can cause unsteady levels of T3 in the bloodstream. Even taking Cytomel several times a day can't guarantee their regulation because of the relatively short lifespan of T3 (compared to T4).

Unsteady T3 levels can give rise to symptoms including arrhythmia, anxiety, and insomnia. Treating hypothyroidism with liothyronine can diminish the body's ability to regulate T3 according to the body's needs via T4 conversion.

Still, liothyronine is appropriate in some cases. In patients who have undergone ablation therapy with radioactive iodine to treat conditions such as thyroid cancer or Graves' disease, for example, the medication may be prescribed on a temporary basis until TSH levels return to normal, and a T4-only medication becomes the best course. Also, in patients who suffer from impaired peripheral-tissue conversion of T4 to T3, liothyronine may also be the best course.

SYNTHETIC T3 AND T4 (LIOTRIX)

Branded as Thyrolar, liotrix is a synthetic T3/T4 combination designed to increase the body's levels of T3 beyond what natural conversion would create. Liotrix comes some of the same risks associated with liothyronine, and because the medication is administered only once a day, it can be difficult to rebalance T3 levels once they drop off. Physicians who want to augment synthetic T4 with T3 in customized doses can also prescribe specially compounded medications. Synthetic T4/T3 combinations are often prescribed for patients suffering from an enlarged thyroid.

NATURAL T4/T3

Marketed as Armour Thyroid, NP Thyroid, Nature-Throid, and WP Thyroid, natural T3/T4 is made from desiccated porcine thyroid gland. The most popular form of thyroid hormone replacement before synthetic medications were developed, this medication remains popular with women searching for a nonsynthetic alternative to T4-only or T4/T3 combination hormone replacement therapy.

As with the synthetic T3/T4 combination, a risk of unsteady T3 levels is associated with Armour Thyroid. In order to offset this, I recommend patients take half a dose twice a day to avoid the spikes and sudden depletions of T3. Also, this form of medication can contain certain porcine proteins and hormones that, while not necessarily harmful, are foreign to the human body.

INFOCEUTICALS

For both the Overachiever (see page 407), an archetype character-ized primarily by hyperthyroidism, and the Underdog, Energetic Integrator 9 (EI9) is the infoceutical I recommend to help restore and realign the fields of energy that surround the thyroid.

EI9 operates along your "triple warmer meridian." This begins at the tip of your ring finger, running through your knuckles and into your wrist, between the two bones of your forearm (radius and ulna), and up through your shoulder, pericardium (the sac that surrounds the heart), and collarbone before ultimately looping around to the back of the ear. You can think of the meridian as an energetic high-way of sorts, connecting the heart with the energy-center "furnace" of the thyroid.

In addition to energetically addressing disrupted metabolic function and immune failure, EI9 is also associated with the emo-tions of confidence and courage and the ability to verbalize. Similar to spiritual exercises that can help open the throat chakra, EI9 can help release energetic blockages and disruptions that can not only negatively impact physiological functioning of the thyroid, but also keep you from accessing the inner strength that will help you move forward along your journey toward balance.

As we discuss at various points in this book, including in the appendix dedicated to a discussion of energetic integrators, EI9 con-tains no hormones or medication of any type. But given its power to help restore the balanced flow of energy in the field surrounding the thyroid, it can be a helpful complement to other elements of the Underdog's SHINES protocol. This can be particularly important if/when your thyroid activity begins to increase, bringing about a series of physiological and psychological changes.

I have also stated earlier that the energetic aspect of the thy-roid comes from the throat chakra. Energetically, this chakra is open when you are speaking your truth and saying things that are energetically loving and open. Therefore, if you are engaging in gossip or angrily speaking with others, there is the potential that this gland may be affected in a negative manner.

ESSENTIAL OILS

Essential oils that may be beneficial for low or low-normal thyroid (which can cause issues with energy and metabolism) include:

Cedarwood	Pine
Geranium	Spearmint
Myrrh	Wintergreen
Peppermint	

NUTRITION

No one type of diet, whether it's Mediterranean, vegetarian or vegan, paleo, or ketogenic, is an Underdog diet. For this archetype, the primary focus is on key nutrients the body needs for healthy thyroid function and trying to ensure you consume sufficient amounts of these each day. Two secondary objectives are weight loss where warranted and incorporating gut-health-friendly foods into your daily routine. Particularly in those cases where hypothyroidism is linked to an autoimmune disorder, such as Hashimoto's thyroiditis, gut sensitivity and health become critically important to restoring overall hormonal balance and well-being.

NUTRIENTS TO EMBRACE

Iodine

As discussed, iodine is required for the conversion of T4 to T3. Iodine is also an "essential nutrient," meaning that your body does not produce it on its own and it must be consumed from exogenous sources.

In 1924, American food manufacturers began adding iodine (in the form of potassium iodide) to salt to help resolve what had become an epidemic of thyroid goiters. For a time, this measure helped keep the general population's iodine levels sufficiently high. In recent decades, however, Americans' increased consumption of processed foods has caused a decrease in iodine intake (primarily noniodized salt is used in the manufacture of processed foods). Certain popular types of salt such as sea salt and Himalayan salt generally contain less iodine than conventional table salt to which the mineral has been added.

Given the various cardiovascular health risks associated with salt, eating more of it is not the healthiest way to increase or maintain your iodine levels. In the following pages, we consider the best sources of iodine for the Underdog, including protein and nonprotein options.

For Underdogs, I recommend a daily intake of 150 mcg of iodine per day. Remember: Too much iodine can overstimulate thyroid function just as too little can. Keep this in mind as you consider which foods may make sense for you, taking into account the iodine you are consuming from other sources.

For the Underdog, I recommend the following sources of iodine (and have included their average iodine content per serving):

MEAT AND FISH[*]
Turkey (34 mcg/serving)
Cod (132 mcg/serving)
Scallops (135 mcg/serving)
Sardines (36 mcg/serving)
Shrimp (46 mcg/serving)

---

[*] Whenever possible, seek out organic and wild-caught options, as these tend to contain higher levels of various nutrients, including iodine.

DAIRY*

Cage-free eggs (27 mcg/egg)

Unpasteurized cheese (Brie, Camembert, feta, goat, Montrachet, Neufchatel)

Raw milk (56 mcg/cup)

Unpasteurized yogurt (70 mcg/cup)

OTHER SOURCES

Cranberries

Navy beans

Organic potatoes

Sea vegetables (750 mcg/tablespoon)

Strawberries (13 mcg/cup)

Vitamin D

Recent studies have taken a closer look at the link between vitamin D deficiency and thyroid disorders including Hashimoto's thyroiditis, Graves' disease, and thyroid cancer, and concluded that there is a correlation between these and a moderate to severe vitamin D deficiency.[65] Although a specific causal link remains unclear, some research indicates a link between vitamin D deficiency and increased production of thyroid antibodies.[66] For the Underdog, I recommend having your vitamin D levels checked along with your thyroid and other hormones at the outset and consulting with your physician regarding daily intake for raising/sustaining your levels as necessary.

Sunlight promotes the synthesis of vitamin D, and so long as it's absorbed safely, it can be an effective means of sustaining adequate levels of the steroidal hormone. Certain foods are also good sources of vitamin D. For the Underdog seeking to maintain healthy levels of vitamin D, I recommend the following foods:

---

* I recommend seeking out organic, cage-free dairy options whenever possible, as these tend to be more nutrient-dense.

Raw milk (98 IU/cup)
Cod liver oil (440 IU/teaspoon)
Salmon (400 IU/3-ounce portion)

Selenium

Selenium is a necessary component of a number of enzymes that are critical to thyroid function. (In the body, the highest concentration of the mineral is found in the thyroid.) Selenium also plays an important role in immune function, cognition, and fertility.

Selenium is an essential mineral, meaning the body does not produce it on its own. While consuming too much selenium can cause gastrointestinal distress, for the Underdog, incorporating sufficient amounts of the mineral into your diet is important.

I recommend the following food sources:

Brazil nuts (544 mcg/ounce)
Crab (41 mcg/3-ounce portion)
Lobster tail (41 mcg/3.5-ounce portion)
Shrimp (34 mcg/3-ounce portion)
Yellowfin tuna (92 mcg/3-ounce portion)

Mushrooms

Though their nutritional and medicinal benefits are often overlooked, certain types of mushrooms, including cremini, oyster, shiitake, and portobello, can be a meaningful source of nutrients for the Underdog. Among these nutrients are iodine, vitamin D, and a series of antioxidants.

Paul Stamets, a leading expert on medicinal mushrooms, has created Host Defense, a line of mushroom-based supplements designed to support energy levels, immune system health, and hormonal balance.

FOODS TO AVOID

Soy

Recent studies have indicated that the phytoestrogens contained in soy may contribute to and/or exacerbate hypothyroidism. Mimicking the effects of estrogen, phytoestrogens can prompt the liver to produce thyroid hormone binding globulin (THBG), sometimes in excess amounts. THBG can then bind T4 and T3, reducing the amounts of each in the bloodstream and limiting their impact.

For the Underdog, I recommend consuming little to no soy. While a few edamame beans with your sushi every once in a while is unlikely to have any negative impact on your thyroid hormone levels, consuming 20 to 40 g of soy milk or soy other products on a more regular basis certainly may.

For the Underdog, I recommend looking out for soy in foods you regularly eat and, in general, avoiding it until your thyroid functioning improves.

Cruciferous Vegetables

Although they can yield certain health benefits, cruciferous vegetables such as broccoli, Brussels sprouts, cabbage, cauliflower, and kale can also interfere with the production of thyroid hormone. They do this by limiting the thyroid's ability to absorb iodine, which is critical to its ability to make the hormone. Again, when I talk about the avoidance of these items, it is in larger amounts. In most cases the health benefits outweigh the potential issues with thyroid, but are included here for the purists.

Cooking cruciferous vegetables can help reduce their negative effects on the thyroid. But even with this, for the Underdog, I recommend limiting your total intake of cruciferous vegetables to 5 ounces or less per day.

Gluten

For Underdogs who also suffer from gluten sensitivity or celiac disease, gluten can damage the wall of the small intestine. This damage can hamper absorption of thyroid hormone replacement medication. It can also cause the small intestine to become permeable, a condition known as leaky gut.

Permeability of the small intestine can result in the release of gluten into the bloodstream. And due to the similarity between the molecular structures of gluten and thyroid tissue, an immune response to gluten can trigger an autoimmune response that results in the destruction of thyroid tissue. For Underdogs whose hypothyroidism has arisen out of an autoimmune disorder, including those who have been diagnosed with Hashimoto's thyroiditis, restricting or eliminating gluten can therefore be an important step.

Sugar

If you're trying to lose weight, minimizing or eliminating sugar is an important aspect of your diet. Given that your metabolism has slowed, consuming sugar is likely to make you gain weight at a faster rate.

A little sugar (particularly unrefined sugar) now and again is unlikely to have a significant effect. But in general, for Underdogs, I recommend avoiding all sugar as much as possible.

Alcohol

Alcohol can have toxic effects on a variety of tissues, including the thyroid. Studies have shown that in addition to its direct impact on the thyroid's functioning, alcohol also suppresses the pituitary gland's release of TSH and decreases the levels of T3 and T4 in peripheral tissues.[67]

FOODS AND MEDICATIONS THAT CAN INTERFERE WITH THYROID HORMONE REPLACEMENT MEDICATION

High-Fat Foods

While monitoring fat intake may be advisable for any Underdog, it is particularly important for those taking thyroid hormone replacement medication. This is because even "good fats" such as coconut oil can interfere with the absorption of the medication by the intestine.

To help ensure proper absorption, I recommend taking medication one to two hours before or after consuming food or beverages that contain fat.

Excessive Fiber

Fiber yields a series of benefits, but excessive amounts of fiber can diminish absorption of your thyroid medication. If you are on a high-fiber diet, your physician may need to adjust your dose. Thyroid hormone-level testing will confirm this.

Current recommendations for an adult's daily intake of fiber is 20 to 35 g per day. For an Underdog who is taking thyroid medication, I recommend 25 g/day. I also suggest waiting at least an hour after taking your medication before consuming fiber-containing foods.

Caffeine

Even relatively small amounts of caffeine can block the absorption of your thyroid medication. I recommend taking your medication with water and waiting at least 30 minutes before drinking coffee, tea, or other caffeinated drinks.

Calcium Supplements and Chromium Picolinate

Over-the-counter calcium and chromium picolinate supplements can also interfere with the absorption of thyroid medication. Although you may continue taking these supplements when you're also taking thyroid medication, I recommend ingesting either of these at least four hours before or after taking your thyroid medication.

EXERCISE

For the Underdog who constantly feels depleted of energy, exercise can feel like a chore—and an impossible one. But the reality is that even small amounts of exercise—particularly when combined with other elements of this SHINES protocol—can improve your overall energy levels, raise your metabolic rate, and elevate your mood by releasing endorphins. For the Underdog, I recommend starting slow, with easy, low-impact exercise routines 10 to 15 minutes in duration.

WALKING

If you're just embarking on a workout routine, walking is one of the best exercises to start off with. Whether you walk indoors or outdoors, begin at a comfortable pace and work toward gradually increasing both your speed and the length of time you spend walking. Any number of apps can help you track your progress, including those that monitor the number of steps you take, your heart rate, and how many calories you burn. Using these can also help keep you motivated and accountable, which is key—whatever your workout, a consistent commitment to it is critical to your success.

For the Underdog who wants to move past walking and try running, I recommend an app called Couch to 5K. Promising to get "just about anyone from the couch to running 5 kilometers or 30 minutes in just 9 weeks," the program provides a series of resources, including outdoor and indoor workout plans and online progress reporting.

TAI CHI

Tai chi is a practice that can help restore the flow of the body's energy along its meridians. And for Underdogs who nearly always report feeling that their energy feels both depleted and blocked, this gentle and graceful form of exercise that incorporates breathing, stretching, and mindful movement can be a very effective means of addressing both.

Tai chi is a practice you may undertake with a group or on your own. Classes are commonly offered at tai chi, yoga, martial arts, and other studios, as well as at many gyms, and there are also many online classes available for practitioners at every level. Once you're familiar with the practice, it becomes one you can do anytime, anywhere, increasing the intensity and duration of your practice at your pace.

ROWING

Whether outside on the water in a sculling boat or kayak, or inside on an erg (a rowing machine), rowing can be a great form of exercise for the Underdog. A cardiovascular exercise you can take at your pace, rowing also uses all your major joints, including your hips, knees, and shoulders, and works all the major muscle groups of your upper and lower body, including the abdominal muscles, pectoral muscles, triceps, and biceps, in addition to the hamstrings and glutes.

As with tai chi and some of the spiritual practices recommended here, rowing involves restoring the flow of energy along the body's major energy "highways." It also incorporates a meditative element, requiring focus on the body's fluid movements and continuous deep breathing.

SUPPLEMENTS

For the Underdog, the role of supplements is fourfold: ensuring the thyroid has adequate iodine to produce T3 and T4, supporting conversion of T4 to T3, helping sustain a healthy gut, and decreasing inflammation, which is often associated with hypothyroidism.

IODINE

Iodine is an essential mineral required for the production of T3 and T4. The thyroid stores iodine for this purpose, and maintaining sufficient levels of the mineral is essential for its healthy functioning. Excess iodine can also harm the thyroid, however, which means that while iodine can be an important supplement for the Underdog, it must be used carefully.

An adequate iodine intake is 150 mcg/day. One option for a dietary supplement is Lugol's solution, a mixture of potassium iodide and elemental iodine in water. Used to treat iodine deficiency, the solution is also used to disinfect minor wounds and in certain types of cancer screenings.

While Lugol's solution is available over the counter, I strongly recommend consulting with your physician before incorporating it or any of the other iodine-supplement options discussed here. Again, while sufficient iodine intake is critical for thyroid health, excessive dosing of Lugol's solution can be toxic to the thyroid, interfering with its function and potentially giving rise to hyperthyroidism.

Another iodine supplement option is colloidal iodine, also known as atomic or nascent iodine. Because it contains isolated iodine atoms in a state in which they are inactive and therefore not toxic, colloidal iodine is generally considered a safer alternative to Lugol's solution. The body can absorb colloidal iodine, however, and break it down into a form in which it can make use of it as necessary.

Colloidal iodine is available over the counter and is generally sold in glycerin form. (Some brands incorporate alcohol into their solutions, which can cause unpleasant burning sensations. I recommend seeking out alcohol-free options.) Although there are fewer risks associated with colloidal iodine than there are with Lugol's solution, a single drop of a colloidal iodine solution can contain 246 mcg of iodine, or 170 percent of the recommended daily allowance, and I recommend you use it only with a physician's approval and supervision.

CONVERSION PROCESS SUPPORTERS: ZINC, SELENIUM, AND GLUTATHIONE

Conversion of T4 to T3 involves the release of a single iodine atom and relies on a group of enzymes called deiodinases, which make use of zinc and selenium, among other minerals.

Underdogs who are low in zinc are likely to benefit from a zinc supplement. (Consuming excess zinc can cause nausea, vomiting, and diarrhea as well as stomach and kidney damage.) For an Underdog whose levels are low, I recommend a daily intake of 15 to 20 mg. Being mindful of the zinc contained in the foods you eat, I suggest supplementing with zinc picolinate with the approval of your physician.

As with zinc, Underdogs whose selenium levels are low are likely to benefit from a dietary supplement of the mineral. (Consuming excess selenium is unlikely to help boost the conversion process, and may cause such side effects as gastrointestinal distress, hair and nail loss, skin rashes, and a garlicky taste in the mouth.) If tests reveal that your selenium levels are low, I recommend a supplement of 55 mcg/day. Again, remain mindful of the selenium contained in the foods you eat and consult with your physician regarding potential interactions or side effects.

One of the most powerful antioxidants in the body, glutathione aids in reducing oxidative stress and cellular toxicity by destroying free radicals and assisting the body in detoxifying metals, chemicals, xenobiotics, and carcinogens. It is also one of the major factors influencing the conversion of T4 to T3, so incorporating a glutathione supplement into your daily regimen can help boost the effectiveness of the conversion process. Although glutathione supplements are available over the counter, I recommend consulting with your physician before beginning to take them.

SUPPLEMENTS THAT SUPPORT DIGESTIVE HEALTH

The health and proper functioning of your digestive system are important to both medication absorption and immune system fitness. Each of these can play a role in alleviating the symptoms of hypothyroidism and/or restoring your thyroid to health, and a few supplements I recommend for the Underdog can help support them.

Vitamin B12

Underdogs suffering from low iodine levels often also suffer from low levels of vitamin B12. Associated with your stomach's ability to absorb nutrients, some of the symptoms of vitamin B12 deficiency echo those of hypothyroidism. Among these are tiredness, weakness, light-headedness, constipation (and diarrhea), and mood disorders, including depression. Underdogs taking proton pump inhibitors such as Protonix or Prilosec are particularly at risk for this deficiency.

Also known as methylcobalamin or cyanocobalamin (its synthetic form), vitamin B12 is available over the counter. Although naturally occurring high levels of vitamin B12 in the system may be a sign of an underlying disorder, there are no known risks associated with ingesting excessive amounts of cyanocobalamin. Still, as with any supplement, I recommend confirming with your consulting healthcare practitioner before incorporating it into your daily routine.

PROBIOTICS

Probiotics' support of gut health helps the Underdog on two fronts. The first is improved absorption of thyroid hormone medication. As we considered earlier in this section, when the walls of the small intestine are weakened, their ability to absorb medications into the bloodstream is compromised.

The second is a strengthened immune system. According to leading experts on hypothyroidism, including Izabella Wentz, author of *Hashimoto's Protocol*, Underdogs whose symptoms are tied to auto-immune dysfunction generally suffer from intestinal permeability and low levels of certain strains of probiotic gut bacteria such as *Lactobacillus* and *Bifidus*. To improve these and protect the strength of the intestinal wall, Wentz recommends that Hashimoto's and hypo-thyroidism sufferers consume (living) probiotics and/or incorporate foods such as fermented vegetables, kefir, or certain kinds of yogurt into their diets.

SUPPLEMENTS THAT DECREASE INFLAMMATION

Certain fatty acids have been shown to reduce inflammation associated with hypothyroidism. One is guggul (also sold under the brand name Gugulipid), a resin extract from the *Commiphora myrrha* (myrrh) tree. Used for centuries in Ayurvedic medicine, guggul is commonly used in modern Western medicine to lower cholesterol levels. Recent studies have shown that guggul may also have anti-inflammatory effects that can help support healthy thyroid function.

Turmeric is another agent that can help reduce inflammation throughout the body in addition to helping heal the gut and detoxify the body of heavy metals. The spice's most active constituent, curcumin, can help protect the intestinal wall from bacterial infections.

It has also shown tumor-inhibiting activity in the thyroid in addition to protecting against genetic damage and the side effects of radioactive iodine (treatment for hyperthyroidism), each of which can give rise to hypothyroidism.

BOOK RECOMMENDATIONS FOR UNDERDOGS

Izabella Wentz, PharmD, FASCP, *Hashimoto's Protocol: A 90-Day Plan for Reversing Thyroid Symptoms and Getting Your Life Back* (New York: HarperOne, 2017)

See also: Izabella Wentz's nine-part docuseries, *The Thyroid Secret* (http://thethyroidsecret.com/trailer/)

UNDERDOGS

"Cosette" Euphrasie Tholomyes (fictional character from Victor Hugo's novel *Les Misérables*) is the daughter of Fantine and Felix Tholomyes, the former of whom—after Felix leaves her—places Cosette in the care of the cruel, thieving, inn-owning Thenardiers. In their care, she is abused—made to wear rags, go barefoot, and she is malnourished and neglected. A chance encounter leads a later hospitalized Fantine to meet escaped convict Jean Valjean, who, at her dying request, manages to free Cosette from the Thenardiers' grip, and begins to care for her as his own daughter.

Valjean takes Cosette to Paris and begins her education, but is still running from Inspector Javert, who eventually learns his whereabouts. Together, he and Cosette escape to a convent. There, they shelter for several years, and Cosette meets Marius Pontmercy as a teenager, with whom she soon falls in love. Eventually, after Marius has a close brush with death, they marry, and though Marius bars Valjean from seeing Cosette, he later learns the extent to which he is to thank for rescuing her, and they reconcile on Valjean's deathbed.

Katherine Johnson (née Coleman, August 26, 1918–February 24, 2020) *African American mathematician and celestial scientist.* Katherine Johnson worked at NASA from 1953 until 1986, and was instrumental to the success of such legendary missions as the 1969 Apollo 11 mission to the moon and the early journeys of astronauts John Glenn and Alan Shepard. In 1970, Johnson's work on the ill-fated Apollo 13 mission contributed significantly to the crew's safe return to Earth. As Johnson described her and her colleagues' work at that time, "Everybody was concerned about getting them [to the moon]. We were concerned about getting them back."[68] Johnson's work was also critical to later NASA endeavors, including the Space Shuttle program.

Demonstrating her prowess for geometry helped Johnson ascend into the all-male flight research team, but gender and racial barriers imposed on her from all sides. In accordance with state-based racial segregation laws and federal workplace segregation guidelines instituted by President Woodrow Wilson in 1913, Johnson and her African American colleagues were mandated to work and eat separate from their white peers, in addition to using separate washrooms. The office in which she worked was labeled "Colored Computers." Adding to this, early in her tenure at NASA, Johnson's name did not appear on any of the reports she had authored or coauthored. While Johnson has downplayed the impact of these barriers on her work at NASA, claiming "[y]ou had a mission and you worked on it, and it was important to do your job . . . and play bridge at lunch," and "I knew [segregation] was there, but I didn't feel it," she has also acknowledged the necessity of speaking up.[69] "We needed to be assertive as women in those days," she has said. "[A]ssertive and aggressive—and the degree to which we had to be that way depended on where you were. I had to be."[70]

During her thirty-plus-year career at NASA, Johnson authored or coauthored a total of twenty-six scientific papers in addition to continuing her work on the agency's various missions. The recipient of a number of honorary degrees and the Daughters of the American Revolution's Medal of Honor, among other awards, Johnson was presented with the Presidential Medal of Freedom by President Barack Obama in 2015. In 2017, the eighty-nine-year-old attended the dedication of the Katherine G. Johnson Computational Research Facility at the NASA Langley Research Center in Hampton, Virginia. The grandmother of six and great-grandmother of eleven continued until her death to support aspiring young scientists in their pursuits of science, technology, engineering, and mathematics and was the subject of the bestselling book and successful film *Hidden Figures*.

The SHINES Protocol: How Do You Reward the Overachiever?

The Overachiever's SHINES protocol centers on restorative practices on every front. Whether it's a calming spiritual or physiological exercise or a nutritional element that can help replenish your tissues' depleted stores of key vitamins and minerals, the goal of each aspect of the Overachiever's SHINES method is to gently rebuild your physical, psychological, and spiritual strength as you also address your thyroid's overactivity and the impact it has had on your body and your overall well-being.

SPIRITUAL PRACTICE

Similar to the Underdog's spiritual practice (see page 385), the Overachiever's practice centers on the throat (fifth) chakra, or Vishuddha, as it is known in Hindu tradition. The throat chakra is closely associated with the endocrine system, and the thyroid gland in particular.

For the Overachiever, spiritual practices designed to help restore the flow of energy through the throat chakra can help bring ease and calm to this region of the body, helping to restore equilibrium and exerting a restorative and rebalancing effect. These practices involve using the voice, breath, and body more generally.

BREATHING EXERCISES

From yogic tradition comes the following breathing exercise that can gently help restore the flow of energy through the throat chakra and among the organs associated with it. For the Overachiever, I recommend:

Simple Deep Breathing

As its name suggests, this breathing exercise is simple. But it can also be a powerful means of relaxing the body, slowing your heart rate, and diminishing the tension that drives anxiety and panic.

Sitting in a straight-backed chair, rest your forearms on the arms of the chair or, if there are none, relax your arms and place your hands facedown on your thighs, allowing your elbows to fall naturally to your sides. You may close your eyes if you wish, or leave them open. From this position, breathe in slowly and deeply through your nose. Allow this to last 5 or 6 seconds, filling your belly and allowing it to expand before filling your chest. Next, pause for 3 or 4 seconds, holding on to your breath. Then relax your jaw, open your mouth slightly, push your lips slightly forward as though you're saying the word "two," and *slowly* exhale through your mouth for a count of 7.

At first, try 10 breaths. As your comfort level increases, try for a higher number of breaths per session. The maximum number of breaths appropriate for this exercise is 20.

HUMMING AND SINGING

Something as simple as humming along to a tune can help exercise your voice and restore the flow of energy through your throat chakra. Do this intentionally, paying attention to the vibration, and you will feel the ease it can inspire.

Singing can have a similar effect. Whether it's in the car, in the shower, or onstage at karaoke night, try out your voice. Without hesitation or self-consciousness, let your voice out—let it carry forth unimpeded and induce a sensation of release.

YOGA POSES

Certain yoga poses are particularly helpful for restoring the energetic flow and circulation along the throat chakra, helping to regulate the thyroid and bring its activity back into balance. Poses I suggest for the Overachiever include Matsyasana (Fish Pose), Setu Bandha Sarvangasana (Bridge Pose), and Marjaryasana/Bitilasana (Cat/Cow Pose).

Matsyasana (Fish Pose)

Begin seated, either in easy pose (with your knees bent and pointing outward and your feet under opposite thighs) or lotus, and gently lie down on your back. Rest your palms on your thighs and lift your chest toward the sky, allowing your head to fall backward and your throat to relax and open. With the top of your head on your mat, breathe deeply and slowly through your nose, allowing your chest to lift a little with each breath and your throat chakra to open a little more.

As it opens the throat and front of the body, Fish Pose helps relax your neck and shoulders. It can also help lower your stress level and diminish the intensity of mood swings.

Setu Bandha Sarvangasana (Bridge Pose)

Well suited to both Underdogs and Overachievers, Bridge Pose helps release tension from the back of the neck and reduce anxiety in addition to exerting a positive impact on digestion.

Begin by lying on your back on the mat, with the palms of your hands flat on the mat next to you and your legs outstretched. Next, bend your knees, bringing your feet closer as you keep the soles of your feet on the mat. From here, gently press your heels into the mat as you lift your lower back as high as possible and hold it aloft for 10 seconds. (You may also try supported Bridge Pose, performed with bolsters under your middle and upper back.) For maximum opening of the front of the throat and chest, you may also bring your palms together under your back (unsupported Bridge Pose only).

Marjaryasana/Bitilasana (Cat/Cow Pose)

Performed together, the "cow tilt" and "cat stretch" can yield significant mental and physical benefits for the Overachiever. Associated with emotional equilibrium and peace, these poses focus on the breath and increased flexibility of the spine, helping to release tension and alleviate stress. These poses also stretch the muscles of the hips, abdomen, and chest, increasing the circulation throughout the upper body and addressing disruptions in the digestive tract and reproductive systems.

This pose begins in "tabletop" position, with your knees bent on the floor and your palms facedown on the mat. With your weight evenly distributed between your arms and upper legs and your spine straight, begin with the "cow tilt," inhaling through your nose and letting your belly expand toward the floor as you look up toward the ceiling, allowing your eyes to walk backward along it as your throat opens to the sky. Now begin to exhale, pulling your belly button toward your spine as it begins to return to neutral and your eyes walk forward along the ceiling and then the wall in front of you, eventually looking in toward your chest as your spine lifts toward the ceiling, stretching from its base all the way up to the top of your neck.

Repeat as you wish, inhaling into the cow tilt and exhaling into the cat stretch.

SPEAKING YOUR TRUTH

In addition to its association with the thyroid and other organs in the region of the head and neck, the throat chakra is also associated with creativity and personal expression. For this reason, a reluctance or inability to speak out on your own or others' behalf—to speak your truth—can cause a "closure" or blockage of the throat chakra that corresponds to a series of health problems rooted in the neck, throat, and mouth, including thyroid dysfunction.

In order to clear energetic blockages that may be negatively influencing your thyroid's functioning, I recommend exercises involving speaking your truth—even to yourself. Often, this can involve acknowledging emotional or physical injuries others have knowingly or unknowingly inflicted on you and honoring the pain you suffered. It can also involve making the decision to let go of the resentment, fear, and/or anger others' actions have inspired, and forgiving them, if only to yourself. Speaking your truth can also entail self-forgiveness. If an inventory of your emotional attachments reveals guilt or regret, you may consider giving yourself the time and space to consider these without judgment and acknowledge the pain they've caused you and the ways in which they've diminished your self-concept and/or compromised your relationships with others.

A religious practice may help here, as may talk therapy with a trained professional. You may also embark on this process on your own, however. If the idea of this practice resonates with you but you're not sure where to begin, try a guided meditation by Reiki master and spiritual teacher Wendy Irene. Called "Speak Your Truth (Throat Chakra Healing)," this meditation is designed to help you open your throat chakra in order to speak clearly and authentically about your true feelings and experiences of the world around you. Irene recommends returning to the minutes-long meditation when you are suffering from a sore throat or pain in or near your neck, as emotional and energetic blockages can manifest in physical discomfort and dysfunction.[71]

HORMONE MODULATION

If you're an Overachiever, there is no "hormonal fix" that can act directly on your thyroid or thyroid hormone to offset or reverse your too-high levels of T4 and T3. A characteristic of hyperthyroidism is that it gives rise to other hormonal imbalances, however. Where these cause certain symptoms, I recommend using hormone-based treatments to address them.

NON-HORMONE-BASED TREATMENTS FOR THE OVERACHIEVER

Depending on the severity and root cause of your symptoms, certain non-hormone-based medications or treatment measures may be appropriate to address your thyroid's overactivity and related side effects.

Methimazole is an oral medication that can stop the thyroid from producing excess thyroid hormones, for example. Propylthiouracil (PTU) is another oral medication often used in patients with Graves' disease and/or when methimazole has proven ineffective. PTU both decreases the amount of thyroid hormone produced by the thyroid and blocks the conversion of T4 to T3.

In addition to medications that act directly on the thyroid and thyroid hormone, beta-blockers that help slow down the heart rate are appropriate in some cases. Where the Overachiever's symptoms cannot be managed with medication, diet, and lifestyle changes, treatment with radioactive iodine or surgery may be necessary.

Finally, some with hyperthyroid traits are actually hypothyroid and are taking too much medication. This shows why it is important for women who are having symptoms of the Overachiever to seek out medical assistance, and if you are taking any thyroid medications, please always consult your prescribing provider first.

HORMONE-BASED TREATMENTS TO ADDRESS DOWNSTREAM IMBALANCES

Hyperthyroidism can result in the body acting like a furnace, burning through healthy tissue—including muscle and bone—and disrupting various systems and processes along the way. Hormonal imbalances, including deficits of estrogen, testosterone, and progesterone, are all common. And helping bring these closer to equilibrium can offset certain downstream effects of your excess thyroid hormone production and release.

Of all the hormone imbalances to which an overactive thyroid is likely to give rise, progesterone deficiency may be the most significant in terms of its impact on your overall well-being.[72] The hormone that yields the most calming effects on the body, progesterone also helps regulate sleep. For the Overachiever who is tense and anxious, and often struggles with insomnia, increasing progesterone levels even temporarily can bring a significant measure of relief.

When I treat Overachievers, I check their progesterone levels and their estrogen-progesterone ratio. When a woman's hormones are in balance, this ratio is roughly 10 to 1. But in Overachievers, I often supplement with progesterone for a short period of time, reducing this ratio to 5 to 1 or even 2 to 1.

There are some side effects of raising progesterone in this way, including intermittent spotting from the endometrial lining and risk of dehydration (since progesterone is a diuretic). But when taken as a temporary measure to help an Overachiever to get her thyroid hormone production under control, the benefit of progesterone's calming effects can outweigh the risks associated with it.

INFOCEUTICALS

For both Underdog (see page 391) and the Overachiever, Energetic Integrator 9 (EI9) is the infoceutical I recommend to help restore and realign the fields of energy that surround the thyroid.

EI9 operates along your "triple warmer meridian." This begins at the tip of your ring finger, running through your knuckles and into your wrist, between the two bones of your forearm (radius and ulna), and up through your shoulder, pericardium (the sac that surrounds the heart), and collarbone before ultimately looping around to the back of the ear. You can think of the meridian as an energetic highway of sorts, connecting the heart with the energy-center "furnace" of the thyroid.

In addition to energetically addressing disrupted metabolic function, EI9 is also associated with the emotions of confidence and courage and the ability to verbalize. Similar to spiritual exercises that can help open the throat chakra, EI9 can help release energetic blockages and disruptions that can not only negatively impact physiological functioning of the thyroid, but also keep you from accessing the inner strength that will help you move forward along your journey toward balance.

EI9 contains no hormones or medication of any type. But given its power to help restore the balanced flow of energy in the field surrounding the thyroid, it can be a helpful complement to other elements of the Overachiever's SHINES protocol. This can be particularly important if/when your thyroid hormone levels begin to decrease, bringing about a series of physiological and psychological changes.

I have also stated earlier that the energetic aspect of the thyroid comes from the throat chakra. Energetically, this chakra is open when you are speaking your truth and saying things that are energetically loving and open. Therefore, if you are engaging in gossip or angrily speaking with others, there is the potential that this gland may be affected in a negative manner.

ESSENTIAL OILS

While essential oils may not directly affect your circulating levels of thyroid hormone, they may be able to help with the symptoms experienced with high thyroid levels. I suggest trying these:

Evergreen	Sandalwood
Frankincense	Spearmint
Lemongrass	

NUTRITION

For the Overachiever, supportive nutrition involves consuming a sufficient number of calories—and sufficient nutrients—each day.

Lean proteins are a key element of the Overachiever's diet. These help offset the body's catabolic processes and sustain the health of muscle, bone, and organ tissues (see page 120 for more on catabolism). Complex carbohydrates (from natural sources, not processed foods) are another important source of fuel for the Overachiever. Cruciferous vegetables and certain fruits are particularly valuable. Omega-3 and omega-6 essential fatty acids are a third beneficial source of calories. Important building blocks of cells and tissues, these fatty acids also help support the body's immune and circulatory systems and reduce inflammation throughout the body.

FOODS TO EMBRACE

Protein

For the Overachiever, whose body is consuming its own tissues to sustain its rapid metabolism, I recommend 1 g of lean protein per pound of body weight per day. Good sources of lean protein for the Overachiever include:

Fish, including salmon and tuna

Lean meats, including ground beef and pork loin

Beans and lentils

Nuts and nut butters

Protein powders, such as vegan pea, rice, or
powdered peanut options

Cruciferous Vegetables

Known as "goitrogens"[73] for their ability to disrupt and diminish thyroid activity, cruciferous vegetables interfere with the thyroid's uptake of iodine, reducing its production of T4 and T3. However, cooking them significantly diminishes their impact on the thyroid's iodine uptake. Cruciferous vegetables I recommend for the Overachiever include:

Broccoli

Brussels sprouts

Kale

Berries

Certain kinds of berries can yield benefits for the Overachiever. Some of the phytonutrients they contain can help support the Overachiever's cardiac health by moderating cholesterol levels. Others are antioxidants that can help offset the destructive effects of free radicals, which often plague the Overachiever. The nutrients contained in berries can also help moderate inflammatory cytokines, molecules excreted by immune cells that circulate through the bloodstream, promoting inflammation. I recommend the following:

Blackberries

Blueberries

Raspberries

Omega-3 and Omega-6 Essential Fatty Acids

Omega-3 and omega-6 essential fatty acids can be a great source of energy for the Overachiever. Rather than breaking down muscle, collagen, or other tissue, the body can break these fatty acids down for fuel. They have also been shown to decrease inflammation. Once broken down into ketone bodies (the brain's preferred fuel source), omega-3 and omega-6 can also help support memory and mental clarity. Among the sources of these fatty acids that I recommend for the Overachiever are:

OILS

Coconut oil

Olive oil

Oil blends, including Udo's Oil Omega 3-6-9 Blend, a mixture of omega-3, -6, and -9 fatty acids

NUTS AND SEEDS

Walnuts, almonds, and pistachios

Nut and seed butters, including almond, cashew, and sunflower seed

Chia seeds

Flaxseed

Sunflower seeds

OTHER FOOD SOURCES

Avocados

Fish, including salmon and tuna

Olives

Water

In addition to ensuring proper calorie and nutrient consumption, the Overachiever also needs to stay hydrated. According to Ayurvedic medicine, drinking water also cleanses the throat chakra and maintains the flow of energy through it.

FOODS TO AVOID

Iodine-Rich Foods

For the Overachiever, it's important to monitor and/or reduce the levels of iodine in your system. The thyroid holds on to the mineral, using it to produce T4 and T3. Over time, reducing the amount of iodine available to the thyroid can help decrease the levels of thyroid hormone in your system. Iodine may be found in various protein and nonprotein sources. Among the most important for the Overachiever to avoid are:

MEAT AND FISH

Turkey
Cod
Scallops
Sardines
Shrimp

DAIRY

Eggs
Cheese
Yogurt

OTHER SOURCES

Cranberries
Navy beans
Organic potatoes
Sea vegetables, including seaweed and kelp
Strawberries

EXERCISE

When it comes to exercise for the Overachiever, the goal of any practice is to calm and restore. Given the accelerated pace of your metabolism and the likelihood that your body is already in a catabolic state, burning more calories is not only unnecessary but also unadvisable. Exercising too vigorously puts you at risk of additional destruction of healthy tissue and, even more dangerously, thyroid storm (see page 175).

That said, gentle exercise can help maintain your flexibility, improve your circulation, and reduce stress, anxiety, and tension. All these are significant benefits to the Overachiever that can complement the other supportive aspects of the SHINES protocol.

CYCLING

Biking at a gentle pace is another exercise you may do inside or outside. It can be psychologically restorative. Even at subaerobic levels, it can help improve circulation and respiration, increasing the flow of blood, energy, and nutrients throughout your system.

YOGA

Also a spiritual exercise for the Overachiever, yoga can feature prominently into your exercise regime. Gentle and restorative yoga practices are those that will yield the most benefit. I recommend avoiding any type of hot yoga, including Bikram, hatha yoga, or a vinyasa flow class held in a heated room, and suggest that you check in with a studio or instructor to learn about how physically demanding any given class may be. Certain practices such as Ashtanga are too rigorous for the Overachiever, even when performed in a cooler environment.

If you are interested in practicing on your own, I suggest searching for classes on Glo.com. The site offers thousands of classes based in different styles, which require different levels of experience, ability, and energy output; you may try some free of charge. You may also experiment with one or more of the simple, spiritually and physically fortifying postures I recommended earlier (see page 407) or those that follow.

Savasana (Corpse Pose)

Known to some as the "easiest pose to perform and the most difficult to master," Savasana is both a deceptively simple and powerful pose. Advocated for its ability to help increase awareness of physiological experiences, lower blood pressure, and diminish symptoms of anxiety and depression, Savasana can be a highly beneficial pose for Overachievers.

Savasana involves lying flat on your back on the mat with your arms at your sides and palms facing upward, your legs outstretched, each of your heels near one edge of the mat, and your feet relaxed outward. With your eyes closed, breathe naturally as you systematically relax every part of your body from the soles of your feet upward. Deepen your breath as feels comfortable for you, releasing all tension from your muscles, joints, and organs as you go.

If lying flat is uncomfortable for you, try placing a pillow or bolster under your knees.

You may remain in Savasana as long as you choose. If the pose is part of a series, experts recommend remaining in it for 5 minutes for every 30 minutes of your practice.

Balasana (Child's Pose)

A popular beginner's pose, Child's Pose may be practiced on its own or as part of a series. (In the latter case, it provides an opportunity for rest and rejuvenation between more challenging poses.) As an Overachiever, your yoga practice should be generally calming and restorative, and Child's Pose can play an important role in it.

Recommended for its power to reduce stress and fatigue by soothing the brain and nervous systems, Child's Pose involves relaxing into a comfortable position, breathing deeply and calmly, and maintaining an awareness of the breath throughout. Beginning with your hands and knees on the mat, bring your big toes to touch and spread your knees wide apart. (If your hips and/or thighs are very tight, you may keep your knees together.) Then sit back on your heels. If this is uncomfortable for you, try placing a blanket or pillow between your calves and your thighs. Doing this will not diminish the benefits of the pose.

Now sit up straight, stretching your spine, and then slowly bring your torso forward toward the mat, resting it between (or on) your thighs. Your forehead should rest on the mat. You may let your arms relax out in front of you with your palms on the mat, or you may choose to bring them alongside your body, letting them rest with your palms facing up.

In this position, close your eyes and breathe softly, increasing the depth of your breath as feels comfortable and as you release any tension from your neck, shoulders, and upper back as you allow this to broaden with each inhale. Relax your arms, letting these sink deeper into the mat. Remain in this pose for 1 minute or longer as you wish.

SUPPLEMENTS

For the Overachiever, the role of supplements is to help offset the negative effects of hyperthyroidism on bone health. Subclinical and clinical hyperthyroidism are both associated with bone degradation.[74] Some of this may be reversible with multifaceted treatment. In concert with other aspects of your SHINES protocol, supplementing with vitamin D and calcium can help maintain bone density levels.

VITAMIN D

In addition to helping regulate the immune and neuromuscular systems, vitamin D is also responsible for helping the body absorb calcium and promoting bone growth. Studies have linked vitamin D deficiencies in people with hyperthyroidism to increased rates of bone metabolism (breakdown) and decreased bone density.[75]

Vitamin D deficiencies are also commonly found in people suffering from autoimmune conditions. For the Overachiever whose hyperthyroidism is linked to Graves' disease, early-stage Hashimoto's thyroiditis, or other autoimmune condition, supplementing with vitamin D can be particularly critical.[76]

L-CARNITINE

It is known in the medical community that carnitine is depleted in women who have hyperthyroidism. Carnitine is similar to an amino acid and in the body is responsible for aiding metabolism, and when the metabolism is in overdrive it is utilized at a greater rate.

GLUCOMANNON

Glucomannon is a dietary fiber made from the root of the konjac plant. There is some evidence to show that supplementation with this could lower levels of circulating thyroid hormones if given early on in the treatment paradigm

BOOK RECOMMENDATIONS FOR OVERACHIEVERS

Izabella Wentz, PharmD, FASCP, *Hashimoto's Protocol: A 90-Day Plan for Reversing Thyroid Symptoms and Getting Your Life Back* (New York: HarperOne, 2017)

Alan Christianson, ND, *The Thyroid Reset Diet: Reverse Hypothyroid-*

ism Hashimoto's Symptoms with a Proven Iodine-Balancing Plan (New York: Rodale Books, 2021)

Datis Kharrazian, DHSc, DC, MS, *Why Do I Still Have Thyroid Symptoms? When My Lab Tests Are Normal* (Carlsbad, CA: Elephant Press, 2010)

For more information on chakras and chakra healing: Anodea Judith, PhD, *Eastern Body, Western Mind: Psychology and the Chakra System as a Path to the Self* (San Francisco: Celestial Arts Press, 2004)

OVERACHIEVERS

Golda Meir (née Goldie Mabovitch, May 3, 1898–December 8, 1978), *Israeli teacher, stateswoman, and the country's fourth prime minister (1969–1974).* Born in Ukraine to a homemaker and a carpenter, Golda Meir was one of eight children, only three of whom survived into adulthood. At the age of seven, she immigrated with her family to Milwaukee, and by the age of eight she was helping her mother run a small grocery store on the city's north side. She displayed natural leadership abilities early on, organizing a fund-raiser to pay for her own and her fellow students' textbooks when she was still in grade school.

During her adolescence, Meir was exposed to various religious and political ideologies, including Zionism, women's suffrage, and trade unionism, all of which fueled her drive to live in a kibbutz in Palestine and later take up residence in Jerusalem. There, she began her career in politics, and by 1946, she had advanced in the ranks to become the head of the political department of the Jewish Agency. In advance of Israel's declaration of independence in 1948, she managed to raise $20 million—three times what her colleagues had anticipated—to help bolster the country's armed forces in preparation for what became the Arab-Israeli War. For this effort, Israel's first prime minister, David Ben-Gurion, called Meir that "Jewish woman who got the money which made the state [of Israel] possible."[77]

In 1949, Meir was elected to the Knesset (Israeli legislature). She served as minister of labor and foreign minister before retiring briefly in 1966 due to illness, but returned to government and became prime minister in 1969. During her tenure as prime minister, Meir kept company with some of the most influential cultural and political leaders of her time, including Eva Perón, John F. Kennedy, Richard and Pat Nixon, Nicolae Ceaușescu (former president of Romania), Pope Paul VI, and Henry Kissinger. Following her retirement from the government in 1974, Meir continued to play an important role in international politics, including welcoming Egyptian president Anwar Sadat to the Knesset and praising his efforts to bring an end to the persistent violence of the Arab-Israeli conflict. (As of the writing of this book, Meir remains the only woman to ever have held the post of prime minister in Israel.)

Meir was the recipient of a series of awards, including the Israel Prize for her contributions to that country, the designation of World Mother by the American Mothers organization, and Princeton University's James Madison Award for Distinguished Public Service. She died in Jerusalem at the age of eighty following a battle with lymphatic cancer.

Margaret "Meg" Whitman (b. August 4, 1966), *American business executive and philanthropist.* Meg Whitman is perhaps best known for the decade she spent as CEO of eBay, a company she took from thirty employees and $4 million in revenue to 15,000 employees and $8 billion in annual earnings. Born in Huntington, New York, Whitman graduated from Princeton and Harvard before embarking on a career that would see her serve in high-ranking executive positions at the Walt Disney Company, DreamWorks, Procter & Gamble, Hasbro, and, of course, eBay. In 2008, the *New York Times* declared Whitman one of the women most likely to become the first female president of the United States, and in 2014, *Forbes* named her the twentieth most powerful woman in the world.

Whitman, one of the richest women in California (with a current net worth of nearly $3 billion), ran for governor of that state in 2010, investing more than $140 million of her own money in the race. She lost relatively narrowly to her Democratic opponent, Jerry Brown, but continued her involvement in state and national politics. During the 2016 presidential race, she initially supported Chris Christie before throwing her support behind Hillary Clinton once Donald Trump had secured the nomination. Calling Trump a "threat to democracy," Whitman wrote on Facebook, "To vote Republican out of party loyalty alone would be to endorse a candidacy that I believe has exploited anger, grievance, xenophobia and racial division. Donald Trump's demagoguery has undermined the fabric of our national character."[78]

Since February 2018, Whitman was the CEO of Hewlett Packard and Quibi, and had an unsuccessful run as a presidential candidate.

The SHINES Protocol: How Do You Organize a Chairwoman?

For the Chairwoman, the focus of the SHINES protocol is making space for herself in which she is not working, not ruling, and not running herself ragged. Space in which she remains accountable but is so—first and foremost—to herself. For her physical body as well as her spiritual and emotional experiences of herself and the world around her.

SPIRITUAL PRACTICE

For the Chairwoman, the goal of a spiritual practice is to relax and restore in a space where you are free from the demands that typically press upon you. The actual exercises or routines you may engage in are less important than the environment in which you engage in them and the mindset you maintain while doing so.

Practices including meditation, massage, and acupuncture can all help slow your rapid thoughts, subdue your emotional reactivity, and leave you feeling more centered and less cast about by the turmoil that has plagued your inner life. But in order for any of these practices to be effective at reducing stress and helping your body recover from symptoms such as weight gain, fatigue, and headaches, as well as anxiety and depression, you must surrender control, relinquishing your inner Queen's and Workaholic's desires to "run the show" and dictate the outcome.

EMPLOY HELP

Whether you rely on your spouse or partner, or a real or virtual assistant, delegating some of your responsibilities to a trusted aide can provide critical logistical and emotional support that can help lower your stress level and interrupt the estrogen dominance and cortisol excess feedback loop that has contributed to the rise of your collection of symptoms. I recommend leveraging others' help organizing the various aspects of your life at home or work, including arranging appointments, preparing meals, managing home improvement projects, or even planning social engagements.

The most important aspect of any type of help you may employ is the freedom from managing the various details of your life that the help can provide. Even technology can provide this. Instead of shopping for groceries, consider home delivery. Stores now offer extensive choices as well as some automatic reordering, a feature that can save you time, energy, and checklist bandwidth.

SPEND TIME OFFLINE

For all that technology can make your life easier and more efficient, as a Chairwoman, it's important that you also give yourself time offline. Detaching from all your devices, eliminating your exposure to email, social media, and news of all types, creates a space in which you can enjoy uninterrupted silence—where you can be alone and focus entirely on yourself. The relatively straightforward act of disconnecting from your phone, computer, and television can help you decompress and recharge your physical and emotional batteries that your busy life is always drawing upon.

As simple as this sounds, you may find it difficult to do. Many of the Chairwomen I've treated have told me that disconnecting makes them feel invisible. Lonely. If this happens, it's important to remember two things. The first is that being alone in silence becomes easier over time. And if you continue to practice it, being in silence can have significant calming and restorative effects. The second is that drawing these lines in the sand makes your family, friends, and colleagues aware that you need time for you, and that they need to honor that. It also makes the time you are available for them more important, making it less likely that they will take you or your time for granted.

To start, I recommend setting aside 20 to 30 minutes each week, preferably the same time, and working up to one to two hours at a stretch. (Ultimately, detaching for half a day is ideal.) Some of my patients choose early weekend mornings, when their houses are quiet and work is more or less at bay. Others choose late evenings during the week or weekend, again, a time when the people who rely on them are least likely to need their help. The important thing is to set the time aside and honor your plan to eliminate your exposure to any of your electronics during it.

In the silence, the questions become: What do you hear? What is the message your body is sending you? Can you heed it? Will you? For so many of my patients, silence has revealed important secrets they were withholding even from themselves. Of course, this can take time. But if you remain open to the possibility of discovery and healing, a message will come.

HORMONE MODULATION

For the Chairwoman, the goal of hormone modulation is to diminish estrogen dominance and reduce cortisol levels. Distinct approaches can help achieve each of these objectives.

COUNTERACTING ESTROGEN DOMINANCE

If you are taking any form of estrogen replacement therapy, adjusting your dose may be an important first step. Because your absorption rate of oral or transdermal medications varies according to your tissues' permeability and your sensitivity to the medication's active ingredients, it is important to remember that even a relatively low-dose estrogen replacement medication may be driving your symptoms.

Your birth control medication may also be at the root of your estrogen dominance. If you are taking a medication that contains synthetic estrogen and progesterone, you may want to consider a birth control medication that contains *only* progestin (synthetic progesterone). Because this type of medication contains no estrogen, making the change to it may help bring your estrogen and progesterone closer to balance. At the same time, however, synthetic progesterone may not have the same effects as the progesterone produced by your own body or a bioidentical replacement.

If you are not taking an estrogen replacement or birth control medication, a progesterone supplement may be an effective method of counteracting your estrogen dominance. I recommend bioidentical progesterone replacement medications. There are several forms available, including tablets, gels, suppositories, and injectables.

If you and your physician decide that a progesterone medication is right for you, make sure he or she closely monitors your progesterone and estrogen levels during the period of time you are taking it. Changes normally require between one and three weeks to take hold, so it's best to test your levels at this point and then every several weeks after that.

REDUCING CORTISOL LEVELS

In the Chairwoman (as in the Workaholic), cortisol excess can give rise to a debatable phenomenon that has become known as the "pregnenolone steal." Pregnenolone is an endogenous steroid that is a precursor to a series of hormones, including estrogen, progesterone, and cortisol, and when the body is overproducing cortisol, it is likely to "steal" pregnenolone in order to keep these levels high. In the Chairwoman, supplementing with pregnenolone may provide the body with raw material critical for producing a series of hormones and thus help restore balance among all of them. Supplementing with DHEA can also help offset cortisol excess.

INFOCEUTICALS

For the Chairwoman, the two most important Energetic Integrators (EI) are EI8 and EI10.

EI8 exerts its effects along the liver meridian, influencing the energy fields in and around the liver. The liver is responsible for breaking down and eliminating excess hormones, including estrogen, as well as exogenous toxins, including phtyoestrogens that can contribute to estrogen dominance. Clearing energetic disruptions along this meridian can help regulate these processes and diminish the estrogen dominance aspect of the Chairwoman archetype.

As for EI10, this integrator bioenergetically influences the hypothalamus, which helps control the ovaries' production of estrogen. (Nerve cells in the hypothalamus release gonadotrophin-releasing hormone, sending messages to the pituitary gland to produce luteinizing hormone [LH] and follicle-stimulating hormone [FSH], each of which plays a role in estrogen production.) Adding to this, EI10 operates along the circulation/pericardium meridian, influencing the energy fields surrounding the neuroendocrine and circulatory systems, and contributes to overall hormonal balance.

Energetically, as a Chairwoman you have the power to move mountains, but you could also be a bit headstrong and feel as though things will only be done correctly if you do them yourself. A Chairwoman can also struggle with migraines and headaches because she can be blocked in the sixth chakra. So how does she energetically balance? Sound therapy is a good way to unblock this chakra and some say that a vibration of 288 Hz is optimal. For Chairwomen, I recommend some time with singing bowls, which are actually bells that are slightly bowl-shaped, and when they are tapped or rubbed with a special mallet create different sounds. They are used in many spiritual and religious rituals. And the Chairwoman should use not just any singing bowl, but a singing bowl that is at 288 Hz or bass note D. Sit in your quiet place (as a Chairwoman, make sure you have a quiet space), and make that bowl sing while you focus your thoughts on letting go.

ESSENTIAL OILS

The power of the Chairwoman comes from her being the Queen of her domain and a Workaholic. Obviously a very powerful, maybe the most powerful, archetype but also the one most likely to burnout and fatigue. Try these essential oils:

Chamomile	Patchouli
Frankincense	Vetiver
Lemon	

NUTRITION

For the busy Chairwoman who is accustomed to meals on the go, adhering to a diet that can help ameliorate her symptoms and bring her estrogen, cortisol, and other hormones into balance can pose a challenge. But this is far from impossible. Small adjustments such as preparing a week's worth of meals in advance or incorporating important vitamin, mineral, fat, and protein elements into shakes you can consume on the go can go a considerable distance toward making your ideal diet easier to embrace and adhere to over the long term. The key is to commit to planning, so you have nutritious foods at the ready.

FOODS TO EMBRACE

Antioxidant-Containing Fruits and Vegetables

Vegetables rich in antioxidants, including vitamins A, C, and E and beta-carotene, as well as minerals such as copper, zinc, and selenium, can yield benefits for the Chairwoman. These unrefined carbohydrates are also a healthy source of fiber, which can help diminish estrogen dominance by aiding the excretion of excess estrogen via the bowel. I recommend seeking out colorful—and different-colored—fruits and vegetables. Among good choices for the Chairwoman are:

Bell peppers in yellow, orange, and red
Broccoli
Brussels sprouts
Cantaloupe
Carrots
Eggplant (including the skin)
Sweet potatoes
Butternut squash

Lean Proteins

Lean proteins comprise an important part of the Chairwoman's diet. In addition to helping improve your body composition (by reducing your body fat percentage), a diet containing lean proteins provides the body with the amino acids lysine and threonine. These help the body metabolize estrogen in addition to supporting liver function, both of which can help reduce estrogen dominance.

A diet containing lean proteins can also help repair and restore tissues that the catabolic processes associated with cortisol excess have likely damaged. Once your body burns through its sugar-based energy reserves, it begins breaking down tissues, including muscle and bone. Consuming lean proteins helps provide the building blocks necessary for repairing them. Good sources of lean protein for the Chairwoman include:

> Fish, including salmon and tuna
> Lean meats, including ground beef and pork loin
> Eggs
> Low-fat or nonfat dairy products, including milk, yogurt, and cottage cheese
> Beans and lentils
> Nuts and nut butters
> Seeds
> Protein powders, such as vegan pea, rice, or powdered peanut options

Healthy Fats

Healthy fats—omega-3 and omega-6 monounsaturated and poly-unsaturated fats—can be a great source of fuel for the Chairwoman whose cortisol excess is driving catabolic processes. They can also help diminish symptoms of "foggy brain." Broken down into ketone bodies, the brain's preferred energy source, healthy fats can help with memory and mental clarity. Healthy fats have also been shown to decrease inflammation, which excess cortisol tends to cause, and improve the health of your skin. Good sources of healthy fats:

OILS

Coconut oil

Olive oil

Oil blends, including Udo's Oil Omega 3-6-9 Blend,
    a mixture of omega-3, -6, and -9 fatty acids

NUTS AND SEEDS

Walnuts, almonds, and pistachios

Nut and seed butters, including almond, cashew,
    and sunflower seed

Chia seeds

Flaxseed

Sunflower seeds

OTHER FOOD SOURCES

Avocados

Eggs

Fish, including salmon and tuna

Olives

Tofu

Fiber

Excess estrogen is excreted via the bowel. This means that depressed function of your digestive tract can lead to reabsorption of estrogen into the bloodstream, which can contribute to estrogen dominance. Cruciferous vegetables such as broccoli, cabbage, celery, and kale are all great sources of fiber. (Because these contain phytoestrogens, however, I recommend restricting your consumption of cruciferous vegetables to one serving every other day.) Seeds such as flax and sunflower are also good sources of fiber for the Chairwoman, as are beans, berries, fruits such as apples and pears, and nuts, including almonds, pecans, and walnuts.

To protect against estrogen dominance, I recommend the Chairwoman consume 25 mg of fiber per day. Although I always recommend food sources rather than supplements, if you find that you cannot consume 25 mg of food-based fiber per day, I recommend that you add a fiber supplement. Regardless of the source, I recommend slowly increasing the amount of fiber you consume. Doing this too quickly can trigger your body to produce excess gas and cause mild to severe stomach pain.

Cruciferous Vegetables

In addition to providing fiber, cruciferous vegetables such as broccoli, Brussels sprouts, cabbage, kale, mustard greens, and turnips contain a compound called indole-3-carbinol (I3C). Studies have indicated that this compound impedes estrogen receptor cell proliferation (at least in breast tissue). This may help reduce estrogen dominance. I3C may also help lower the risk of breast, cervical, endometrial, and/or colorectal cancers.

When you consume cruciferous vegetables, your body naturally produces another compound called diindolylmethane (DIM). Research has shown that DIM can help break down estrogen and convert it to its safer metabolites. DIM has also been shown to have a weak estrogenic effect, meaning that it can bind to estrogen receptors and block the potentially carcinogenic impact of stronger forms of estrogen. DIM may also help ease the Chairwoman's symptoms of PMDD and jump-start weight loss.

FOODS TO AVOID

Exogenous Estrogens and Phytoestrogens

Because exogenous estrogens and phytoestrogens can exacerbate estrogen dominance, I recommend the Chairwoman limit or eliminate her intake of each. Common sources of exogenous estrogen include beef, poultry, and dairy products as well as plastics and certain cosmetics. In recent years, many producers of these products have introduced hormone-free options. For the Chairwoman, it is worth seeking these out.

The most common source of phytoestrogens is soy. Although there are positive health benefits associated with soy, I recommend the Chairwoman limit her intake of soy (fermented and nonfermented) to two to three servings per day. If you enjoy soy milk, I recommend you consider switching to almond or rice milk.

Caffeine

Among the Chairwomen I've treated, dependency on caffeine is common. Unfortunately, it also tends to exacerbate their symptoms, particularly those related to cortisol excess. Caffeine increases cortisol production, raises your heart rate, and drives up your blood pressure. Caffeine also escalates diuresis, which leaves you chronically dehydrated. In addition to headaches, long-term dehydration can also weaken the skin and other tissues.

If you are reliant on caffeine, suddenly eliminating it from your diet can have adverse effects of its own. I recommend decreasing your caffeine intake over time both by consuming lower amounts of highly caffeinated drinks such as coffee and exchanging these for lower-caffeine alternatives. As difficult as these changes may feel at first, as the SHINES protocol takes hold and your symptoms abate, you may expect any cravings for caffeine to wane. This will make substituting lower-caffeine or caffeine-free options that much easier.

EXERCISE

While exercise is an important aspect of the Chairwoman's protocol, it is also one that requires caution. As we've discussed at various points in this chapter, a Chairwoman's cortisol excess is already stressing the body, driving catabolic processes that exercise can intensify. The majority of the Chairwomen I've treated have unexpectedly gained weight and looked to an exercise regime to them lose it. While weight loss can be one of the goals of your exercise routine, improved circulation and muscle and joint health are all equally important objectives. Physical and psychological relaxation and restoration are also critical objectives. The simple act of slowing down during and after a workout can help ameliorate a number of your physiological and psychological estrogen-dominance—and cortisol-excess-related symptoms.

YOGA

For the Chairwoman, I recommend a moderately cardiovascular 60- to 90-minute yoga practice. Whether you participate in a class or practice on your own at home, it is important that you remain detached from your electronic devices during this time. This ensures your practice serves the dual purpose of helping improve your physical health and providing an opportunity for psychological rest.

WALKING

Similar to yoga in the way it gently bestows physical and psychological benefits, walking or hiking for an hour or more in a landscape you find calming can help improve your cardiovascular fitness, improve your muscle tone and joint health, and provide an opportunity to detach from the demands of your hectic daily life.

For some archetypes, I recommend guided walks. But for the Chairwoman, I recommend walking in silence. At first, you may find the quiet uncomfortable, even difficult to bear. Over time, however, giving yourself a space in which you can hear only your thoughts can help you listen to these more closely and honor them more effectively.

SUPPLEMENTS

For the Chairwoman, the role of supplements is to help diminish the symptoms of estrogen dominance on the one hand and help the body recover from the impact of cortisol excess on the other. The supplements I recommend are divided along these lines. Which of these you choose to try may depend on which of the underlying causes of your archetype is more prominent. As such, the supplements that are most beneficial may change over time as certain of your symptoms improve.

SUPPLEMENTS THAT HELP DIMINISH ESTROGEN DOMINANCE

Indole-3-Carbonyl (I3C) and Diindolylmethane (DIM)

Earlier in this section, we discussed the benefits associated with I3C, a compound found in cruciferous vegetables, and DIM, a compound the body produces when it breaks down I3C. Studies have indicated that the compound impedes estrogen receptor cell proliferation, at least in breast tissue. In recent years, researchers have become interested in I3C as a possible preventative of breast, cervical, endometrial, and colorectal cancers.

From I3C, your body naturally produces another compound called diindolylmethane (DIM). Research has shown that DIM helps break down estrogen and convert it to its safer metabolites. DIM has also been shown to have a weak estrogenic effect, meaning that it can bind to estrogen receptors and block the potentially carcinogenic impact of stronger forms of estrogen. DIM can also ameliorate the Chairwoman's symptoms of PMDD and jump-start weight loss.

A variety of I3C and DIM supplements are available. If you choose to begin taking one of these, I recommend 15 mg/day to start and increasing this as you and your physician deem appropriate.

There are some side effects associated with these supplements. These include skin rashes, abdominal pain, nausea, and an increase in liver enzymes. DIM may be slightly easier on your digestive system than I3C, because I3C is the unstable precursor to DIM and needs to be activated in the stomach before your body can convert it into DIM.

Vitex (Chasteberry)

Vitex agnus-castus, commonly known as chasteberry or vitex, is an herbal supplement that has been used for thousands of years by cultures around the globe to help maintain a healthy balance of estrogen and progesterone. Studies have shown that vitex can inhibit the secretion of follicle-stimulating hormone (FSH) by the pituitary gland, which leads to a decrease in estrogen production by the ovaries. Vitex has also been shown to stimulate the secretion of luteinizing hormone (LH), which triggers the formulation of a corpus luteum and increases progesterone production.

For the Chairwoman, I recommend a dose of 20 to 40 mg of extract each morning.

I do share a few **warnings** about vitex with patients. First, although vitex may begin working in as few as ten days, studies show that women taking the supplement may need to wait for up to six months to experience it benefits. Second, although there are few significant side effects associated with vitex, some of my patients have reported nausea, gastrointestinal upset, skin reactions, and headaches. Women who suffer from menstrual depression or PMDD have also reported an exacerbation of these symptoms. **Vitex is not recommended for women who are pregnant or breastfeeding.**

Maca

An herb grown in Peru, maca has long been used to promote hormone balance (in men and women) as well as reproductive and menstrual health. Each of the thirteen differently colored varieties of maca exerts distinct effects, and many maca-based supplements combine different varieties of the herb. Some of these can raise estrogen levels, which is why it's critical to use a supplement that contains the right types of maca in the right ratios to address your estrogen dominance.

The particular maca supplement I recommend for the Chairwoman is Femmenessence MacaHarmony, a 100 percent organic and vegan mixture of sustainably farmed maca that has been shown to have a balancing effect on women's levels of estrogen, progesterone, and other hormones. I recommend taking the standard dose: two capsules twice daily, taken away from meals. Take the first dose in the morning, before breakfast, and the second dose in the early evening, ideally 30 minutes before you normally experience an energy low. Consider taking half the recommended amount for two weeks, then gradually increase to the standard amount. Assuming your system tolerates the maca well, I suggest continuing to take the supplement at the near-full or full dose.

Two notes of **caution** with regard to MacaHarmony: First, I recommend that a Chairwoman take this supplement for two to three months and then take a week off. This can help upregulate your estrogen receptors and enhance the supplement's benefits. Second, MacaHarmony can amplify the effects of caffeine. So while a Chairwoman is always wise to limit or avoid caffeine, taking extra caution around caffeine when taking this supplement is a good idea.

SUPPLEMENTS THAT AMELIORATE SYMPTOMS OF CORTISOL EXCESS: ADAPTOGENS

Adaptogens are plants and plant-based substances known for their ability to help support the adrenal system and the body's ability to manage stress, fend off fatigue, and counter the normal effects of aging. They take their name from their ability to help the body "adapt" to the ever-changing elements of its environment.

Used for centuries in Chinese and Indian Ayurvedic medicine, adaptogens have significantly increased in popularity in Western cultures during the past several decades.[79] For the Chairwoman, I recommend the adaptogen supplements listed here.

Ginseng

Containing chemical components called ginsenosides, Asian ginseng is known for its power to support physical stamina and the body's immune system. It has also been touted for its ability to slow the aging process and alleviate symptoms of certain respiratory and cardiovascular disorders. Ginseng is also believed to help diminish anxiety and relieve symptoms of depression, and some studies indicate that it also reduces the frequency and intensity of hot flashes.

As with any supplement, I recommend researching your options. Make sure that any supplement you take contains the ingredients you're looking for—and few, if any, others. For ginseng and other adaptogen supplements, I recommend the Nature's Way, Integrative Therapeutics, and Designs for Health brands.

A word of warning regarding ginseng: Make sure you are taking the right type. The terms "red ginseng" and "white ginseng" both refer to preparation of Asian ginseng. "Panax ginseng" refers to American ginseng, and "Siberian ginseng" refers to another adaptogenic herb called eleuthero, which is not actually related to ginseng at all.

Ashwagandha

Sometimes called Indian ginseng (though it is not ginseng at all), ashwagandha has been used for centuries in Ayurvedic medicine for its immune-system-boosting effects. An all-around adaptogen that can help users cope with daily stress and offset the physiological effects associated with it and cortisol excess, ashwagandha has also been shown to help improve sleep and cognitive functioning in addition to reducing inflammation.

Astragalus

Long used in Chinese medicine as an immune booster, this adaptogen is known for its ability to help protect against the physically and psychologically destructive effects of stress.[80] The herb may also minimize the impact of excess cortisol by limiting its ability to bind to cell receptors.

Like holy basil, astragalus is known for its antiviral, anti-inflammatory, antibacterial, and antioxidant properties. It can also help lower blood pressure and strengthen the immune system.

Rhodiola (Golden Root)

After ginseng, rhodiola is perhaps the most widely studied adaptogen. Like some of the other adaptogens we've discussed, rhodiola can help minimize the effects of long-term stress. It has been shown to help restore normal patterns of eating and sleeping in addition to reducing fatigue and oxidative stress (the body's inability to counteract or detoxify the harmful effects of free radicals). Native to the arctic areas of Asia and Eastern Europe, rhodiola has also been found to directly decrease the cortisol response to awakening stress.

Rhodiola can also help burn belly fat. The herb contains a compound called rosavin, which has been shown to stimulate an enzyme called hormone-sensitive lipase. This enzyme can break down fat stores in adipose tissue, such as the fat that builds up in the abdominal area. In one 1999 study, subjects on a restricted-calorie diet who added a daily dose of rhodiola experienced more than twice the weight loss of subjects who did not include the adaptogen, and also showed a significant decrease in body fat.

SUPPLEMENTS THAT ADDRESS BOTH SETS OF A CHAIRWOMAN'S SYMPTOMS

Chrysin

Belonging to a class of chemicals known as flavonoids, chrysin is a naturally occurring compound found in plants, including passion-flower and silver linden, as well as in honey. Chrysin has been shown to inhibit the aromatization of testosterone into estrogen in addition to suppressing cortisol production. Studies have also shown that chrysin possesses strong antianxiety properties and can also reduce hypertension.[81]

BOOK RECOMMENDATIONS FOR CHAIRWOMEN

James Gordon, MD, *Manifesto for a New Medicine: Your Guide to Healing Partnerships and the Wise Use of Alternative Therapies* (New York: Perseus, 1996)

Donald M. Vickery, MD, and James F. Fries, MD, *Take Care of Yourself* (New York: Perseus, 2001)

Brené Brown, PhD, LMSW, *Rising Strong: How the Ability to Reset Transforms the Way We Live, Love, Parent, and Lead* (New York: Random House, 2017)

Don Miguel Ruiz, *The Four Agreements: A Practical Guide to Personal Freedom* (San Rafael, CA: Amber-Allen Publishing, 1997)

CHAIRWOMEN

Barbara Walters (b. September 25, 1929). Born in Boston, Barbara Walters spent her early years in the city before moving with her parents between Miami and New York. After graduating from Sarah Lawrence College with a degree in English, Walters went to work in television, becoming a writer on CBS's *The Morning Show* before joining NBC's *Today* show as a writer and researcher; she would go on to host the show, the first woman in America to do so. From that time, she would go on to host shows including *The View, 20/20*, and the *ABC Evening News*. She has been named as one of *TV Guide's* "50 Greatest TV Stars of All Time" and received a Lifetime Achievement Award from the National Academy of Television Arts and Sciences. Retired from her full-time hosting roles, Walters continues to work as a guest contributor on a series of daytime and evening programs.

Ruth Bader Ginsburg (March 15, 1933–September 18, 2020). Born in New York to Russian Jewish immigrants, Ruth Bader Ginsburg was educated at Cornell, Harvard, and Columbia, where she ultimately earned her law degree, graduating first in her class. Following a career as a civil rights activist and academic, teaching at Rutgers and Columbia, Ginsburg served as one of the ACLU's general counsels before President Jimmy Carter appointed her to the US Court of Appeals for the District of Columbia Circuit. President Bill Clinton nominated her for the Supreme Court in 1993, and she took her seat on the bench in June of that year and served until her death in September of 2020.

The SHINES Protocol: How Do You Enlighten a Philosopher?

For the Philosopher, the SHINES protocol provides opportunities for self-examination and self-care that, when taken together, can help alleviate your physiological, psychological, and emotional symptoms and bring you into balance. Central to the Philosopher's protocol in particular are both grappling with the "big" questions, such as "Who am I?" and "What do I really need to feel fulfilled and happy in this life?," and also imparting her wisdom to others. As we will discuss at various points in the following section, sharing the lessons you've learned can be as important to your journey toward balance as leveraging them in your own life.

SPIRITUAL PRACTICE

As I explain to the Philosophers I treat, the spiritual practices I recommend are akin to walking a labyrinth. Each involves a journey inward toward self-examination and discovery and a journey outward toward using your discoveries to make changes in your life and sharing those discoveries with others.

GENOGRAM

One spiritual exercise I recommend for Philosophers of all ages is creating a genogram. More detailed than a traditional family tree, a genogram is designed to help its creator envisage the patterns of behavior and emotional interactions that have shaped the relationships among relatives. For the Philosopher, the relationships between herself and the other women in her family are the most critical. Graphical depictions of these reveal patterns of discord and communion that can help you better understand how your family history has helped shape your life's path.

JOURNALING

A contemplative practice, journaling serves the dual purpose of focusing a Philosopher's efforts at self-discovery and providing an opportunity to share her wisdom with others. As strongly as I recommend journaling for your own sake first and foremost, recording your experiences and sentiments honestly and without a thought of who may later read what you have written, in reality, your story may come into others' hands and provide them with insight into your life and their own. My mother-in-law kept a journal during the last fifteen years of her life, and after she died, my wife and her siblings took comfort in reading her words. In a way, my mother-in-law maintained a presence among her children and continued to help guide them through her journals.

DRAWING AND PAINTING

In addition to writing, drawing or painting can be a significant intellectual and creative endeavor for the Philosopher. I recommend reaching into your memories and calling forth a single image that you then draw or paint to the best of your ability. The quality of the image is unimportant. What matters are the images themselves and how you choose to construe them. Sometimes, it is helpful to engage in this exercise with someone who knows you well and has some familiarity with your past. How they interpret the image you create can be revealing in itself. Chances are, they will see the image differently from the way you do, and will point things out you would not have noticed on your own.

HORMONE MODULATION

For a Philosopher (as for any of the other eleven archetypes we discuss in this book), hormonal modulation may or may not temporarily or permanently figure into her SHINES protocol. As with any medications, there are risks associated with hormone replacement therapy, and taking these into account is critical.

When deciding whether hormonal modulation is right for you, the question you need to ask yourself is whether and to what extent your symptoms are keeping you from living the life you want to live. If your lethargy, muscle weakness, diminished libido, hot flashes, and irritability are combining to make you miserable and negatively affecting your life at work and home, supplementing your body's estrogen, progesterone, testosterone, and even DHEA with a bioidentical replacement may be right for you.

As I have discussed at various points in this book, in my practice, I tend to prescribe bioidentical hormones. As for estrogen replacement, this comes in custom-compounded and branded formats and may be administered orally or transdermally. (Studies have shown that transdermal estrogen is less likely to break down into the 4-hydroxy or 116α-hydroxyestrone form that may be more carcinogenic, which has made it more popular among some prescribers.) Branded medications are generally covered by insurance, while custom-compounded medications are not. Depending on your insurance company's formulary restrictions and copay structure, however, custom-compounded medications may be the less expensive option.

For the Philosopher and any other archetype for whom estrogen replacement therapy may come into play, I recommend also taking a progesterone replacement medication. While this is necessary for any woman who still has her uterus, I strongly advise women who have had full hysterectomies to add progesterone to their hormone replacement regime. In addition to decreasing the risk of estrogen dominance, progesterone can also help combat insomnia and anxiety more generally. Again, custom-compounded and branded versions of bioidentical progesterone are available.

As of the writing of this book, a female-specific testosterone replacement medication has yet to hit the market. Your physician can prescribe a custom-compounded bioidentical option, however, and a pharmacy can create the individualized dose you and your physician determine is appropriate for you.

Last, Philosophers may benefit from a supplement of DHEA. Known in some circles as "the fountain of youth" for its naturally protective effects on the body's various systems, DHEA is naturally produced by the adrenal glands. In women and men, DHEA levels tend to drop off after the age of thirty. For the Philosopher, replacing DHEA with a bioidentical supplement may help alleviate symptoms including skin dryness and thinning, vaginal atrophy, and osteoporosis.

INFOCEUTICALS AND ESSENTIAL OILS

The two Energetic Integrators (EI) best suited to the Philosopher's needs are EI10 and EI11. Similar to other Integrators, these operate by "echoing" the impact of the hormones as your body has known them, helping to restore the flow of energy along the pathways your estrogen and testosterone deficiencies have disrupted.

Operating along the circulation/pericardium meridian, EI10 is a critical integrator for the neuroendocrine and circulatory systems, and it plays a major role in overall hormone balance. EI10 bioenergetically influences the hypothalamus, which helps control the ovaries' hormone production. (Nerve cells in the hypothalamus send messages to the pituitary gland to produce luteinizing hormone [LH] and follicle-stimulating hormone [FSH], which are carried via the bloodstream to the ovaries, where they help regulate the menstrual cycle.) This integrator also bioenergetically influences manifestations of PMS and/or PMDD, including mood swings, irritability, and depressive symptoms.

EI11 addresses the energetic disruptions associated with testosterone deficiency. Operating along the stomach meridian, it influences digestion and the liver's processing of heavy metals and environmental toxins. EI11 also exerts effects across the pelvic region or sacral chakra, including on the reproductive organs. The sacral chakra corresponds to the domain of emotions, encompassing those related to relationships (with people as well as the material elements of our lives, such as money), sex, and sexuality.

ESSENTIAL OILS

The Philosopher walks the hallways always contemplating because she shares the brain power of the Wisewoman and the Nun. The issue coming from this archetype is that she can suffer from fatigue and lack of desire. Try these essential oils:

Clary sage	Neroli
Fennel	Rose
Frankincense	Sandalwood

NUTRITION

For the Philosopher, the following foods can help alleviate the symptoms associated with estrogen deficiency and low testosterone. In some cases, certain nutrients can even help support the production of each of these hormones.

FOODS TO EMBRACE

Antioxidant-Containing Fruits and Vegetables

Vegetables rich in antioxidants, including vitamins A, C, and E and beta-carotene, as well as minerals such as copper, zinc, and selenium, can yield benefits for the Philosopher. I recommend seeking out colorful—and different-colored—fruits and vegetables. Among good choices for the Philosopher are:

Bell peppers in yellow, orange, and red
Broccoli
Brussels sprouts
Cantaloupe
Carrots
Eggplant (including the skin)
Sweet potatoes
Butternut squash

Soy

When it comes to balancing out estrogen deficiency, one of the foods physicians and other healthcare practitioners focus on most is soy. Rich in isoflavones, including genistein and daidzein, which the body can convert into weak forms of estrogen, soy can help elevate your estrogen levels and diminish the symptoms of deficiency. These may include everything from hot flashes to vaginal atrophy. In order for soy to exert these effects, you need to consume roughly 60 grams of soy protein per day—the equivalent of five to six glasses of soy milk.

Before we dive deeper into the various forms of soy protein and which of those I recommend, it is important to note that consuming large amounts of soy can pose a danger to women who have battled breast cancer or are at increased risk for the disease. As previously noted, even weak estrogens can bind to estrogen receptors, including those in breast tissue, and have stimulatory effects. Be aware, too, that soy is a crop that has been genetically modified, so choose your sources wisely and consume soy in moderation. If you or other women in your family have a history of breast cancer, it is best to discuss the incorporation of soy into your diet with your physician.

In addition to an increased risk of cancer, some studies have shown that soy products containing genetically modified plant material can damage the thyroid. Some of my patients have also tested positive for soy allergies. If you are concerned that you may have a soy allergy yourself, I encourage you to ask your physician to test you for it.

For all that these risks merit consideration, the most important thing to note about soy may be this: Fermented soy products are believed to pose far fewer concerns than unfermented soy, affording consumers more of the benefits and fewer of the risks. Examples of fermented soy, many of which are widely used in Asian cultures, include:

Fermented soy milk
Miso
Natto
Soy sauce
Tempeh

Examples of unfermented soy products include tofu, soy protein isolates (such as those found in bars and shake powders), edamame, soy flour, and processed foods that contain soy derivatives or soybean oil. Many of these products have become increasingly popular during the past decade.

For Philosophers, I recommend consuming fermented soy, including fermented soy milk (which you can mix with berries and other fruits), and making sure any soy product you choose is organic in order to avoid potential hazards associated with genetically modified soybeans.

Foods Rich in Vitamin B12

Vitamin B12 can have a positive impact on sleep. For Philosophers suffering from insomnia due to nighttime hot flashes, a progesterone deficiency, or generalized stress or anxiety, foods rich in cobalamin (vitamin B12) can be a useful complement to other aspects of the SHINES protocol. Among these foods are:

Red meat, including beef, beef liver, and lamb
Fish, including salmon, mackerel, and sardines
Poultry
Eggs
Dairy products, including cheese

One important note is that acid inhibitors such as Zantac, Pepcid, and Prilosec (and their generics) can also inhibit absorption of vitamin B12. If you are taking one of these medications, you may want to eat additional portions of foods rich in B12.

Foods Containing L-Tryptophan

A precursor to melatonin, the amino acid L-tryptophan (commonly referred to simply as tryptophan) can help with sleep and mood more generally. Related to the production of serotonin, tryptophan can help alleviate depression symptoms that can accompany the onset of menopause. Foods high in L-tryptophan I recommend for Philosophers include:

Turkey
Eggs
Cheese
Salmon
Soy (including fermented soy)
Spinach
Seaweed
Pineapple

Foods Containing High Levels of Omega-3 Fatty Acids

During the past several years, I've been pleased to see a medical and cultural shift away from fat-restrictive diets and back toward those containing "good fats," including omega-3 unsaturated fatty acids. These have been shown to help support cardiovascular health, stabilize blood sugar levels, boost immunity, and improve mood, among other benefits. For Philosophers, consuming 2 g of omega-3 fatty acids per day can also help ameliorate symptoms including hot flashes and vaginal dryness as well as hypertriglyceridemia, joint pain, depression, and osteoporosis.

Known as "essential" fatty acids because the body does not produce them on its own, the omega-3 fatty acids ALA (alpha-linolenic acid), DHA (docosahexaenoic acid), and EPA (eicosapentaenoic acid) are found primarily in seafood, sea vegetables, some nuts and seeds, and grass-fed meat. For the Philosopher, I recommend consuming 2 grams (2,000 mg) of omega-3 fatty acids per day, with as much as possible coming from food sources. Among the best of these sources are:

FISH

Wild-caught salmon (and salmon oil) and tuna
White fish, including herring and mackerel
Sardines and anchovies
Cod liver oil

NUTS, SEEDS, AND OILS

Walnuts, brazil nuts, cashews, hazelnuts, butternuts
Flaxseeds (and flaxseed oil—see page 301), hemp seeds, chia seeds
Coconut oil
Fish oil (see page 301)

VEGETABLES

Brussels sprouts

Kale, spinach, watercress

Seaweed, algae

Algal oil (vegetarian)

ADDITIONAL SOURCES

Natto

Egg yolks

Regardless of whether you are actively trying to lose weight, lean protein sources are an important element of the Philosopher's diet. Even for women who are relatively thin, maintaining a healthy body mass index (BMI) of 18.5 to 24.9 is particularly important during and after menopause. Again, your body may tend to hold on to excess fat during and after menopause. But substituting healthy lean proteins for those containing saturated fat and avoiding processed carbohydrates and refined sugars can be a healthy counterbalance.

Water

For the Philosopher, remaining sufficiently hydrated is important. Dehydration can worsen the decreased vaginal lubrication associated with estrogen deficiency, as well as general skin thinning and wrinkling, so ensuring that you drink enough water is important.

The question is, how much is "enough"? When it comes to making these recommendations, I tend to be conservative. I don't encourage my patients to wander around with gallon jugs of spring water, forcing themselves to constantly drink it. I simply advise them to try to drink eight 8-ounce glasses each day, and to increase this amount if they intensify their workout regimens or routinely experience excessive sweating.

Remember, too, that we get water from a variety of sources, including the food we eat. The key is to remain mindful of the potential for dehydration and its negative effects, and to substitute water for juice or soda whenever possible.

Dark Chocolate

Dark chocolate (at least 70 percent pure cacao) can yield a series of benefits for the Wisewoman. Researchers at institutions including the Cleveland Clinic and the American Cancer Society have found that when consumed in moderation, dark chocolate can help boost your mood, improve your cardiovascular health by lowering your blood pressure and improving circulation, and help protect all your body's systems from potentially disease-causing free radicals. These potential benefits arise out of the antioxidant effects of the flavanols found in the chocolate.

For the Philosopher, dark chocolate can be a healthy treat. At roughly 170 calories an ounce, dark chocolate contains 2.2 grams of protein and 3.1 grams of fiber, as well as significant amounts of iron and magnesium.

Foods High in Vitamin D

In women, vitamin D deficiency has been linked not only to low testosterone, but also to osteopenia and osteoporosis. Vitamin D supports the body's absorption of calcium and phosphorus, and it has been shown to improve bone strength after menopause.

Foods rich in vitamin D that I recommend for the Philosopher include:

Egg yolks (also rich in omega-3 "good" fatty acids)
Tuna (also rich in omega-3 "good" fatty acids)
Enriched nondairy milks, such as almond or cashew milk

Foods High in Zinc

Studies have shown that if you have low testosterone, zinc can help boost your body's natural production of the hormone. For the Philosopher whose zinc levels are low, good sources of zinc include:

Oysters and other shellfish, including lobster and
  Alaskan king crab
Grass-fed beef (chuck roast or ground beef patty)
Chickpeas
Cashews
Mushrooms
Spinach

Almonds

Whole almonds contain a set of nutrients vital to testosterone production, including vitamin E, calcium, magnesium, and potassium. They are also rich in arginine, an amino acid that is involved in increasing blood flow to the genitals. Increasing your arginine levels can help ameliorate Philosopher's symptoms including vaginal atrophy and general diminution of sexual desire and arousal.

Although almonds are a source of quality protein and contain high levels of unsaturated fatty acids, they are also a significant source of calories. For the Philosopher, I recommend consuming no more than ten to twenty each day.

Antidepressant Medications and the Philosopher Archetype

Some of the Philosophers I've treated, particularly those who have been menopausal or postmenopausal, have chosen to take an antidepressant to help combat not only depression, but also some of the physiological symptoms of menopause, including hot flashes and night sweats.[82]

This is particularly common among Philosophers for whom estrogen replacement therapy is not a viable option. Examples of popular antidepressant medications include venlafaxine (Effexor), fluoxetine (Prozac), sertraline (Zoloft), paroxetine (Paxil), desvenlafaxine (Pristiq), and citalopram (Celexa). These medications are listed because they are frequently utilized by allopathic and osteopathic providers for symptom relief. While I do not prescribe them for this, I list them here in an effort to be thorough.

Any antidepressant may affect your appetite, and weight gain can be a side effect of taking almost any of them. During menopause, weight gain can be particularly significant and difficult to counteract. Amitriptyline (Elavil) is an example of a tricyclic antidepressant that has been known to produce larger increases in weight gain than others.

If you're interested in antidepressant therapy, certainly discuss this with your physician. Consider your options and be aware of all their potential side effects, including weight gain and decreased libido. Consider also how an antidepressant will integrate into your SHINES protocol and complement its other aspects.

FOODS TO AVOID

Caffeine

Across the board, I recommend that Philosophers try to avoid caffeine. Although your testosterone deficiency can cause your energy to wane, data indicates that caffeine can contribute to an increased frequency in hot flashes and night sweats. Caffeine can make a poor night's sleep that much worse, especially when it's consumed after three o'clock in the afternoon.

Some studies indicate that caffeine consumption can also worsen symptoms of menopause, including anxiety, mood swings, and even bone loss.[83]

Alcohol

I also encourage Philosophers to reduce their alcohol intake. Alcohol is a natural vasodilator and therefore a potential contributor to hot flashes and night sweats, and has also been shown to impair rapid eye movement (REM) sleep cycles. As with caffeine, consuming alcohol later in the day can worsen its impact. Note that different alcohols have a different glycemic index. Fortified wines have the most sugar, and the sweeter the wine the more of a glycemic index. Clear alcohols like tequila, gin, and vodka have a very low glycemic index. Studies have shown that having a high glycemic index four hours before bedtime can prolong the onset of sleep.

EXERCISE

While low-impact cardiovascular exercise plays a role in the Philosopher's exercise regime, yielding significant benefits including reductions in excess fat, blood pressure, and total cholesterol levels, resistance training is at its center. Activities such as yoga, isometrics, and light weight training help improve balance and muscle strength, support joint health, and prevent bone loss. Particularly for a Philosopher who is postmenopausal, exercises that help stave off osteoporosis are critically important.

One note of caution: In advance of any workout, I recommend spending a little time warming up in order to avoid injury. Allot ten minutes to get your blood moving and slightly elevate your heart rate. Walking at a brisk pace is a good option, as is doing some light weights or resistance exercises.

YOGA

Promoting muscle strength, balance, and overall alignment among all the body's systems, yoga can provide significant benefits for the

Philosopher. Yoga is also low-impact, and can be more or less aerobic, depending on the form and pace of the practice.

For Philosophers who are struggling with hot flashes, I recommend hot yoga (Bikram yoga), a practice that consists of 90-minute classes of twenty-six postures in a humid room heated to 95° to 108°F. Bikram yoga can help you learn to breathe through the heat and diminish your body's reaction and resistance to it. Learning to do this can also help alleviate the pain and anxiety associated with frequent hot flashes.

If hot yoga does not appeal to you, any type of yoga, whether practiced in a heated room or not, can provide the critical physiological benefits I've described. If you are interested in taking a class in your neighborhood, I recommend researching local studios and inquiring of instructors there which classes would best serve your goals. If you are inclined to practice on your own at home, you can find thousands of online classes at Glo.com.

SWIMMING

For the Philosopher, swimming can yield physical and psychological benefits alike. A low-impact cardiovascular exercise, swimming can help boost your muscle strength and tone in addition to improving your overall coordination and balance. It can also increase your flexibility and support your joint health.

A calming and solitary form of exercise, swimming also provides a space for peaceful contemplation and spiritual restoration that can help relieve the stress and anxiety that is so often associated with a number of the Philosopher's symptoms.

ISOMETRICS AND RESISTANCE EXERCISES

Isometrics are a low-impact *and* highly effective way of toning your muscles. They moderately elevate your heart rate, increase your blood flow, and burn calories, and depending on what they involve, may help improve your balance. Resistance exercises, such as those that make use of bands or light weights, can yield some of these same benefits.

In order to determine what will work best for you, I recommend working with a personal trainer. As these and other aspects of your workout regimen begin to have a positive impact, a reliable guide can help you adjust certain exercises or add or subtract them from your routine.

GARDENING

For the Philosopher in particular, I recommend gardening as a form of exercise. Low-impact and gently aerobic, gardening can help improve your cardiovascular health while also improving your muscle tone and flexibility. Gardening also involves being outside, an added benefit for the often vitamin D–deprived Philosopher, in addition to affording her the opportunity to focus exclusively on the calm and peaceful activity at hand.

Last, gardening encompasses helping something to grow and mature, a spiritually beneficial experience for the Philosopher who is naturally inclined to leverage her wisdom to do exactly this.

DANCING

A lightly aerobic activity you can perform on your own or with a partner, dancing can yield many of the cardiovascular benefits we've discussed in addition to giving you opportunities for creative self-expression. Even if you have never danced before, learning now can be a physically and emotionally invigorating form of self-expression. Remember the Philosopher who told me that her whole life (see page 201), she'd heard a song playing, and now she was finally dancing to it? Consider taking her lead.

SUPPLEMENTS

For the Philosopher, the role of supplements is to help diminish the symptoms associated with estrogen and testosterone deficiencies in addition to helping you achieve overall hormonal balance.

MACA

Maca, an herb indigenous to Peru, has long been used to promote and protect hormone balance (in men and women), and in certain permutations, maca has also been shown to reduce the intensity of symptoms associated with estrogen deficiency, including hot flashes, night sweats, insomnia, and depression. Although it has not been shown to boost testosterone production, maca is associated with increased energy levels and stamina as well as enhanced sex drive in women and men. Each of the thirteen differently colored varieties of maca exerts distinct effects, and many maca-based supplements combine different varieties of the herb.

For the Philosopher, I recommend two different maca blends. If you are premenopausal, I recommend Femmenessence Maca-Harmony. In addition to supporting overall hormonal balance, this particular maca blend also helps improve energy levels, mood, and bone health. If you are postmenopausal, I recommend Femmenessence MacaPause. This blend helps alleviate common menopause-related symptoms such as hot flashes and interrupted sleep in addition to improving your energy levels and libido, and reducing vaginal dryness. I recommend the standard dose: two capsules twice daily, taken away from meals. Take the first dose in the morning, before breakfast, and the second dose in the early evening, ideally 30 minutes before you normally experience an energy low. (For women who are more sensitive to higher clinical dosages, consider taking just one capsule in the morning and one in the early evening.)

All maca products can cause some level of gastrointestinal distress because they contain fiber. If you decide to give maca a try, I recommend starting off slow in order to give your system time to acclimate to it. Consider taking half the recommended dose for two weeks, then gradually raising this amount. You may find that your symptoms abate when you take less than the full dose. Assuming your system tolerates the maca well, I suggest continuing to take the supplement at the near full or full dose for four to six weeks in order to give yourself enough time to determine whether it is having the intended positive effect.

Two notes of **caution** with regard to MacaHarmony: First, I recommend that a Philosopher take this supplement for two to three months and then take a week off. This can help upregulate your estrogen receptors and enhance the supplement's benefits. Second, MacaHarmony can amplify the effects of caffeine. So while a Philosopher is always wise to limit or avoid caffeine, taking extra caution around caffeine when taking this supplement is a good idea.

FLAXSEED, FLAXSEED OIL, AND FISH OILS

Flaxseeds, flaxseed oil, and fish oil are all good sources of omega-3 essential fatty acids. These yield benefits for the Philosopher including improving your cardiovascular health, stabilizing your blood sugar levels, boosting your immunity, and improving your mood among others. Consuming 1 to 3 g of omega-3 fatty acids each day can also help ameliorate hot flashes and vaginal dryness as well as hypertriglyceridemia, joint pain, depression, and osteoporosis.

You may take flaxseed in one of two ways. The first is to eat the seeds themselves. But eating them whole won't help. Your body cannot digest the shell, which means that unless you grind up the seeds to release their oil, you won't get what you need. Once the seeds are ground, your body can digest the fiber. I recommend that patients add ground flaxseed to their smoothies or salad dressings.

There are several flaxseed oil options available on the market; these come in both lignan (fiber)-free and lignan-rich varieties, and in capsule and pourable-oil forms. I recommend oil over capsules for simplicity. In order to ingest the recommended tablespoon per day, you would need to take between ten and fifteen capsules. Adding the oil to a shake, smoothie, or dressing is easier—and more appealing. You may also take the oil directly, though it does have a bit of a grassy taste.

Taking pure flaxseed oil can give you the recommended amount of omega-3 fatty acids each day. But for Philosophers, I tend to recommend a blend of oils that contains the recommended amounts of both omega-3 and omega-6. It's called Udo's Oil Omega 3-6-9 Blend, which contains the recommended amounts of both omega-3s and omega-6s. Created by Dr. Udo Erasmus, author of the widely popular 1993 book *Fats that Heal, Fats that Kill*, this supplement combines fresh flax, sesame, and sunflower seeds with oils from evening primrose, rice germ, oat germ, and coconut to create an ideally balanced mix of omega-3 and omega-6 fatty acids.

Fish oil is another option for Philosophers who are looking to increase their intake of omega-3. Although this is a good option for women who don't want to incorporate fish into their diets, the most common complaint I hear is that once the capsules are in the stomach, they can release a fishy odor you can taste. To mitigate this, I recommend freezing the capsules. This way, the oil will not be thawed until it has passed through your upper digestive system. I also recommend patients choose a brand called Nordic Naturals. Flavored with lemon, the oil inside these capsules emits a more pleasant aroma.

An alternative to fish oil is krill oil. Made from the tiny crustaceans that comprise most of a whale's diet, krill oil has less of an aftertaste than traditional fish oil and is also more environmentally sustainable. (Only 1 percent of the world's total supply of krill are utilized for oil extraction each year.) Adding to this, krill oil contains an antioxidant called astaxanthin, which prevents the oil from spoiling when stored in your cupboard.

Two important recommendations regarding flaxseed oil, fish oil, and others:

1. With the exception of krill oil, I recommend purchasing only *refrigerated* products. Oils can become rancid, and because they are contained in capsules (or shells, in the case of flaxseed), you will not know. Look for products with expiration dates that are one to two months from the date of purchase.

2. Be mindful that your liver is responsible for processing these oils and that they may cause GI upset, including dyspepsia and diarrhea. Start slow, taking less than the recommended dose in order to give your body a chance to gradually adjust.

CALCIUM AND VITAMIN D

Calcium and vitamin D are important supplements for maintaining bone health and density. But Philosophers need to be wary of taking too high a dose of either.

In the past, physicians have recommended daily doses of calcium as high as 1,200 mg. For the Philosopher, who is at an elevated risk for kidney stones, however, this can be too much. I recommend 600 to 800 mg per day of calcium, with a maximum dose of 1,000 mg.

As for vitamin D, taking too much can result in vitamin D toxicity, symptoms of which include hypercalcemia (a buildup of calcium in the blood), nausea, vomiting, frequent urination, and diminished kidney function. Reaching toxic levels requires taking roughly ten times the dose I recommend, which is 5,000 IU per day. But when my patients are taking vitamin D, I closely monitor their levels. Should you and your physician or healthcare provider decide that a vitamin D supplement is right for you, make sure they closely monitor your levels at this dosage. (A more standard dosage is 1,000 IU per day.)

ST. JOHN'S WORT

Used around the world to treat a variety of medical conditions, in the United States St. John's wort is most commonly used to treat mild to moderate depression, including menopause-related depression. Although research into its efficacy has yielded mixed findings, some studies have shown that a St. John's wort supplement may be as effective as certain tricyclic antidepressants and selective serotonin reuptake inhibitors (SSRIs).

As with any supplement, it is critical that you consult with a physician, naturopath, nutritionist, or other knowledgeable healthcare practitioner before you begin taking St. John's wort. It may interact or interfere with medications or other supplements, which can have a deleterious impact on your physiological or psychological health. The supplement can have negative side effects of its own as well, including anxiety, interrupted sleep, and GI distress. Again, close monitoring is key.

HOPS

For Philosophers struggling with sleeplessness, I recommend hops (*Humulus lupulus*). Hops have long been used in herbal medicine to treat anxiety, restlessness, and insomnia.

Hops are available in capsule form. Alternatively, you may place a sachet of hops in your pillow. Widely regarded as a folk remedy, some of the Philosophers I've treated have reported that this has improved their sleep. I often recommend Nature's Way hops, taken as directed on the label. It is effective and very inexpensive, and I have gotten many patients off prescription sleep medication with this product.

DHEA (AND VAGINAL DHEA)

Known as the "hormone of youth" because its levels of production drop off after we turn thirty, DHEA (dehydroepiandrosterone) is a hormone produced by the adrenal glands that can convert into estrogen and testosterone. Exerting both androgenic and estrogenic effects, DHEA can enhance sexual desire and enjoyment in addition to alleviating symptoms of estrogen deficiency, including hot flashes, vaginal dryness, and weight gain. DHEA's estrogenic effects mean, however, that women with a personal or family history of breast cancer must discuss the relevant risks with their healthcare provider.

For the Philosopher who decides that DHEA is right for her, I recommend a dose of 25 mg/day. In addition to its capsule formulation, DHEA comes in the form of a vaginal cream. Applied directly, it can help with lubrication in the short term as well as vaginal dryness and other symptoms of vaginal atrophy in the longer term. The DHEA dosage in this form typically is around 6.75 mg. As with the capsule formation, I strongly urge you to consult with your healthcare provider before using a DHEA cream.

DHEA is an adrenal hormone that I routinely check in my hormone panel, and I find women with low or low-normal DHEA about 10 percent of the time. If I decide to start a patient on DHEA, I will start with anywhere from 10 to 25 mg, but rarely ever go above 37.5 mg. Remember that DHEA can convert into estrogen and testosterone in the body.

SUPPLEMENTS THAT HELP SUPPORT TESTOSTERONE PRODUCTION/LEVELS

Chrysin

Belonging to a class of chemicals known as flavonoids, chrysin occurs naturally in plants, including the passionflower and silver linden, as well as in honey. Chrysin has been shown to inhibit the aromatization of testosterone into estrogen. Studies have also shown that chrysin possesses strong antianxiety properties and can also reduce hypertension.

Horny Goat Weed

Also known as barrenwort, bishop's hat, and fairy wings, horny goat weed is an herb belonging to the genus *Epimedium*. Native to China, horny goat weed has been used for centuries in Eastern medicine as an aphrodisiac for women and men, and has become popular in the West.[84] Although their specific mechanisms of action are unknown, the flavonoids in horny goat weed have been shown to help increase blood flow, which can enhance sexual arousal in women and men. These compounds have also been shown to help prevent osteopenia and osteoporosis by stimulating the proliferation of cells called osteoblasts, which play a critical role in bone restructuring. Horny goat weed supplements are available in a variety of forms, including liquid extract and capsules.

Yohimbe

Derived from the chemical yohimbine, extracted from the bark of yohimbe trees indigenous to Africa, this supplement may help enhance your libido and levels of sexual arousal. Yohimbe has been shown to increase both blood flow and nerve impulses to the vagina, which can intensify sexual excitement. It has also been shown to counteract the negative sexual side effects of SSRIs. If you're interested in adding a yohimbe supplement to your daily regime, be sure to confirm the ingredients and review them with your physician. Certain ingredients in yohimbe supplements can interact with prescription medications. Also important to consider are the supplement's potential side effects, which include rapid heart rate, anxiety, high blood pressure, cold sweats, vomiting, nausea, stomach pain, and insomnia. If you experience any of these side effects, immediately cease taking the yohimbe and consult your physician.

Tribulus

Commonly found in dry climates around the globe, *Tribulus terrestris* is a weedy plant covered in spines. Chemicals contained in its fruit, leaves, and roots are used in the creation of powder- and capsule-based supplements. Tribulus (also known as cat's-head, puncture vine, and devil's eyelashes, among other names) is used in Eastern and Western medicine to treat kidney, bladder, and urinary tract issues, digestive difficulties, and circulatory problems. Studies have shown that tribulus can also have a positive impact on sexual desire and arousal in women with hypoactive sexual desire disorder.[85]

Tribulus's mechanism of action is unclear. Several studies have indicated that the herb does not directly boost testosterone levels in women or men. Research has shown, however, that the herb may enhance androgen receptor density in the brain, which can amplify the effects of testosterone on libido.

One important side effect of tribulus is its impact on blood sugar levels. If you are diabetic and rely on blood-sugar-regulating medications, taking the supplement may necessitate that your physician adjusts your dose. Also, tribulus should be taken only in the short term. For the Philosopher, I recommend a period of no longer than eight weeks.

Resveratrol

Found in the skins of red grapes, mulberries, and blueberries, and in nuts such as peanuts and pistachios, resveratrol is a chemical compound produced in plants in response to injury, including bacterial and fungal attacks. Although resveratrol's potential benefits for humans remain a matter of debate, recent research suggests it may have a positive effect on testosterone levels.

Like chrysin, resveratrol may help reduce the aromatization of testosterone into estrogen, increasing the levels of free testosterone in the bloodstream. It may also activate the body's androgen receptors, enhancing testosterone's effects. Resveratrol may also reduce inflammation, which has a negative impact on metabolism and contributes to muscle deterioration.

One limitation of resveratrol is its bioavailability. When you consume it via food, drinks, or supplements, resveratrol is absorbed by the intestines and conjugated by the liver. Check each supplement for bioavailability. Standard doses of resveratrol are between 250 and 600 mg per day. For the Philosopher, I recommend a dose of 125 to 200 mg per day. (If you're hoping to get your resveratrol from red wine, I have some bad news: The average bottle contains only 2 mg.)

There are few side effects associated with resveratrol itself. Like other supplements, however, it may interfere with prescription medications that are processed by the liver. Resveratrol supplements can affect circulating amounts of blood thinners, birth control pills, and antibiotics.

BOOK RECOMMENDATIONS FOR PHILOSOPHERS

Jeanne Achterberg, *Woman as Healer: A Panoramic Survey of the Healing Activities of Women from Prehistoric Times to the Present* (Boulder, CO: Shambhala Publications, 1991)

Barbara Dossey and Jeanne Achterberg, *Rituals of Healing: Using Imagery for Health and Wellness* (New York: Bantam, 1994)

Joseph Marshall III, *Walking with Grandfather: The Wisdom of Lakota Elders* (Louisville, CO: Sounds True Publishing, 2005)

Marianne Williamson, *A Woman's Worth* (New York: Random House, 1993)

PHILOSOPHERS

Simone de Beauvoir (January 9, 1908–April 14, 1986). Born in Paris to a wealthy banker's daughter and a legal secretary who aspired to an acting career, Simone de Beauvoir was educated at the Sorbonne, earning undergraduate and graduate degrees in philosophy during the years shortly following the admission of women to French institutions of higher education. Around this time, she became acquainted with a young Jean-Paul Sartre, and the two entered into an intellectual and romantic partnership that would last until Sartre's death in 1980.

Despite resisting being labeled a "philosopher," de Beauvoir nonetheless contributed significantly to modern feminist theory. A devoted social and political activist throughout her life, de Beauvoir was also a prolific writer, producing a series of fiction and nonfiction works. She is perhaps best known for her 1949 treatise *The Second Sex*, in which she famously asserted that "one is not born but becomes a woman." Thus, credited with first articulating what is now known as the sex-gender distinction, the author nonetheless resisted being called a "feminist" until 1972, when she conceded that a gender-neutral socialist revolution could bring about women's civic equality or liberation. Often a controversial and even scandalous figure, de Beauvoir continued to write and agitate for women's liberation until her death.

Margaret Atwood (b. November 18, 1939). Born and raised in Ontario, Atwood was educated at Victoria University and Radcliffe College before launching her career as a poet, novelist, essayist, and creative nonfiction writer. Atwood is also a staunch environmental activist, and the theme of climate change often appears in her fictional dystopian works and her nonfiction writing.

Perhaps best known for her 1985 novel *The Handmaid's Tale*, Atwood has won numerous literary awards, including the Man Booker Prize. She has also been inducted into Canada's Walk of Fame and cofounded the Writer's Trust of Canada, a nonprofit association dedicated to supporting writers across that country.

Hypatia (b. circa 350–370, d. 415). Born in Alexandria in the Province of Egypt to Theon of Alexandria, Hypatia was a philosopher, mathematician, and teacher credited with editing or authoring a series of important scholarly works of her age. A pagan by birth, Hypatia was tolerant of Christians. A number of these ranked among her students, many of whom hailed from privileged backgrounds and came to assume high-ranking government positions. Near the end of her life, Hypatia became involved in a feud between the pagan Orestes, the Roman governor of Egypt, and Cyril, the Christian bishop of Alexandria. A counselor to Orestes, Hypatia was regarded as anti-Christian and a danger to Alexandria, and in 415, she was brutally murdered by a Christian mob. Centuries later, during the Age of Enlightenment, Hypatia became a symbol of opposition to Catholicism. By the twentieth century, the philosopher had become recognized as a historical icon for women's rights, and her life a precursor to the modern feminist movement.

CONCLUSION

The Heroine's Journey

I hope you have embraced your own heroine's journey while reading this book. By approaching your hormones through the lens of your personal health story, you will begin to see the connections between your mind and your internal and external life, and how one inevitably affects the other. My patients usually come to me with a list (sometimes a long one) of symptoms, often highlighted by a primary health concern. But considering this list of symptoms is just the start of our conversation. I take each of my patients through the same discovery process that you have now experienced in this book, in an effort to better understand how their symptoms and needs intersect with strategies and actions they can take not only to feel better, but to live optimally.

The SHINES protocols serve to prompt action. I hope that by now you have identified your archetype and taken action on the related protocol(s). Remember that you have the power, and you can take a proactive approach to alleviating and managing your troubling symptoms. I encourage you to build and add to your heroine's journey by crafting a narrative that is grounded in how you feel, how you want to feel, and how you want to be living your life. Your heroine's journey becomes your story, in all its challenges, triumphs, plot twists, and surprises. You can use the information in this book to direct you on a path of discovery that may expose an early sign of an underlying health condition that, once found, can be addressed. And ultimately, you can use your hormones to optimize your health and life at every stage.

I have always been fascinated by the concept of the labyrinth. Your journey starts as you enter the labyrinth, and you work your way through the maze, never quite sure if you are on the right path because of the twists, turns, and unexpected dead ends. But when you get to the center, you obtain the prize, the secret that makes the journey worth it. I like to think of this book as the secret to vibrant hormonal health. Your great challenge now is to use the tools in this book to find your way back out of the labyrinth, in order to live your life, access your full potential, and use your unique health demands to create the environment that your body, mind, and spirit need at any given time. That is the reason for the comprehensive nature of this book. It is designed to take you through every heroine's challenge and to help you support other women close to you.

Let's return for a moment to that list you wrote on page 9. Just as I ask my patients to do, once again, I want you to make a list of the top five ways, both physically and emotionally, that you would like to feel better. Be as specific as you can be with your answers.

Your Hormonal Balance
Point – Goals

1 ....

2 ....

....

3 ....

....

4 ....

....

5 ....

....

Now take a look at that first list you created and compare them. If they are the same after you've read this book, then you can be sure that you have the direction of your own hormonal balance point that we are working toward together. If they are different, consider if you've already experienced a change that adds to your story.

This book captures so many experiences and scenarios and can guide you to your own aha moments, where the pieces finally fit together and you see a clear path to feeling and living better. You can return to these pages to find answers that encompass all the major and minor health events in a woman's sexual and hormonal health. There exists a larger community of women who are seeking their own answers, and this book serves to elevate not only your own health, but also to help other women find those answers. While many of the suggestions and recommendations here require a health professional, many more are health and lifestyle strategies that you can enact at any time to start feeling better. By approaching your solutions in a narrative way, you can more easily begin to see how all the pieces fit together. Any journey can go off path. There are distractions and blocks along the way, but the spiritual part of the heroine's journey connects you to a larger vision of how you want to be in the world. Hormonal health is often overlooked as we strive for beauty and fitness and disease prevention and regulation. Your hormones sit at the very center of all these endeavors. When you begin to connect with your journey back out of the labyrinth of physical health and learn how to traverse it, it becomes so much more than just a list of troubling symptoms that have to be dealt with and managed. Optimizing your hormonal health takes you to a grand place. It leads you to *you*, in your optimal state, with the full potential of what your body is capable of. That has an enormous span, from something as simple as getting a restful night of sleep to having a long-wished-for baby. The journey to the center of your own well-being is the ultimate heroine's journey.

Being shut down, living with pain, wondering how long a symptom will persist, the feeling of "where is this going," or the worry that it is something more serious—there is no good reason to endure feeling crappy when you can find solutions. As you address the many options in the protocols, you can find methods that work for you. Eighty percent of what is suggested here, you can do on your own. The other 20 percent can be accomplished by finding the right healthcare practitioner, who also becomes part of your story—wisdom leaders such as a knowledgeable physician, a compounding pharmacist, a coach, a trainer, or a yoga instructor will also add their part and keep you going.

Many women have been shut down so many times that they are discouraged. Every phase of your journey is going to have forks in the path, choices about alternate paths that lie before you and which you will take. Lab tests, symptoms, emerging patterns, timetables, they can all be directional, leading you to a better (or worse) place. You are going to change. Your status and your health are going to change. By referring to this book, you can use the messages of your body to discover your best path. You are much more than a group of symptoms . . . there is a message calling out to you. Understanding how your body performs and what it most needs are in those messages. You can listen to your own emerging story and put language to it that helps you find your way. This book is an early and continuing contributor to that effort.

While it is true that my mother inspired my journey to help women find these answers, the amazing thing is that I'm evolving, you are evolving, science is evolving. Where you are today in your understanding, practice, and journey becomes something else with your thoughts, choices, and actions. I hope I have given you much to think about, but more important, things to do that enable and uplift your journey. From sitting with my mom and watching her suffer, to sharing much of what I have learned through caring for thousands of women for the past two decades, I have come full circle. I am honored to be a part of how your story takes shape.

The great storyteller Orson Welles once said, "If you want a happy ending, that depends, of course, on where you stop your story."

I look forward to hearing more about your journey. There is more to come . . .

ACKNOWLEDGMENTS

A book is the culmination of so many ideas and people. This book is no exception, and without the help of many different people who embodied certain strengths, it would never have come to be. Keeping with the theme of archetypes, I am thanking the people below with their corresponding archetype and how they have been a part of my life in bringing this book into existence.

Karen (Tassone) Hvizda (The Mother)—She is literally the mother of my life and the reason you are holding this book. Without her struggles, I would not be the physician I have become. I hope she is proud.

Carrie Thornton (The Visionary)—President and Editorial Director at Harper Dey Street. She is the one who could see the book for what it is and what it will be. Her guidance is immeasurable.

Scott Hoffman (The Creator)—The man who met me as a stranger and decided this book needed to happen. My literary agent and now friend, this is what you've helped create.

Dado Derviskadic (The Expert)—Literary agent at Folio who was a major force behind the proposal. My coach, my sounding board, and friend.

Nancy Hancock (The Alchemist)—So many times you have taken the ore that is this book and turned it into gold. This book is because of you on so many levels.

Kelly McNamara (The Storyteller)—The one who sat on the phone with me for endless hours getting the stories out of my head and onto paper.

Nat Kringoudis (The Best Friend)—You embody all the friends into one and you've been there from the beginning and your light always illuminates the darkness.

J. J. Virgin (The Godmother)—It's been nineteen years since I had an Earthly mother, and you filled that energetic role and so many others, it's hard to place them all. You are a protector and visionary.

Karl Krummenacher (The Integrator)—This man can turn water into wine and on countless occasions simply was there and kept me going. He transformed not only my business, but my life.

Jessica Sindler (The Organizer)—You change what you see and what we can't. With your help and keen eye, this book has become a force.

Ivy McFadden (The Reformer)—A true editor and leader bringing this book as close to perfection as possible.

Hannah, Hunter, Angelo, and Anthony (The Children)—You are why I do what I do.

Wayne Tassone (The Dad)—My dad, always supporting me, and you may not think it, but you are my role model.

Ed Hvizda (The Stepdad)—You were always there for me and Mom, and for that I will be forever grateful.

Mary Agnes Antonopoulos (The Networker)—You introduced me to Scott, my agent, for an impromptu dinner, and that meeting set this all into motion.

Jerry Bailey (The Jester)—You keep me laughing and continue to show me how to assume the best in people.

Anthony Youn (The Renaissance Man)—Physician, marketer, father, husband, dog-lover, and you are unabashedly you. Thanks for being a leader in my life.

My Patients (The Reasons)—Tens of thousands of reasons for me to be here and this book to have a place.

To all my friends in the Mindshare and Mastermind communities, who are too numerous to count, you all have made me the human I am today, and I appreciate your love and support over the last four years of this project.

NOTES

Introduction: Hormones, the Invisible Driving Forces of Women's Lives

1. https://www.questdiagnostics.com/hcp/intguide/EndoMetab/EndoManual_AtoZ_PDFs/Testosterone_Calculated.pdf.
2. R. M. Islam, R. J. Bell, S. Green, and S. R. Davis, "Effects of Testosterone Therapy for Women: A Systematic Review and Meta-Analysis Protocol," *Systematic Reviews* 8, no. 1 (2019): 19, https://doi.org/10.1186/s13643-019-0941-8.

Chapter 2: Our Hormones, Ourselves

1. All patient names have been changed throughout to protect anonymity.
2. A. Gomez-Gomez, J. Miranda, G. Feixas, et al., "Determination of the Steroid Profile in Alternative Matrices by Liquid Chromatography Tandem Mass Spectrometry," *Journal of Steroid Biochemistry and Molecular Biology* 197 (2020): 105520, https://doi.org/10.1016/j.jsbmb.2019.105520.

Chapter 4: Understanding the Twelve Hormonal Archetypes

1. K. Mohammed, A. M. Dabrh Abu, K. Benkhadra, et al., "Oral vs. Transdermal Estrogen Therapy and Vascular Events: A Systematic Review and Meta-Analysis," *Journal of Clinical Endocrinology & Metabolism* 100, no. 11 (2015): 4012–4020, https://doi.org/10.1210/jc.2015-2237.
2. S. E. Walker, "Estrogen and Autoimmune Disease," *Clinical Reviews in Allergy & Immunology* 40, no. 1 (2011): 60–65, https://doi.org/10.1007/s12016-010-8199-x.
3. N. Jardim, *The Period Fix* (New York: Harper Wave, 2019).
4. M. W. Seif, K. Diamond, and M. Nickkho-Amiry, "Obesity and Menstrual Disorders," *Best Practice & Research: Clinical Obstetrics & Gynaecology* 29, no. 4 (2015): 516–27, https://doi.org/10.1016/j.bpobgyn.2014.10.010.
5. S. Ahmadi, M. R. Eshraghian, M. Hedayati, and H. Pishva, "Relationship

Between Estrogen and Body Composition, Energy, and Endocrine Factors in Obese Women with Normal and Low Ree," *Steroids* 130 (2018): 31–35, https://doi.org/10.1016/j.steroids.2017.12.008.

6. J. L. Gordon, D. R. Rubinow, T. A. Eisenlohr-Moul, J. Leserman, and S. S. Girdler, "Estradiol Variability, Stressful Life Events, and the Emergence of Depressive Symptomatology During the Menopausal Transition," *Menopause* 23, no. 3 (2016): 257–66, https://doi.org/10.1097/GME.000 0000000000528.

7. M. Słomczyńska, "Xenoestrogens: Mechanisms of Action and Some Detection Studies," *Polish Journal of Veterinary Sciences* 11, no. 3 (2008): 263–69.

8. M. E. Alliende, J. A. Arraztoa, U. Guajardo, and F. Mellado, "Towards the Clinical Evaluation of the Luteal Phase in Fertile Women: A Preliminary Study of Normative Urinary Hormone Profiles," *Frontiers in Public Health* 6 (2018): 147, https://doi.org/10.3389/fpubh.2018.00147.

9. A. Czyzyk, A. Podfigurna, A. R. Genazzani, and B. Meczekalski, "The Role of Progesterone Therapy in Early Pregnancy: From Physiological Role to Therapeutic Utility," *Gynecological Endocrinology* 33, no. 6 (2017): 421–24, https://doi.org/10.1080/09513590.2017.1291615.

10. R. W. Rebar, "Premature Ovarian Failure," *Obstetrics & Gynecology* 113, no. 6 (2009): 1355–63, https://doi.org/10.1097/AOG.0b013e3181a66843.

11. K. E. Hannibal and M. D. Bishop, "Chronic Stress, Cortisol Dysfunction, and Pain: A Psychoneuroendocrine Rationale for Stress Management in Pain Rehabilitation," *Physical Therapy* 94, no. 12 (2014): 1816–25, https://doi.org/10.2522/ptj.20130597.

12. "A History of Sugar—the Food Nobody Needs, But Everyone Craves," https://theconversation.com/a-history-of-sugar-the-food-nobody-needs -but-everyone-craves-49823.

13. Alice G. Walton, "How Much Sugar Are Americans Eating?" *Forbes*, August 30, 2012, accessed September 1, 2017, https://www.forbes.com /sites/alicegwalton/2012/08/30/how-much-sugar-are-americans-eating -infographic/#49589bfc4ee7.

14. *DSM-5* defines female sexual interest/arousal disorder as a persistent or a recurrently deficient or absent desire for intercourse, sexual fantasies, or sexual activity. The judgment of the deficiency or absence is made by a clinician, taking into account factors that affect sexual functioning, such as age and the context of the person's life, and the disturbance causes marked distress or interpersonal difficulty. The condition is also not better accounted for by another disorder, such as depression or anxiety, and it is not due exclusively to direct physiologic stress of a substance, such as a prescription or nonprescription drug, or chronic illness.

15. L. J. Burrows, M. Basha, and A. T. Goldstein, "The Effects of Hormonal Contraceptives on Female Sexuality: A Review," *Journal of Sexual Medi-*

cine 9, no. 9 (September 2012): 2213–23, https://doi.org/10.1111/j.1743
-6109.2012.02848.x.

16. S. Assad et al., "Role of Sex Hormone Levels and Psychological Stress in the Pathogenesis of Autoimmune Diseases," *Cureus* 9, no. 6 (June 5, 2017): e1315, https://doi.org/10.7759/cureus.1315.

17. M. A. Sargin, N. Tug, O. A. Tosun, M. Yassa, and E. Bostanci, "Theca Lutein Cysts and Early Onset Severe Preeclampsia," *Pan African Medical Journal* 24 (June 14, 2016): 141, https://doi.org/10.11604/pamj.2016 .24.141.7247.

18. American Thyroid Association, "Graves' Disease," Thyroid.org, accessed December 21, 2017, https://www.thyroid.org/graves-disease.

19. Izabella Wentz, "The 5 Stages of Hashimoto's Thyroiditis," Thyroid Pharmacist.com, April 8, 2107, accessed December 5, 2017, https:// thyroidpharmacist.com/articles/5-stages-hashimotos-thyroiditis/.

20. Andrea Janegova et al., "The Role of Epstein-Barr Virus Infection in the Development of Autoimmune Thyroid Diseases," *Endokrynologia Polska* 66, no. 2 (May 1, 2015), https://journals.viamedica.pl/endokrynologia _polska/article/view/39714.

21. G. Tamagno et al., "A Possible Link Between Genetic Hemochromatosis and Autoimmune Thyroiditis," *Minerva Medica* 98, no. 6 (December 2007), https://www.ncbi.nlm.nih.gov/pubmed/18299688.

22. M. Rich, "Hypothyroidism in Association with Systemic Amyloidoisis," *New York Head and Neck Society* 17, no. 4 (July–August 1995), https:// www.ncbi.nlm.nih.gov/pubmed/7672976.

23. Sarcoid lesions may also show up as cold thyroid nodules, which can be mistaken for cancer. See Elaine Moore, "Sarcoidosis of the Thyroid," Elaine-Moore.com, June 2, 2007, accessed December 5, 2017, https:// elaine-moore.com/Articles/SubclinicalOtherThyroidDisordersArticles /SarcoidosisoftheThyroidGland/tabid/141/Default.aspx.

24. Mary E. Turyk et al., "Relationships of Thyroid Hormones with Polychlo-rinated Biphenyls, Dioxins, Furans, and DDE in Adults," *Environmental Health Perspectives* 115, no. 8 (August 2007): 1197–203, https://www.ncbi .nlm.nih.gov/pmc/articles/PMC1940071/.

25. Environmental Protection Agency, "Facts about Dioxin," November 1999, accessed December 11, 2017, https://www.epa.gov/sites/production/files /documents/r8_dioxinfacts.pdf.

26. National Institute of Environmental Health Sciences, "Dioxins," https:// www.niehs.nih.gov/health/topics/agents/dioxins/index.cfm.

27. Chris Kresser, "How Environmental Toxins Harm the Thyroid," Kresser Institute for Functional and Integrative Medicine, September 6, 2017, ac-cessed December 11, 2017, https://kresserinstitute.com/environmental -toxins-harm-thyroid/.

28. Environmental Protection Agency, "Learn about Polychlorinated Biphe-

nyls (PCBs)," EPA.gov, accessed December 11, 2017, https://www.epa.gov /pcbs/learn-about-polychlorinated-biphenyls-pcbs.

29. Silvia Martina Ferrari et al., "Environmental Issues in Thyroid Diseases," *Frontiers in Endocrinology* 8, no. 50 (March 2017), https://www.frontiersin .org/articles/10.3389/fendo.2017.00050/full; Kresser, "How Environmental Toxins Harm the Thyroid."

30. Mara Ventura et al., "Selenium and Thyroid Disease: From Pathophysiology to Treatment," *International Journal of Endocrinology* (January 2017), article ID: 1297658, https://www.hindawi.com/journals/ ije/2017/1297658/.

31. Kresser, "How Environmental Toxins Harm the Thyroid."

32. Environmental Illness Resource, "Natural Hypothyroid Treatment," May 5, 2016, accessed December 10, 2017, http://www.ei-resource.org /treatment-options/treatment-information/natural-hypothyroid-treat ment/?tmpl=component.

33. The thyroid also produces a hormone called calcitonin, which helps regulate the amount of calcium circulating in the blood.

34. I. Subekti and L. A. Pramono, "Current Diagnosis and Management of Graves' Disease," *Acta Medica Indonesiana* 50, no. 2 (April 2018): 177–82, PMID: 29950539.

35. American Thyroid Association, "Graves' Disease."

36. American Thyroid Association, "Graves' Disease."

37. Richard Carroll and Glenn Martin, "Endocrine and Metabolic Emergencies: Thyroid Storm," *Therapeutic Advances in Endocrinology and Metabolism* 1, no. 3 (June 2010), https://www.ncbi.nlm.nih.gov/pmc/articles /PMC3475282/.

38. National Institute of Diabetes and Digestive and Kidney Diseases, "Graves' Disease," National Institutes of Health website, accessed December 20, 2017, https://www.niddk.nih.gov/health-information/endocrine -diseases/graves-disease.

39. C. E. Hargreaves et al., "*Yersinia enterocolitica* Provides the Link Between Thyroid-Stimulating Antibodies and Their Germline Counterparts in Graves' Disease," *Journal of Immunology* 190, no. 11 (June 2013), https:// www.ncbi.nlm.nih.gov/pubmed/23630351.

40. *Encyclopædia Britannica*, "Plummer Disease," Britannica.com, accessed December 20, 2017, https://britannica.com/science/Plummer-disease.

Chapter 5: The SHINES Protocol, with Recommendations for Each Archetype

1. Xpill, https://www.xpill.com/testimonials/.

2. Jack Canfield, Xpill.com, accessed November 15, 2017, https://www .xpill.com/testimonials.

3. J. H. Ko and S. N. Kim, "A Literature Review of Women's Sex Hormone

Changes by Acupuncture Treatment," *Analysis of Human and Animal Studies, Evidence-based Complementary and Alternative Medicine* 10 (November 15, 2018), https://doi.org/10.1155/2018/3752723.

4. Examples of safer, fermented soy are tempeh, miso, and natto.

5. Hutch News, "Regular Exercise Lowers Estrogens," May 6, 2004, accessed April 2, 2017, https://www.fredhutch.org/en/news/center-news/2004/05/excercise.html.

6. Stephanie L. Brown, "Social Closeness Increases Salivary Progesterone in Humans," *Hormones and Behavior* 56, no. 1 (June 2009): 108–11.

7. HeartMath, "The Science Behind the emWave® and Inner Balance™ Technologies," HeartMath.com, accessed August 1, 2017, https://www.heartmath.com/science-behind-emwave/.

8. Hirofumi Henmi, MD, et al., "Effects of Ascorbic Acid Supplementation on Serum Progesterone Levels in Patients with a Luteal Phase Defect," *Fertility and Sterility* 80, no. 2 (August 2003).

9. G. E. Abraham, "Nutritional Factors in the Etiology of the Premenstrual Tension Syndromes," *Journal of Reproductive Medicine* 28, no. 7 (July 1983); A. G. Ronnenberg, "Preconception B-Vitamin and Homocysteine Status, Conception, and Early Pregnancy Loss," *American Journal of Epidemiology* 1, no. 3 (August 2007).

10. C. J. Chuong, "Zinc and Copper Levels in Premenstrual Syndrome," *Fertility and Sterility* 62, no. 2 (August 1994).

11. Akihisa Takasaki et al., "Luteal Blood Flow and Luteal Function," *Journal of Ovarian Research* 2, no. 1 (January 2009).

12. Morihei Ueshiba, as quoted in Nick Waites, *Essential Aikido: An Illustrated Handbook* (Durham, UK: Koteikan Press, 2014), xi.

13. James Endredy, *Earthwalks for Body and Spirit: Exercises to Restore Our Sacred Bond with the Earth* (Rochester, VT: Bear, 2002), Kindle edition, loc. 1463.

14. Chuong, "Zinc and Copper Levels in Premenstrual Syndrome."

15. Abraham, "Nutritional Factors in the Etiology of the Premenstrual Tension Syndromes"; Ronnenberg, "Preconception B-Vitamin and Homocysteine Status, Conception, and Early Pregnancy Loss."

16. Paul Grant and Shamin Ramasamy, "An Update on Plant Derived Anti-Androgens," *International Journal of Endocrinology and Metabolism* 10, no. 2 (Spring 2012), https://www.ncbi.nlm.nih.gov/pmc/articles/PMC3693613/.

17. National Institutes of Health, "Valerian," accessed August, 1, 2017, https://ods.od.nih.gov/factsheets/Valerian-HealthProfessional/.

18. National Institutes of Health, "Valerian."

19. This is an approximation. Joan of Arc was born on or around January 6, 1412.

20. Chuong, "Zinc and Copper Levels in Premenstrual Syndrome."

21. As quoted in Terry Hardy Olsen, *Blending Two Hearts into One: Tools to*

Help Safeguard Your Marriage Against Divorce (Phinish Line Enterprises, 2012), 24.

22. Nell Painter, *Sojourner Truth: A Life, A Symbol* (New York: W. W. Norton, 1996), 3.

23. BBC News, "The Panorama Interview with the Princess of Wales," November 20, 1995.

24. Stacy Simon, "Is Chocolate Good for You?," American Cancer Society, June 2, 2020, https://www.cancer.org/latest-news/can-chocolate-be-good-for-you.html; Cleveland Clinic, "Heart Healthy Benefits of Chocolate," https://my.clevelandclinic.org/health/articles/benefits-of-chocolate-heart-health.

25. Prema B. Rapuri, J. Christopher Gallagher, H. Karimi Kinyamu, and Kay L. Ryschon, "Caffeine Intake Increases the Rate of Bone Loss in Elderly Women and Interacts with Vitamin D Receptor Genotypes," *American Journal of Clinical Nutrition* 74, no. 5 (November 2001), http://ajcn.nutrition.org/content/74/5/694.full.

26. Mayo Clinic, "St. John's Wort (*Hypericum perforatum*)," accessed May 21, 2017, http://www.mayoclinic.org/drugs-supplements/st-johns-wort/background/hrb-20060053.

27. Deepak Chopra: https://www.youtube.com/watch?v=gYm_p9BHykM; Tara Brach, "Guided Meditations," TaraBrach.com, https://www.tarabrach.com/guided-meditations/.

28. S. Hosseini, A. Heydari, M. Vakili, S. Moghadam, and S. Tazyky, "Effect of Lavender Essence Inhalation on the Level of Anxiety and Blood Cortisol in Candidates for Open-Heart Surgery," *Iranian Journal of Nursing and Midwifery Research* 21, no. 4 (2016): 397–401, https://doi.org/10.4103/1735-9066.185582.

29. See David Winston and Steven Maimes, *Adaptogens: Herbs for Strength, Stamina, and Stress Relief* (Rochester, VT: Healing Arts Press [Inner Traditions], 2007), and Dr. Frank Lipman, "Adaptogens: Nature's Miracle Anti-Stress and Fatigue Fighters," November 13, 2012, accessed July 12, 2017, https://www.bewell.com/blog/adaptogens-natures-miracle-anti-stress-and-fatigue-fighters/.

30. D. Kiefer and T. Pantuso, "Panax Ginseng," *American Family Physician* 68, no. 8 (October 15, 2003): 1539–42, PMID: 14596440.

31. National Institutes of Health/National Center for Complementary and Integrative Health, "Asian Ginseng," September 2016, accessed August 1, 2017, https://nccih.nih.gov/health/asianginseng/ataglance.htm.

32. K. Yamada, P. Hung, T. K. Park, P. J. Park, and B. O. Lim, "A Comparison of the Immunostimulatory Effects of the Medicinal Herbs Echinacea, Ashwagandha and Brahmi," *Journal of Ethnopharmacology* 137, no. 1 (September 1, 2011): 231–35, https://doi.org/10.1016/j.jep.2011.05.017.

33. K. I. Block and M. N. Mead, "Immune System Effects of Echinacea, Ginseng, and Astragalus: A Review," *Integrative Cancer Therapies* 2, no. 3 (2003): 247–67, https://doi.org/10.1177/1534735403256419.

34. Erik Olsson, "A Randomised, Double-Blind, Placebo-Controlled, Parallel-Group Study of the Standardised Extract Shr-5 of the Roots of Rhodiola rosea in the Treatment of Subjects with Stress-Related Fatigue," *International Journal of Natural Products and Medicinal Plant Research* 75, no. 2 (February 2009).

35. Dr. Zakir Ramazanov and Dr. Maria del Mar Bernal Suarez, *New Secrets of Effective Natural Stress and Weight Management Using Rhodiola rosea and Rhododendron caucasicum* (Sheffield, MA: Safe Goods Publishing, 1999). See also Dr. Josh Axe, "Rhodiola Benefits: Burning Fat for Energy & Beating Depression," accessed August 1, 2017, https://draxe.com/rhodiola-benefits-burning-fat-for-energy-and-beating-depression/.

36. Dr. Andrew Weil, as quoted on DrWeil.com, accessed September 2, 2017, https://www.drweil.com/health-wellness/body-mind-spirit/stress-anxiety/breathing-three-exercises/.

37. Eckhart Tolle, *The Power of Now: A Guide to Spiritual Enlightenment* (Novato, CA: New World Library, 1999), 88.

38. N. Singh, M. Bhalla, P. de Jager, and M. Gilca, "An Overview on Ashwagandha: A Rasayana (Rejuvenator) of Ayurveda," *African Journal of Traditional, Complementary and Alternative Medicines* 8, suppl. 5 (2011): 208–13, https://doi.org/10.4314/ajtcam.v8i5S.9.

39. A. Ismaeel, "Effects of Betaine Supplementation on Muscle Strength and Power: A Systematic Review," *Journal of Strength & Conditioning Research* 31, no. 8 (August 2017): 2338–46, https://doi.org/10.1519/JSC.0000000000001959.

40. A. K. Baltaci, R. Mogulkoc, and S. B. Baltaci, "Review: The Role of Zinc in the Endocrine System," *Pakistan Journal of Pharmaceutical Sciences* 32, no. 1 (January 2019): 231–39, PMID: 30772815.

41. "Testosterone Levels by Age," Healthline, https://www.healthline.com/health/low-testosterone/testosterone-levels-by-age#adolescence3.

42. "Addyi Approval History," Drugs.com, accessed October 10, 2017, https://www.drugs.com/history/addyi.html.

43. Federal Drug Administration, "FDA Approves First Treatment for Sexual Desire Disorder: Addyi Approved to Treat Premenopausal Women," press release, August 18, 2015, accessed October 19, 2017, https://www.fda.gov/NewsEvents/Newsroom/PressAnnouncements/ucm458734.htm.

44. N. S. Chauhan, V. Sharma, V. K. Dixit, and M. Thakur, "A Review on Plants Used for Improvement of Sexual Performance and Virility," *BioMed Research International* 2014 (2014): 868062, https://doi.org/10.1155/2014/868062.

45. N. Sokoloff Cano, M. Misra, and K. E. Ackerman, "Exercise, Training,

and the Hypothalamic-Pituitary-Gonadal Axis in Men and Women," *Frontiers of Hormone Research* 47 (2016): 27–43, https://doi.org/10.1159/000445154.

46. In Chinese folklore, horny goat weed was a favorite of the sexually hyperactive mythical creature Yin Yang, who enjoyed more than one hundred orgasms a day.

47. See X.-X. Yin et al., "Icariine Stimulates Proliferation and Differentiation of Human Osteoblasts by Increasing Production of Bone Morphogenetic Protein 2," *Chinese Medical Journal* 120, no. 3 (February 5, 2007): 204–10.

48. The prescription form of yohimbine is called yohimbine hydrochloride. Sold under the brand names Aphrodyne and Yocon, it cannot legally be sold as a dietary supplement.

49. See, for example, Elham Akhtari et al., "*Tribulus terrestris* for Treatment of Sexual Dysfunction in Women: Randomized Double-Blind Placebo-Controlled Study," *DARU Journal of Pharmaceutical Sciences* 22, no. 40 (April 2014), accessed October 21, 2017, https://darujps.biomedcentral.com/articles/10.1186/2008-2231-22-40.

50. S. Galiniak, D. Aebisher, and D. Bartusik-Aebisher, "Health Benefits of Resveratrol Administration," *Acta Biochimica Polonica* 66, no. 1 (February 28, 2019): 13–21, https://doi.org/10.18388/abp.2018_2749.

51. *Encylopaedia Britannica*, "Saint Teresa of Ávila: Spanish Mystic," accessed October 20, 2017, https://www.britannica.com/biography/Saint-Teresa-of-Avila.

52. "Mother Teresa," Wikipedia, accessed October 20, 2017, https://en.wikipedia.org/wiki/Mother_Teresa.

53. "Mother Teresa," Wikipedia.

54. "The essence of warriorship, or the essence of human bravery, is refusing to give up on anyone or anything." Chögyam Trungpa, *Shambhala: The Sacred Path of the Warrior* (Boulder, CO: Shambala Publications, 2007).

55. Paul Grant and Shamin Ramasamy, "An Update on Plant Derived Anti-Androgens," *International Journal of Endocrinology and Metabolism* 10, no. 2 (Spring 2012), https://www.ncbi.nlm.nih.gov/pmc/articles/PMC3693613/.

56. M. Ghazanfarpour, R. Sadeghi, R. Roudsari Latifnejad, K. Najmabadi Mirzaii, M. Bazaz Mousavi, S. Abdolahian, and T. Khadivzadeh, "Effects of Red Clover on Hot Flash and Circulating Hormone Concentrations in Menopausal Women: A Systematic Review and Meta-Analysis," *Avicenna Journal of Phytomedicine* 5, no. 6 (November–December 2015): 498–511, PMID: 26693407; PMCID: PMC4678495.

57. N. Kakadia, P. Patel, S. Deshpande, and G. Shah, "Effect of *Vitex negundo* L. Seeds in Letrozole Induced Polycystic Ovarian Syndrome," *Journal of Traditional and Complementary Medicine* 9, no. 4 (October 11, 2018): 336–45, https://doi.org/10.1016/j.jtcme.2018.03.001.

58. V. Unfer et al., "Effects of Myo-inositol in Women with PCOS: A Systematic Review of Randomized Controlled Trials," *Journal of Gynecology and Endocrinology* 28, no. 7 (July 2012), https://www.ncbi.nlm.nih.gov/pub med/22296306; D. Constantino et al., "Metabolic and Hormonal Effects of Myo-inositol in Women with Polycystic Ovary Syndrome: A Double-Blind Trial," *European Review for Medical and Pharmacological Sciences* 13, no. 2 (March–April 2009), https://www.ncbi.nlm.nih.gov/pubmed/194 99845.

59. Grant and Ramasamy, "An Update on Plant Derived Anti-Androgens."

60. Debra Nowak et al., "The Effect of Flaxseed Supplementation on Hormonal Levels Associated with Polycystic Ovarian Syndrome: A Case Study," *Current Topics in Nutraceutical Research* 5, no. 4 (2007), https://www.ncbi.nlm.nih.gov/pmc/articles/PMC2752973/.

61. Grant and Ramasamy, "An Update on Plant Derived Anti-Androgens."

62. Grant and Ramasamy, "An Update on Plant Derived Anti-Androgens."

63. Grant and Ramasamy, "An Update on Plant Derived Anti-Androgens."

64. Michelle Fondin, "Speak Your Inner Truth with the Fifth Chakra," Chopra Center, accessed December 12, 2017, https://chopra.com/articles/speak-your-inner-truth-with-the-fifth-chakra#sm.001cjchdg1byvf1wy1a1 xopt6k3rf.

65. G. Muscogiuri et al., "Vitamin D and Thyroid Disease: To D or Not to D?," *European Journal of Clinical Nutrition* 69, no. 3 (March 2015), https://www.ncbi.nlm.nih.gov/pubmed/25514898; S. A. Muyesser, "Isolated Vitamin D Deficiency Is Not Associated with Nonthyroidal Illness Syndrome, but with Thyroid Autoimmunity," *Scientific World Journal*, 2015, https://www.ncbi.nlm.nih.gov/pmc/articles/PMC4306373/?report=classic.

66. Muyesser, "Isolated Vitamin D Deficiency Is Not Associated with Nonthyroidal Illness Syndrome."

67. P. Yatan et al., "Impact of Alcohol Use on Thyroid Function," *Indian Journal of Endocrinology and Metabolism* 17, no. 4 (July–August 2013), https://www.ncbi.nlm.nih.gov/pmc/articles/PMC3743356/.

68. As quoted in Meghan Bartels, "The Unbelievable Life of the Forgotten Genius Who Turned Americans' Space Dreams into Reality," *Business Insider*, August 22, 2016, accessed December 15, 2017, http://www.businessinsider.com/katherine-johnson-hidden-figures-nasa-human-computers-2016-8.

69. Katherine Johnson, interview with WHRO-TV, "What Matters," February 25, 2011, accessed December 15, 2017, at https://youtu.be/r8gJqKy IGhE.

70. Wini Warren, *Black Women Scientists in the United States* (Bloomington, IN: Indiana University Press, 200), 143.

71. Wendy Irene, "Guided Meditation: Speak Your Truth (Throat Chakra Healing)," GiveLoveCreateHappiness.com, accessed December 20, 2017,

http://www.givelovecreatehappiness.com/blog/guided-meditation-speak
-your-truth-throat-chakra-healing.

72. M. H. Jacobson, P. P. Howards, L. A. Darrow, J. W. Meadows, J. S. Kes-
ner, J. B. Spencer, M. L. Terrell, and M. Marcus, "Thyroid Hormones and
Menstrual Cycle Function in a Longitudinal Cohort of Premenopausal
Women," *Paediatric and Perinatal Epidemiology* 32, no. 3 (May 2018):
225–34, https://doi.org/10.1111/ppe.12462.

73. E. Gaitan, "Goitrogens," *Baillière's Clinical Endocrinology and Metabolism*
2, no. 3 (August 1988): 683–702, https://doi.org/10.1016/s0950-351x(88)
80060-0.

74. Dominika Tuchendler and Marek Bolanowski, "The Influence of Thyroid
Dysfunction on Bone Metabolism," *Thyroid Research* 7, no. 12 (December
2014), https://thyroidresearchjournal.biomedcentral.com/articles/10.1186
/s13044-014-0012-0.

75. D. K. Dhanwal et al., "Hypovitaminosis D and Bone Mineral Metabolism
and Bone Density in Hyperthyroidism," *Journal of Clinical Densitometry*
13, no. 4 (October–December 2010), https://www.ncbi.nlm.nih.gov/pub
med/20663698.

76. Alam Mohammed Husein Mackawy et al., "Vitamin D Deficiency and Its
Association with Thyroid Disease," *International Journal of Health Sciences*
7, no. 3 (November 2013), https://www.ncbi.nlm.nih.gov/pmc/articles
/PMC3921055/.

77. Francine Klagsbrun, "The Pitch That 'Made the State of Israel Possible,'"
New York Jewish Week, October 10, 2017, accessed December 27, 2017,
http://jewishweek.timesofisrael.com/the-pitch-that-made-the-state-of
-israel-possible/.

78. Amanda Becker, "Hewlett Packard's Meg Whitman Joins CEOs Endorsing
Clinton," Reuters.com, August 2, 2016, accessed December 28, 2017, https://
www.reuters.com/article/us-usa-election-clinton-whitman/hewlett-packards
-meg-whitman-joins-ceos-endorsing-clinton-idUSKCN10E08K?il=0.

79. Winston and Maimes, *Adaptogens: Herbs for Strength, Stamina, and Stress
Relief*, and Lipman, "Adaptogens: Nature's Miracle Anti-Stress and Fatigue
Fighters."

80. Y. Qi, F. Gao, L. Hou, and C. Wan, "Anti-Inflammatory and Immunostimulatory Activities of Astragalosides," *American Journal of Chinese
Medicine* 45, no. 6 (2017): 1157–167, https://doi.org/10.1142/S0192415X
1750063X.

81. Robert Rogers, *My Journey with Plant Medicine* (Berkeley, CA: North
Atlantic Books, 2017), 89.

82. Northwestern University Women's Health Research Institute, "Antidepressant May Have Role in Treating Menopause Symptoms," 2014, http://
menopause.northwestern.edu/content/antidepressant-may-have-role
-treating-menopause-symptoms.

83. Prema B. Rapuri, J. Christopher Gallagher, H. Karimi Kinyamu, and Kay L. Ryschon, "Caffeine Intake Increases the Rate of Bone Loss in Elderly Women and Interacts with Vitamin D Receptor Genotypes," *American Journal of Clinical Nutrition* 74, no. 5 (November 2001), http://ajcn.nutri tion.org/content/74/5/694.full.

84. Yin et al., "Icariine Stimulates Proliferation and Differentiation of Human Osteoblasts by Increasing Production of Bone Morphogenetic Protein 2."

85. See, for example, Elham Akhtari et al., "*Tribulus terrestris* for Treatment of Sexual Dysfunction in Women: Randomized Double-Blind Placebo-Controlled Study," *DARU Journal of Pharmaceutical Sciences* 22, no. 40 (April 2014), accessed October 21, 2017, https://darujps.biomedcentral .com/articles/10.1186/2008-2231-22-40.

INDEX